DONATION

DATE DUE

			PRINTED IN U.S.A.

Intuition in Medicine

Intuition in Medicine

A Philosophical Defense of Clinical Reasoning

HILLEL D. BRAUDE

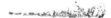
The University of Chicago Press
Chicago and London

Hillel D. Braude completed his medical education and training at the University of Cape Town Medical School and his PhD at the University of Chicago. Since completing further studies as a postgraduate fellow and research assistant in McGill University's Biomedical Ethics Unit and Religious Studies Faculty, his main area of research is neuroethics.

The University of Chicago Press, Chicago 60637
The University of Chicago Press, Ltd., London
© 2012 by The University of Chicago
All rights reserved. Published 2012.
Printed in the United States of America

21 20 19 18 17 16 15 14 13 12   1 2 3 4 5

ISBN-13: 978-0-226-07166-4 (cloth)
ISBN-10: 0-226-07166-9 (cloth)

Publication of this book has been aided by a grant from the Bevington Fund.

Library of Congress Cataloging-in-Publication Data

Braude, Hillel D.
   Intuition in medicine : a philosophical defense of clinical reasoning /
Hillel D. Braude.
       p. cm.
   Includes bibliographical references and index.
   ISBN-13: 978-0-226-07166-4 (hardcover : alkaline paper)
   ISBN-10: 0-226-07166-9 (hardcover : alkaline paper)   1. Intuition   2. Ethi
intuitionism. 3. Medical ethics. 4. Clinical medic e.   I.   le.
   BJ1472.B73 2012
   174.2—dc23   110 35

♾ This paper meets the requirements of ANSI/NI (z3 .4   992 (P   ian n
of Paper).

To the memory of my late father,
Barney Braude z"l

Contents

Acknowledgments

This study is the culmination of many years of reflecting on the nature of clinical reasoning. I began this personal and intellectual odyssey studying medicine at the University of Cape Town. Working as a doctor in South African urban and rural settings I was struck by the crisis of humanistic care, which I perceived to be the result of both the former apartheid regime on South African healthcare and a more widespread internal malaise within Western medicine. I realized that the problem of medical dehumanism represented a crisis of thought as much as practice. The remedy to this malaise lay deeper than simply reintroducing more humanities and ethics into medical school curricula or even focusing on human rights, as important as these activities are. The first part of the cure for medicine must lie in proper reflection on the nature of clinical reasoning and praxis. I was fortunate to be able to follow this intellectual thread as a graduate student in the University of Chicago's then program on History and Culture. My theoretical research was complemented by practical training as a clinical ethicist with the MacLean Center for Clinical Medical Ethics.

My study of intuition in clinical reasoning presents the fruit of this theoretical research and clinical involvement. I explore my own hunch borne out of clinical practice and philosophical reflection that intuition presents a means of uniting the ethical and epistemological elements of clinical reasoning and provides the basis for reconceptualizing the ancient art of medical practice. It is my hope that this book will be useful to physicians and other healthcare practitioners, philosophers, healers, and anyone interested in the vital task of rehumanizing contemporary medicine.

Having roots in three continents and spanning more than a decade, the influences on the development of this book are too tacit and numerous to mention. Nonetheless, there are a number of people to whom I owe an explicit debt of gratitude. Firstly, to the members of my dissertation committee: Sander Gilman, Jean Comaroff, Robert Richards, David Tracy, and Richard Zaner, who each contributed in different and significant ways to the unfolding of this work. Their presence speaks to the fundamentally interdisciplinary nature of this work. Others too were important touchstones on this personal and intellectual journey. Gerhard Baader first introduced me to the writing of Hans Jonas, who has left a deep impression on my thinking. Mark Siegler facilitated my practical immersion in clinical ethics through generous fellowships and teaching opportunities at the MacLean Center for Clinical Medical Ethics. During a fellowship at Northwestern University's Medical Ethics and Humanities Program, Kathryn Montgomery and Todd Chambers actively encouraged the development of my own ideas on how doctors think—thank you, Kathryn, also for your invaluable editorial assistance. Leon Kass introduced me to Aristotle's *Nicomachean Ethics* and encouraged this philosophical defense of clinical reasoning. David Ben Nahum affirmed the clinical relevance and importance of this book. The University of Chicago Center in Paris provided a welcome space to write, and exposure to the city where the modern clinic first developed. Through her invitation to help develop the Centre d'Éthique Clinique, Véronique Fournier facilitated my exposure to clinical ethics in France. The program for philosophy of biology and medicine at the Collège de France directed by Anne Fagot-Largeault also provided a "home away from home." Her seminal study *Les causes de la mort histoire naturelle et facteurs de risque* presages some important insights in my own work. I fondly remember my weekly French-English translation sessions with Jean Paul Amman. Conversations with Dor Abrahamson contextualized the debate about the place of mathematics in practical reasoning. Schirin Nowrousian aided my translations from French into English, and kept my spirits raised through recitations of Beckett in three languages. Patrizia D'Alyssio's enthusiasm for philosophy of biology inspires my own.

My postdoctoral fellowships at McGill University have provided the ideal intellectual environment for the final editing of this manuscript. Kathy Glass and Eugene Bereza have been convivial colleagues in the Biomedical Ethics Unit. Matthew Hunt, James Andersen, and Avi Craimer in the "Pubs and Pubs" reading group have been keen and critical appraisers of my writing process. My present research in neuroethics extends many of the intellectual threads followed in this study. I value Allan Young's engaged support. Katherine Young, my postdoctoral supervisor in the Religious Studies faculty, has been most encouraging of my personal and professional development. I wish to thank the wonderful book team at the University of Chicago Press: Karen

ACKNOWLEDGMENTS   xi

Darling, Susan Karani, Abby Collier, and Micah Fehrenbacher; as well as Siobhan Drummond for creating the index. Finally, I am grateful to my family for their support from afar. My mother nurtured my interest in medicine from my earliest years. My sister Claudia has been a source of unwavering love and support. My wife Ita, an unseen presence during the gestation of this book, has brought her own intuitive insights to our unfolding life project. I dedicate this book to the memory of my late father, Barney Braude z"l, who supported this foray out of clinical medicine into philosophy. May we all have the courage to validate our intuitive wisdoms and help others to do the same.

Introduction

All men are mortal
Socrates is a man
Therefore Socrates is mortal.

This classical logical syllogism often attributed to Aristotle encapsulates an existential dilemma. With irrefutable logic this syllogism demonstrates that Socrates is mortal. What is not addressed, however, is the very scandal of Socrates's mortality, his death at the hands of the Athenians or by whatever means, and furthermore the scandal of every human death. Philosophy has always been concerned with death, but only to attempt to overcome it through universal reason[1] and this is nowhere more obvious than in this famous "Aristotelian" syllogism.[2] The eternal and universal nature of the truth of reason behind the syllogism renders the death of Socrates meaningless.

Medical ethics, which deals with individual persons, provides philosophy a way to escape the impersonalism of universal reason. Medicine as a passion-full area of human engagement attracts philosophers concerned with concrete issues. Indeed, the association between passion and disease is basic to the very language of medicine. The word *pathology*, according to the medical historian Georges Canguilhem, implicitly maintains the notion of disease as a state of passion: "Pathological implies pathos, the direct and concrete feeling of suffering and impotence, the feeling of life gone wrong" (1989, 137). The philosophical engagement with medicine offers a remedy for the lack of existential meaning within rationalistic philosophy. The unique context of medicine, concerned as it is with treating disease, healing the sick, and easing human suffering, offers a means for philosophy to concern itself with the scandal of mortality. In short, the incorporation of the medical field into philosophy presents an opportunity for the latter to deal in a significant way with the questions of human morality and mortality.

The application of moral philosophy to medicine in the discipline of medical ethics is timely. Contemporary moral philosophy faces a crisis of authority, described by Alasdair MacIntyre (1981) in his well-known book, *After Virtue: A Study in Moral Theory*. MacIntyre argues that this crisis of authority is a breakdown of the Enlightenment attempt to justify morality in purely secular rationalistic terms. The result is "emotivism," or the doctrine that "all evaluative judgments and more specifically all moral judgments are nothing but expressions of preference, expressions of attitude or feeling, insofar as they are moral or evaluative in character" (11). In consequence, secular pluralist societies are ultimately unable to choose between divergent moral positions. The immediacy of case-based clinical medical ethics presents an opportunity for philosophy to address this crisis of moral authority.

However, medicine too is in need of philosophy. The widely perceived crisis of humanistic values within medicine has acted as a stimulus for the reuniting of medicine and the humanities. The contemporary crisis of medicine is epitomized in the fallen status of the physician from demigod to mere technician, as well as in the burgeoning alternative health-care industry. This distrust in the authority of the physician occurred, paradoxically, at the same moment that medical technology appeared most powerful.[3] Despite their undeniable benefits, remarkably successful modern biological technologies, such as genetic engineering, have generated anxiety by threatening to change the nature of humanity and have placed in question the benevolence of the modern medical project.[4] Questioning the *ends* of the technological advances of modern biosciences pertains also to clinical medicine. Modern medical practices have, therefore, been criticized for "objectifying" or "reifying" patients.[5] In the face of this perceived crisis in medical and moral authority medical ethics has been developed by physicians, philosophers, and others, in order to rehumanize medicine through a renewed engagement with the humanities.[6]

There is disagreement about the particular founding date or event of American medical ethics.[7] There are, however, two important factors in its development. Firstly, the Nuremberg Code following the Second World War, a legal code written in response to the medical atrocities, such as the mass euthanasia of the physically and mentally disabled and the medical assistance in genocide, perpetrated by German physicians under the Third Reich.[8] The code explicitly delimited the moral boundaries of medical experimentation. Secondly, medical ethics crystallized around the problems posed by new life-sustaining medical technologies, such as the artificial respirator, which enabled newborns to be kept alive earlier and people in vegetative states to be kept alive longer. The possibility of prolonging life through mechanical ventilation and the pressure to procure transplantable organs resulted in the medical redefinition of death in the concept of brain death.

These limit cases—the dehumanization of medicine during the epoch of Nazi medicine and the redefinition of death—exemplify the moral dilemmas associated with the modern medical project that the discipline of medical ethics attempts to address. Both of these limit cases represent to some extent a rupture in human experience in general, and in the traditional conception of the medical project in particular.[9] In the first example, society's trust in the physician as a moral figure was greatly damaged.[10] In the second instance, the institutionalization and mechanization of death through artificial life support meant that medicine became perceived in the public imagination as standing in the way of allowing patients death with dignity. Mechanical ventilation was, therefore, an important medical technology associated with the separation between medical treatment and care. In both cases the Enlightenment project of scientific and technological progress has been put into question. The discipline of medical ethics tries to restore this rupture of trust in the medical profession through the establishment of a watch-guard discipline over medical technologies and practice. For this reason, the application of moral philosophy to medical technology in the discipline of medical ethics may be perceived as an important attempt to salvage the Enlightenment's rational values brought into crisis through the advances of technological modernity.[11]

One important consequence of the nascent discipline was to replace doctors as primary adjudicators of difficult ethical decisions with professional medical ethicists, and primarily with philosophers.[12] Philosophy as the so-called queen of the sciences dominates the nascent field of medical ethics. Philosophical rational and analytic skills are generally considered to provide the best means to consider the ends of medicine. Physicians, in contrast, are often perceived by philosophers to be mere technicians equipped to achieve the ends of health but not to define them. This contemporary prejudice against medicine resuscitates an ancient tension between physicians and philosophers. The classicist Ludwig Edelstein has argued that ancient medicine was influenced by philosophy, and not vice versa. Against philosophy, the Hippocratic author of *On Ancient Medicine* famously claimed that it is physicians and not philosophers who best understand the nature of man.[13] The biological information that modern medicine elicits about the nature of the self appears at last to reverse the ancient reliance of medicine on philosophy. Genetics and neuroscience in particular are of central importance to understanding fundamental questions such as the physiological underpinnings of human freedom, and the nature of subjective consciousness.

In summary, the relation between medicine and philosophy in the discipline of medical ethics is nowadays characterized by a mutually beneficial symbiosis. Philosophy needs medicine to become more relevant, while philosophy restores to medicine an alliance with the human sciences, perceived to have been lost when medicine assumed the mantle of a science modeled on seventeenth-century physics. Medical ethics, as the discipline that unites medicine and philosophy, attempts to overcome the internal weaknesses of each professional discipline. Moreover, both medicine and philosophy each have specific historical traditions and concerns that are inherently ethical. In other words, moral philosophy is traditionally concerned with determining the right and the good, while medicine is concerned with healing.[14]

Is it possible, however, to revive the ancient medical practice of skepticism regarding this new symbiosis? Does not this resuscitated alliance of medicine and philosophy in the emergent discipline of medical ethics merely paper over their respective internal crises?[15] Both medicine and philosophy suffer from the same tendency of reducing the singular, the unique, and the particular to the universal: philosophy, by reducing everyday phenomena to the forms of universal logic; and medicine, through its objectification of the unique person to the generalizable forms of anatomical structure and physiological processes. Where, therefore, between the cracks of universal logic and reifying medicine is there place for the individual patient, for a response to the cry of pain to which medicine responds, or to the voice of injustice upon which moral philosophy is founded?

The Invisible Thread of Intuition

In this book I respond to this question by analyzing the place of the individual in professional structures of clinical reasoning—medical and philosophical. The main focus of my analysis is intuition in medical and moral reasoning. As a form of embodied reasoning that is prereflexive and therefore has not yet been formulated into theoretical language, intuition provides an ideal prism through which to reflect on the nature of clinical reasoning.

Intuition is central to discussions about the nature of scientific and philosophical reasoning and what it means to be human. For example, the Frankfurt school philosopher Jürgen Habermas makes human intuition central in his reflections on the moral hazards of genetic engineering. In *The Future of Human Nature* Habermas claims:

> Many of us seem to have the intuition that we should not *weigh* human life, not even in its earliest stages, either against the freedom (and competitiveness) of research, or against the concern with safe-guarding an industrial edge, or against the wish for a healthy child, or even against the prospect (assumed *arguendo*) of new treatments for severe genetic diseases. What is it that is indicated by such an intuition, if we assume that human life does not from the very beginning enjoy the same absolute protection of life that holds for the person? (2003, 69)

For Habermas, even though our intuitions may change, for example, along with the development of the embryo, our basic moral intuitions are indissociable from our human nature. Jettisoning our moral intuitions, Habermas implies, would be to jettison what it means to be human.

Similarly, the analytic philosopher Hilary Putnam argues that what we require first and foremost in moral philosophy is a "moral image of the world," deeply associated with a reliance on moral intuitions (1987, 52). Putnam, however, rejects an essentialist philosophical conception of reality claiming that any specific entity must possess a specific set of characteristics or properties. He similarly does not take for granted the validity of our reliance on moral intuitions as a kind of given a priori. Putnam notes that the great problem for philosophy since the scientific revolution of the seventeenth century has been "having to philosophize without 'foundations,'" that is, without a commonly accepted set of foundational beliefs upon which our moral claims are based (29). Yet the answer for Putnam does not lie in abandoning all our human intuitions:

> If claiming to abandon *all* our "intuitions" is mere show, retaining all of them would require us to philosophize as if the phenomena I reminded you of did not exist. The task of the philosopher, as I see it, is to see *which* of our intuitions we can responsibly retain and which we must jettison in a period of enormous and unprecedented intellectual, as well as material change. (29–30)

To speak of practicing philosophy with a moral image of the world in mind is to argue for a philosophical anthropology derived from philosophical reflection on human nature in which moral intuitions are central.[16] Skepticism toward the reliability of moral intuitions is therefore often indissociable from the attack on a human centering of scientific and moral reasoning.[17]

This philosophical insight that intuition is central for clinical reasoning fundamentally informs this study of epistemological, ontological, and ethical structures in relation to medicine and medical ethics. However, intuition is notoriously difficult to define. Intuition has a long history in philosophy as a direct perception of things. It is also used to refer to a kind of commonsense reasoning. Contemporary medical science, particularly neuroscience with its imaging techniques allowing visualization of brain function, is beginning to make inroads into the subjective processes of cognition, including intuition. For example, neuroscientist Antonio Damasio has investigated the neurological underpinnings of intuitive reasoning. In his book *The Feeling of What Happens: Body and Emotions in the Making of Consciousness*, Damasio distinguishes between the "core self" at the visceral level and the "autobiographical self" at the conscious level. For Damasio core consciousness "provides the organism with a sense of self about one moment—now—and about one place—here" (1999, 15–16). On the other hand, "extended consciousness . . . provides the organism with an elaborate sense of self—an identity and a person, you or me" (ibid.). The sense of lived time at a conscious level, of personal narrative, is built on the strata of visceral rhythms at an unconscious level. The simplest form of consciousness, where wordless knowledge emerges, is described as "the feeling of knowing" (26). This "feeling of what happens when an organism is engaged with the processing of an object" precedes and engenders the occurrence of "inferences and interpretations" (ibid.). This core consciousness is analogous to intuition in preceding language, and like intuition it is also associated with the later formation of inferences and theoretical formulations.

Rather than defining and using a single concept of intuition—philosophical, practical, or neuroscientific—this study examines intuition as it occurs at different levels and in different contexts of clinical reasoning. Intuition codes for divergent meanings that become manifest in particular philosophical arguments and practical contexts. The task at hand is to flesh out these meanings in order to develop a full theory of clinical reasoning. Investigating the relation between clinical and philosophical conceptions of intuition in relation to medicine provides a method of developing a coherent theory of clinical reasoning. This analysis is necessarily interdisciplinary, drawing on material from philosophy, history of medicine, and medical epistemology. A key historical moment occurred in the seventeenth and eighteenth centuries, with the transition to modern critical thinking, and as medicine incorporated techniques from the modern inductive sciences. This transition also heralded a shift away from reliance on intuition and a rupture of medicine from the humanities associated with Cartesian dualism separating body and mind that this present work seeks to redress.

A return to uniting medicine and the humanities begins with Aristotle. Aristotle' conception of practical reasoning or *phronesis* is paradigmatic for this study of clinical reasoning. Aristotle's insight in the *Nicomachean Ethics* that practical reasoning requires a form of proof sufficient for its context, not necessarily mathematical, informs every clinical situation.[18] It opposes the prejudice in modern thought against intuitive reasoning in favor of quantitative and statistical positivism. In agreement with Aristotle, this study attempts to account for the individual, and the contingent and variable in a theory of clinical reasoning.

Focusing on intuition in medical and moral reasoning presents both an opportunity and a challenge. The advantage is that the analysis of intuition as a form of cognition that is not yet formulated into theoretical language allows for a dissection of the epistemological, logical, ontological, and ethical foundations of clinical reasoning. By focusing on tacit elements of clinical reasoning, this approach challenges a positivist notion of medical science that privileges only that which is directly observable and quantifiable. Besides positivism, rationalism is another philosophical school that this study opposes through relating medicine and philosophy. Rationalism in its more formal definition refers to the belief that ultimate knowledge is gained independently from sense experience. Intuition as a form of direct certainty is often associated with rationalist theories of knowledge. However, paying attention to intuition as an element of practical reasoning acknowledges the reasonableness of commonsense reasoning. Similarly, in emphasizing the importance of a prereflexive but not irrational element within practical reasoning, the approach in this study challenges a purely rationalist view of medical epistemology and ethics.

As a form of cognition resisting abstraction, intuition is necessarily difficult to theorize. For example, how does one put into language that which by definition is presymbolic? What is the relation between the preflexive and symbolic dimension of clinical reasoning? How does one ascertain the validity or truth of assertions when one is relying on intuition? And finally, by privileging intuition how does one not fall into the trap of idealism, the philosophical claim that mind forms the basis of ultimate reality? As with all of these philosophical isms—positivism, rationalism, idealism—my approach in this book is to combine medical and philosophical structures and categories in order to deal with philosophical questions that, because they refer to human practice, cannot be resolved through reflection alone. Intuition, in its philosophical and practical forms, provides the bridge between medical and moral reasoning in clinical reasoning. Intuition also links the epistemological, ontological, and ethical structures inherent in clinical reasoning. In each chapter of this book I use intuition to analyze how these structures relate to each other at different levels of clinical reasoning, from the individual to the

epidemiological. Unpacking the foundational role of intuition in clinical reasoning explains why clinical reasoning remains a uniquely human endeavor
and deservedly remains a paradigm linking science with the humanities.

Chapters

The first chapter discusses intuition as it has been used in a debate about
the nature of clinical medical ethics that occurred in the United States in the
1970s and 1980s. This debate demonstrates the distinction between intuition
as a form of practical reasoning and its philosophical use as a form of direct
perception. In general terms, the intuitions possessed by physicians and
philosophers in regard to medical ethics, and their intuitions about intuitions,
are revealing about the epistemological, ethical, and ontological foundations
of clinical reasoning. This analysis of key figures in the nascent phase of
American medical ethics, through their reliance on philosophical and moral
intuitions, establishes the basis for this study of clinical reasoning. In particular, this chapter begins to demonstrate the importance of the ethical face-to-
face encounter for a moral theory of clinical reasoning.

The second chapter continues to follow the thread of the philosophical
understanding of intuition in the examination of moral intuitionism, the
philosophical theory that relies on moral intuitions. Moral intuitionism as
espoused by British philosopher G. E. Moore is associated with a nonnaturalistic approach that does not consider moral concepts of the Good as natural
categories. Moral intuitionism as applied to medical ethics has been most
rigorously developed by another American philosopher-ethicist Baruch
Brody. Brody is singular in developing a modified theory of moral intuitionism to ground his casuistic, or case-based, approach to medical ethics. While
Brody's theory has some very strong aspects to it, I argue that his strict analytic approach results in philosophical gaps that become obvious from a clinical perspective and that are better accounted for through phenomenological
approaches. Instead, philosopher-ethicists can bring their reflections closer
to the clinical life world through an increased awareness of temporal and
narrative horizons of patients' lives provided more adequately by philosophical approaches rooted in hermeneutics and phenomenology. In other words,
closer attention to narrative and lived experience is important in developing
a moral theory for medicine that does not abstract personal lived experience
from philosophical reflection on hard moral issues.

If moral intuitionism refers to philosophical intuitions, intuition as an
element of practical reasoning occurs in relation to Aristotle's well known
concept of *phronesis*. The idea that clinical reasoning should be modeled on

phronesis has been articulated by two influential philosophers of medicine, Edmund Pellegrino and David Thomasma. While Pellegrino and Thomasma's intuitions are correct in modeling clinical reasoning on *phronesis*, their modernist reworking of *phronesis* departs from my own reading in chapter three of Aristotelian *phronesis*, in not accounting for the presence of intellectual *nous*. This omission of *nous* from Pellegrino and Thomasma's understanding of *phronesis* has real moral relevance. The recognition of the place of *nous* within *phronesis* provides a means of avoiding Cartesian dualism, separating body and mind, in a renewed theory of clinical reasoning. A rehumanization of medicine through alliance with the humanities can only be ultimately successful if it pays attention to the variable and contingent in human experience. Only by recognizing the delicate relation between *nous* and *phronesis* can Aristotelian *phronesis* become a resource for the modeling of clinical reasoning. *Phronesis* serves as the model for clinical reasoning because it is both an intellectual and emotional virtue. Similarly, analyzing *phronesis* allows for the transition from moral to epistemological aspects of clinical reasoning. The great medical epistemological themes discussed in the following chapters include the problems of induction, causality, and statistical correlation—all of which possess deep epistemological associations with intuitive reasoning.

The fourth chapter continues the examination of practical reasoning and action in Aristotle by focusing on the structure of his practical syllogism. This analysis deepens my reading of the corporeal structure within *phronesis*. Rather than being absent from Aristotle's practical syllogism, its anthropomorphic substrate is too present to be mentioned explicitly, and therefore risks being neglected in reflections about Aristotle's theory of action. This discussion of the practical syllogism provides a basis for the further comparison in the fifth chapter between *phronesis* and physiognomy, the ancient art of interpreting character from facial characteristics. While physiognomy is rightfully considered a pseudoscience, it played a vital historical role in the development of medical statistics. Two influential European figures in the history of statistics, Adolphe Quetelet and Francis Galton are central for the application of statistics to the medical sciences. However, as I shall argue, their revolutionary achievement was contingent on inverting the intuitive structure of Aristotelian practical reasoning. In their respective sciences of the contingent, Quetelet and Galton hypostatize the corporeal substrate of physiognomy into mathematical abstraction. This conceptual move made possible the application of statistics to medicine, but also established the tension between intuition and statistical reasoning in clinical medicine that continues up to and including the present.

The tension between clinical intuition and statistical reasoning is epitomized in the modern medical statistical movement of evidence-based medicine. Evidence-based medicine provides an influential critique of clinical expertise and intuition. However, as demonstrated in chapter six, the development of evidence-based medicine's statistical epistemology is premised on ignoring the clinical context. Evidence-based medicine should be distinguished from its precursor discipline, clinical epidemiology, as developed by American physician Alvan Feinstein. Feinstein's theory of clinical epidemiology was characterized by a more nuanced understanding of clinical reasoning, including clinical intuition. Feinstein did not eschew the use of statistics in clinical epidemiology. Instead, for Feinstein statistics was meant to be used as a tool to aid clinical reasoning. The analysis of clinical epidemiology in this chapter suggests that the dichotomy between clinical intuition and statistical reasoning established by proponents of evidence-based medicine is a false one.

Galton's discovery of statistical correlation finally made possible the application of statistics to the medical sciences. However, as seen with Galton himself, and the evidence-based medicine movement, the success of statistical correlation was often at the expense of intuitive reasoning. In order to understand better the significance of modeling clinical reasoning on statistics, chapter 7 compares Galton's discovery of statistical correlation with the anatomo-pathological correlate initiated by the nineteenth-century French clinician Xavier Bichat. The analysis of Galton in relation to Bichat, and other physicians' attitudes toward the application of statistics to medicine during the eighteenth and nineteenth centuries, leads to the conclusion that the relation between intuition and statistics is not one of inherent opposition. Both intuitive and statistical inferences share a common thread in their epistemological association with human corporeality. As will be explained in greater detail, the hypostasis of an anthropomorphic essence through Galton's discovery of statistical correlation indicates that intuitive and statistical inferences are different poles of a single spectrum, rather than dichotomous entities.

The eighth chapter concludes this analysis of intuition and statistics through the problem of induction, well known to philosophers of science. The responses of two influential twentieth-century philosophers, Hans Reichenbach and C. S. Peirce, to Hume's problem of induction and the place of intuition in scientific reasoning is of especial interest in relation to clinical reasoning. For both philosophers there is a close relation between inductive and probabilistic reasoning. The role of abduction is especially important for Peirce in providing intuitive support for inductive reasoning. Peirce's theory of abduction, provides the subconceptual mechanism behind clinic equipoise, a key concept for clinical research ethics. Clinical equipoise maintains a similar tension found within clinical reasoning, between intuition and statistics, the individual and the group, and moral and epistemological values. Additionally, it is fitting to conclude this study with Peirce's theory of abductive reasoning, since it unites elements which will appear throughout this study (i.e., intuition, induction, anthropomorphism, physiognomy, and *phronesis*).

Concluding Chapter

The main purpose of this book is to demonstrate, through an analysis of intuition, the epistemological, ontological, and ethical structures pertaining to clinical reasoning. While most of the examples and arguments in this book are drawn from medicine and analytic philosophy, key aspects of this study are phenomenological. In the concluding chapter I trace the formative influence of phenomenological conceptions on this analysis. Specifically, I examine Edmund Husserl's phenomenological conception of intuition in relation to medical empiricism, and the ethical phenomenological critique of Emmanuel Levinas. A key idea within this book adapted from Levinas is that the presence of the human face as an ethical structure may rupture the causal chain of inference within clinical reasoning. Levinas's ethical critique limits the ability of phenomenological intuition to grasp ethical difference, or what he calls alterity, that which grounds intersubjective responsibility. This insight may also be applied to Aristotelian intuition. If Aristotelian intuition acts as the model for clinical reasoning, then the analysis of intuition in the face-to-face encounter in medicine provides a means of determining whether Aristotelian intuition does in fact account adequately for the individual in medicine. In other words, medicine provides a means of critiquing the philosophical model upon which clinical reasoning is based.

This ethical conception is implicit in many of the chapter-length analyses of aspects of clinical reasoning. The ethical obligation within medicine is shown to occur in the divergent contexts in which intuition is used in medicine, both philosophical and practical. There is rhetorical value in allowing this ethical insight to emerge from within different epistemological and ontological domains, for example, within analytic philosophical arguments or statistical texts, rather than being seen as a purely phenomenological perspective, and being categorized accordingly—despite the increased cross-fertilization between analytic and phenomenological philosophers. In the concluding chapter these phenomenological and ethical concerns are finally brought into the foreground through examining the concepts of intuition and correlation in Husserl and the concepts of temporality, the face-to-face relation and the trace in Levinas. Levinas's critique of Husserlian phenomenology may be used to reconceptualize the ethical foundations of clinical reasoning. There is, in other words, a radical ethical alterity underlying the epistemological and ontological structures of clinical reasoning. This ethical structure explains the rupture of theoretical philosophical principles and categories in the clinical context. However, this infinite obligation in Levinas does not preclude the necessity for practical interventions to alleviate suffering and reduce harm. Levinas's ethical philosophy helps explain the primacy of beneficence as the "principle of principles" of medical ethics. The physician's task is to constantly overcome the gap between various supposed dichotomies, such as between reason and practice, the individual and the group, statistics and intuition, principles and cases, and concrete facts and the moral imperative, in order to relieve the suffering of a particular person. In the face-to-face relation of the clinical encounter, the individuality of the physician and patient breaks through the abstracting medical generalizations and philosophical universalisms. Intuition, sometimes described as the art of medicine, lies at the heart of this face-to-face relation.

Intuition in Medical and Moral Reasoning

There are, however, certain physicians and scientists who say that it would be impossible for anyone to know medicine who does not know what man consists of, this knowledge being essential for him who is to give his patients correct medical treatment. The question that they raise, however, is a matter for philosophy, for those who, like Empedocles, have written about natural science, what man is to begin with, how he came into being at the first, and out of what constituents he was constructed. For my part, I consider first, that all that has been said or written by scientists or physicians about natural science has less to do with medicine than it has with the art of writing. Next, I consider that clear knowledge of nature can be derived from no source except medicine; that it can be learnt when medicine itself has all been correctly comprehended, but till then I am convinced that this knowledge is far from possible—I mean, by this "learning," to know what a man is, through what causes he derives his being, and the rest of it accurately. For this at least about nature I am convinced that a physician must know, and devote himself to knowing, if he is going to do anything of his duty, the nature of man in relation to what he eats and drinks, and in relation to his habits generally, and what will be the effect of each on each individual.

HIPPOCRATIC AUTHOR, *On Ancient Medicine*

The relation between theory and practice characterizes the history of reason in the West. In this relation, at least since Plato and even with his student Aristotle, theoretical reflection has occupied a privileged place. Medicine, as the combination of both theory and practice to promote the end of health, provides an important model that reverses this relation between theory and practice. In the well-known passage from *On Ancient Medicine* cited above, the Hippocratic author opposes medical to philosophical knowledge. His argument affirms the Hippocratic empiricism that was suspicious of universal philosophical laws being applicable to the individual. Yet the antagonism toward philosophy on the part of Hippocratic physicians did not mean that ancient medicine was oblivious to philosophical argument. As classics scholar Werner Jaeger has argued, it was only through coming into conflict with philosophy that ancient medicine "reached a clear understanding of its own purpose and methods, and worked out the classical expression of its own particular conception of knowledge" (1944, 4).[1] Jaeger adds that the craft of healing in ancient Greece only became a methodical science once it had internalized the Ionian philosophical concept of universal laws that are understandable through observation and reason. Thus, the idea of human nature developed by Greek medicine was itself an extrapolation of the prior Ionian philosophical concept of the great *physis* (φύσις), or nature of the universe.[2]

This relation between ancient medicine and philosophy is of more than mere historical interest as a marker in the centuries-old tension between reason and practice in Western epistemology, but has a contemporary analogy in the debate between physicians and philosophers about the nature and scope of medical ethics that occurred during the nascent period of American medical ethics in the 1970s and 1980s.[3] This seminal period of clinical medical ethics was characterized by a heated professional and epistemological conflict in which physicians and philosophers both claimed that the discipline they represented was most qualified to lead the nascent profession. This conflict was not all that surprising in the sense that medical ethics was then primarily conceived as a combination of clinical medicine with moral philosophical reflection. At the very least, the terrain was open for professional turf wars where personal ambition and professional livelihood were at stake. Yet, to limit this conflict to material interests alone would be to miss the more fundamental issue of the nature of clinical medical ethics itself. This debate between physicians and philosophers over the nature of medical ethics represents in its extremes a schism between two positions rooted respectively in clinical experience and philosophical reflection. Moreover, the philosophical and clinical attitudes crystallize in the divergent uses and understanding that physicians and philosophers have of intuition.

Philosophical Intuition

In philosophy, the word "intuition," derived from the Latin word *intuitus* meaning "to look or to gaze," denoted from Plato to Descartes a direct perception which presented a concept that was then made intelligible through cognitive understanding. Thus for Plato, who probably originated the concept, intuition is the image of the ideal truth able to be perceived by the mind (*nous*).[4] Aristotle appropriated and transformed this Platonic idealistic notion of *nous* to refer to the capacity of the mind to abstract universals from corporeal reality known empirically by the senses. According to Aristotle the intuitive mind simply "knows" without constructing its proof on prior knowledge.[5] This notion of intuition as direct perception is retained by most modern philosophers. For example, Descartes (1596–1650) utilized a notion of intuition to help overturn the classical order. Intuition for Descartes possessed incorrigible certitude, not of the outside world as with Aristotle, but rather of the internal, subjective mind. In other words, intuition for Descartes is the inner certitude that accompanies the perception of relations between clear and distinct ideas:

> By *intuition* I understand, not the fluctuating testimony of the senses, nor the misleading judgment that proceeds from the blundering constructions of imagination, but the conception which an unclouded and attentive mind gives us so readily and distinctly that we are wholly freed from doubt about that which we understand . . . *intuition* is the undoubting conception of an unclouded and attentive mind, and springs from the light of reason alone. (1968, 7)

Descartes's use of intuition as direct and infallible characterizes the philosophical interpretation of intuition.

Spinoza (1632–77), while otherwise critical of Cartesian dualism, also incorporated a concept of intuition into his philosophy of conception. For Spinoza, intuition, or the *scientia intuitiva*, constituted a third kind of cognition, different from the knowledge of individual objects and reason. "This kind of knowledge proceeds from an adequate idea of the formal essence of certain attributes of God to an adequate knowledge of the essence of things," Spinoza wrote in part 2 of his *Ethics* (proposition 40).[6] Spinoza claimed that the highest virtue of the mind is to "understand things by the third kind of knowledge" (part 5, proposition 27). Logico-mathematical understanding provides an exemplary instance of intuitive knowledge. Thus, Spinoza argued that for simple numbers, such as one, two, and three, it is obvious that the fourth proportional is six. This is seen all the more clearly, "because we infer in one single intuition the fourth number from the ratio we see the first number bears to the second" (part 2, proposition 40). This kind of intuition is the highest form of human cognition in leading to the "highest state of human perfection," and is "affected by the highest pleasure" (ibid.). Despite its divine associations, this third category of intuition is practical in being a kind of quick inference often aided by the two prior forms of human cognition, physical signs, and inferential reason. Spinoza's conception of intuition as containing both divine and practical elements is of particular interest here, since it is precisely this contradiction between intuition as infallible certainty or an error prone form of practical reasoning that, as will be seen, characterizes debates about intuition in medicine.

Intuition also occupied a central place in the Enlightenment philosopher Immanuel Kant's (1724–1804) epistemology. In his celebrated *Critique of Pure Reason* Kant outlined a theory of synthetic a priori judgments. According to Kant's conception, pure intuition of space and time made possible knowledge of first truths, as well the possibility of outer experience. Thus, space and time are the "two pure forms of sensible intuition, serving as principles of a priori knowledge" (*B*35–36).[7] While "space is a necessary a priori representation, which underlies our outer intuitions," time is the form of the inner sense, and "is a necessary representation that underlies all intuitions."[8]

While other modern philosophers have privileged intuition, such as Henri Bergson, the final philosophical perspective on intuition important to mention is that of Edmund Husserl (1859–1938), founder of the philosophical movement called phenomenology.[9] It is useful to describe Husserl's conception of intuition in some detail here, since Husserl's phenomenological method has an important, albeit indirect, influence on this analysis of intuition in clinical reasoning. Even though Husserl has been accused of being an idealist philosopher, his conception of intuition was intended to provide a philosophical method to understand everyday reality. This alone gives reason to take phenomenology seriously in developing a theory of clinical reasoning.[10] Intuition for Husserl, as in the history of philosophy more generally, provides the foundation stone upon which knowledge of the world is possible. Despite the complexity of Husserl's writing and his continuous reworking of the phenomenological method, it is possible to summarize a few relevant points relating to Husserl's concept of intuition.

Intuition occupied a central place within Husserl's unfolding phenomenological project, whose task was to elucidate core philosophical questions concerning the nature of reality.[11] The phenomenological method emphasized the subjective way in which objects and ideas are mentally determined. Intuition is a central aspect of intentionality, as it is the process through which objects are presented or given to consciousness. Intuitive acts include perception, imagination, and memory.[12] Despite this emphasis on subjectivity, Husserl was not a strict idealist in that intuitions are not possible without the prior or simultaneous existence of an external world. As Emmanuel Levinas notes in his study of Husserlian intuition, intuition for Husserl is an act that possesses its object.[13] In other words, intuitions are inconceivable without the prior natural object, which intuitions conceptually contain. Intuition is a determinate structure through which we enter into contact with being.[14] Husserlian intuition is an intentionality that "consists in reaching its object and facing it as existing" (1973, 84).[15] For Husserl, intuition is the source of all knowledge.[16] Truth is achieved when there is a correspondence between "an object as it is thought in an act of signification with an object as it is seen intuitively" (88–89). Or as Husserl claims, truth occurs when there is an identity between the meant and the given[17] (Hua 19/53, 566;

Zahavi, 31–32).[18] Fulfilled intuitions refer to intentions that attain an object, and correspond to both perceptual and categorical intentions.

These examples highlight the role of philosophical intuition in providing direct evidence to the understanding mind. Whether in Platonic idealism, Aristotelian empiricism, Spinozistic divination, or Cartesian and phenomenological subjectivism, these theories share the understanding that intuition is fundamental in bridging the relation between the world and the mind.

Practical Intuition

Philosophical conceptions of intuition do not exhaust its entire signification. Intuition, besides its philosophical understanding, refers, of course, to a type of instinctual certainty. Clinicians often use intuitions in this sense to describe their own processes of clinical reasoning. Intuition as an element of commonsense reasoning has an old association with clinical reasoning. Medical historian Arturo Castiglioni has noted the role of intuition for Hippocratic clinical reasoning in his study of the neo-Hippocratic tendency in modern medicine. Castiglioni describes Hippocratic intuition as "a keen critical observation, a logical analysis followed by a rapid synthesis, exact proportion of measures and moderation in the balance between the various opposite tendencies" (1943, 120).

This Hippocratic skill is not, however, simply a historical phenomenon. One finds this notion of intuition, or the art of medicine, affirmed by modern-day clinicians. For example, physician Alvan Feinstein argues that "without intuition, imagination, or esthetics, the 'scientist' is a dullard." On the other hand, "without rationality, discipline, or logic, the 'artist' is a dawdler" (1967, 295).[19] Feinstein emphasizes intuition within clinical judgment as part of his broader attempt to apply the scientific method to clinical and bedside medicine. Rather than affirming intuition in a nonscientific manner, Feinstein attempts to raise the subjective element within clinical reasoning to the light of day for scientific examination.

Popular medical writer Jerome Groopman refers to his own use of intuition as a clinical skill that he can turn on and off at will.[20] This modern-day sense of intuition used by clinical practitioners seems, then, to posses both aspects of "high" and "low" intuition.[21] In other words, clinical intuition is possessed by an elite group of clinicians and associated with a sophisticated body of reasoning akin to philosophical reasoning; and yet, clinical intuition also maintains its connection to the Hippocratic craft, resembling the kinds of gut thinking associated with the experienced navigator and equestrian breeder.[22]

Unsurprisingly, the notion of intuition as infallible perception and as instinctual certainty are not synonymous. As philosopher Mary Midgley notes, the status of intuition has fallen in the modern period from something considered direct and certain to something considered unscientific and unverifiable—a form of common sense. Thus, for Midgley an intuition in the contemporary sense, a sense influenced by the physical sciences, means any view that does not require special methods of verification:

> For physics, all common-sense views on the nature of matter are equally "intuitions," whether they spring from the complexities of accepted culture, from folklore, or directly from our natural muscular perceptions. The term intuition used, till lately, to mean always a direct perception, and would only have allowed (at most) the last of these meanings. (1989, 55–6)

The main reason for intuition's fall from grace is that in the light of the modern scientific revolution in which inductive logic is king, intuition is derided as not possessing the processes of inferential logic. Intuition therefore has been lumped together with sources of knowledge considered irrational, particularly mysticism. The dismissal of intuition as unscientific can be considered to be part of a broader sweep against particularistic knowledge traditions by the rationalistic forces of scientific Enlightenment beginning in the seventeenth century. Conversely, intuition as a form of embodied knowledge resists the clear subject-object dichotomy upon which the modern scientific project is premised.

The philosophical and clinical understandings of intuition are central for medical ethics, which exists on the borderline between clinical medicine and moral philosophy. The appeal of Leon Kass, former chair of the United States Presidential Bioethics Commission, to the "wisdom of repugnance," or so-called "yuck" factor in order to ban human cloning, is arguably a kind of moral intuitionism.[23] However, barely noted in the heated discussion that Kass's concept generated around the "wisdom of repugnance" was the fact that Kass does not rely on a philosophical notion of intuition as a faculty of moral reasoning. Instead Kass appears to refer to moral intuitions as a kind of moral instinct more akin to a psychological perception. Rationalist models that emphasize explicitly conscious aspects of moral reasoning have characterized most philosophical writing on moral decision making. Recently, psychological research has emphasized the intuitive dimension of moral decision making.[24] Moral intuition has been defined as the "sudden appearance in consciousness of a moral judgment, including an affective valence (good-bad, like-dislike), without any conscious awareness of having gone through steps of searching, weighing evidence, or inferring a conclusion" (Haidt 2001).

This psychological theory of moral reasoning is also analogous to the psychological process of intuition in clinical reasoning. One wonders whether the conflict about human cloning and the associated stem-cell debate is not the result of two different conceptions of intuition—the one arising from clinical practice, and the other from philosophical reflection. In other words, the controversy around the stem-cell debate is indebted to a basic binary distinction between divergent kinds of moral intuitions generated from clinical experience and philosophical reasoning and paralleled in the distinction between clinical and philosophical forms of intuition. If so, the divergence between philosophical and clinical intuitions represents a structural dichotomy within medical ethics itself. This would explain why philosophical intuitions arising purely from the realm of philosophical reflection abstracted from any concrete situation often result in surprisingly different conclusions than those reached by physicians relying on clinical intuition. Similarly, clinical intuitions arising from interactions with individuals, and epistemologically associated with practical reasoning, often give rise to moral intuitions that do not make sense to the analytically trained philosopher. Generally speaking, the different life structures of medicine and moral philosophy may be said to characterize two sides of the spectrum of ethical thinking that can be divided into such categories as theoretical reflection versus clinical experience, reasoned argument versus authority, principalism versus case-based reasoning or casuistry, and, perhaps, most significantly autonomy versus beneficence.

Medical principalism, as espoused most prominently by Tom Beauchamp and James Childress, famously advocates four principles upon which medical ethics is based: autonomy, beneficence and nonmaleficence, and social justice.[25] Autonomy refers to the ability of a person to make informed personal decisions free from the control of others. Beneficence and its negative corollary, nonmaleficence, refers to the moral obligation arising from medicine as a profession to contribute to patient welfare through positive beneficial actions and the removal of harm. Justice refers to larger social equity issues, such as the distribution of scarce health resources and the respect for human rights. The two principles of autonomy and beneficence are the overarching principles arising in the treatment of individuals, and they are often in tension with each other. While our Western society privileges autonomy over beneficence, exemplified in the legal rulings granting autonomy over the right to refuse treatment, for example, in validating the right of Jehovah's Witness adherents to refuse life-sustaining blood transfusions, the principle of beneficence is correctly regarded as the fundamental ethics principle arising from within the practice of medicine. Medical beneficence arises from the physician's acknowledgment of the duty to heal and not to harm vulnerable patients. Medical beneficence was already formulated in the statement within the Hippocratic Oath, obligating physicians to use medical regimens only for the benefit of the ill, and to keep away from causing harm. The principle of autonomy is derived from the duty for moral self-determination, expressed most fully by the Enlightenment philosopher Immanuel Kant. A tension between medical beneficence and autonomy characterizes many actual clinical medical ethics cases. For example, does one respect the autonomy of an individual refusing a life-saving intervention? Does it matter whether the individual is being treated in an emergency center, or in an alternative context? Casuistic medical ethicists evaluate the effect of factual details on the application of accepted ethics principles to individual cases. Another related approach, the one I pursue in this chapter, is a reexamination of the foundations of moral and epistemological foundations of clinical reasoning through a closer analysis of the relation between philosophical and clinical intuitions.

The Scope and Nature of Medical Ethics

The debate and sometimes low-level conflict that simmered during the nascent period of American medical ethics in the 1970s and 1980s provides a fertile resource with which to think about the nature of medical ethics through the reliance on philosophical and clinical intuitions by philosophers and physicians.[26] The list of academic leaders whose arguments I shall examine includes Mark Siegler, Leon Kass, Robert Veatch, Baruch Brody, Tristram Engelhardt, and Stephen Toulmin.[27] This approach is given weight by the observation that not only do physicians and philosophers tend to have divergent moral intuitions, but that this is reflected in their conception of the importance of intuition itself as an element of clinical reasoning. Examining and comparing the use of clinical intuition with moral intuition provides, therefore, a vantage point from which to analyze the tension, if not outright dispute, between physicians and philosophers during the early period of American medical ethics, specifically as to whether clinical medical ethics was a medical subdiscipline, or whether the moral reflection in clinical medical ethics was best left to philosophers.

Clinical Medical Ethics as a Medical Subdiscipline

Articulating a clinician's perspective, Mark Siegler has argued for the place of clinical intuition to help resolve particularly difficult cases in medical ethics.[28] In the difficult instance of acute, critically ill patients who refuse therapy, they claim that "physicians must utilize clinical intuition, *an inductive form of reasoning*, to appreciate what clinical intuition is suitable to the situation" (1978, 18). Thus, for Siegler clinical intuition, as a form of inductive reasoning, provides the model for ethical reasoning. Similarly, Siegler argues elsewhere that clinical ethics should be considered a subdiscipline of medicine.[29] Siegler distinguishes here between the philosophical foundations of clinical ethics and "traditional medical ethics," presumably an applied form of moral philosophy, that he argues does not have significant applicability to individual patient care. Siegler's claim presupposes the existence and validity of a professional ethic intrinsic to medicine upon which clinical medical ethics is based. As such, an intelligent and caring physician possessed with good common sense should be able to deal with most clinical ethics issues that arise in the daily practice of medicine. Siegler's handbook of clinical ethics, coauthored by Al Jonsen and Bill Winslade, epitomizes this conception of medical ethics as a subsection of medicine, analogous to other specializations, such as cardiology and nephrology.[30]

Leon Kass has also argued that the medical profession is unique in being intrinsically moral and in possessing its own special norms and duties. These are derived from the dignity and precariousness of the healing goal of medicine, from the meaning-laden experience of human illness, and from the mutually shared self-consciousness of the doctor-patient relationship.[31] Kass's argument for an ethics intrinsic to medicine can be associated with his 1990 critique of the "hyper-rationality" found in contemporary philosophical ethics. At the twentieth anniversary symposium to commemorate the founding of the Hastings Center for medical ethics, Kass, one of the center's founders, berated much of biomedical ethics for being "all talk and no action" that has "at best, improved our speech." He continued his criticism by claiming that

> philosophical ethics today is *rationalist*, I would say "hyper-*rational*," and, I would allege, unreasonably so. The dominant mode of American philosophizing remains analytic. It concerns itself with the analysis of concepts, the evaluation of arguments, and the criticism of justifications, always in search of clarity, consistency, coherence. It spends little time on what genuinely moves people to act—their motives and passions: that is, loves and hates, hopes and fears, pride and prejudice, matters that are sometimes dismissed as nonethical or as irrational because they are not simply reducible to *logos*. Repugnances and their correlative taboos are also overlooked; since they cannot give incontrovertible logical defences of themselves, they tend to fall beneath the floor of ethical discourse. As a result, ethical discourse focuses almost exclusively on matters conceptual and logical. (1990, 7)

Perhaps, what is most interesting in Kass's critique of philosophical reflection is not that philosophers fail to understand the reality of clinical responsibility, but that professional philosopher-ethicists have lost their capacity for emotional reasoning, a vital element of moral reflection. In any event,
it is apparent from these examples that there is a link between arguing for
a naturalistic ethic intrinsic to medicine, posited notably by Kass and Pellegrino, and advocating a reliance on forms of moral intuitions best possessed by physicians and other health-care professionals that are not attained
through expert philosophical reflection. Yet, one wonders how it is possible
to avoid the analytical tools of reflection on our moral intuitions provided
by philosophy. Is not an appeal to intuition, as MacIntyre claims, an appeal
one makes when one has no further reasonable argument to make?[32] Is it
possible to pay attention to repugnances and taboos and not fall into a form
of irrationalism?

Medical Ethics as Applied Philosophy

As with the physicians just mentioned, one finds the parallel assumption by
philosophers that *they* are most qualified to represent the discipline of medical ethics. For example, R. M. Hare has dismissed the philosophical challenges to medical-ethical questions, claiming that if philosophers cannot
analyze medical ethics cases, they might as well close up shop.[33] While all
analytical philosophers share the same basic trust in the ability of rational
reflection and argument to evaluate moral dilemmas in medicine, obviously
not all philosophers share the same philosophical approaches and methods.
Mirroring this diversity, one finds a spectrum of attitudes toward the value of
clinical medical experience.

Robert Veatch is a philosopher and medical ethicist noted for his flagrant
opposition to physician-centered medical ethics. Veatch represents the arche-
typal philosophical gadfly against medical paternalism. Veatch defines ethics
as the "enterprise of disciplined reflection on the *moral intuitions* and moral
choices that people make," and medical ethics is the "analysis of choices in
medicine" (1997, 1; italics mine). By disciplined reflection, Veatch presumably refers to a systematic philosophical reflection on the moral intuitions
we have regarding difficult medical decisions. It is precisely this predominant
reliance on reason by philosopher-ethicists that has been criticized by Kass as
a form of hyper-rationalism." Veatch for his part is critical of the attempt by
physician to have hegemony over medical ethics. He continues his definition
of medical ethics by claiming that it covers choices made most importantly

by nonmedical people, such as patients, parents, legislators, public officials, and judges. In a later article, Veatch states that "claiming that deciding the moral goals of life is the province of a professional cadre called physicians is hubris of the worst form" (1999, 164).

One can trace Veatch's position to an early article of his regarding the nature of the medical model. In this article Veatch (1973) argued that physicians have the authority to diagnose as illness social deviancies, for example, drug addiction, generally accepted to be within the medical realm, but that physicians do not possess the authority to arbitrate over whether these medical conditions are morally normative or not. More recently, in an autobiographical article describing his career as a medical ethicist, Veatch (2002) has clarified his fiercely antimedical position. Veatch begins this confessional article by stating that

> the single most important intellectual event in my career in medical ethics occurred the day I realized that the Hippocratic ethic for medicine was not merely outdated and irrelevant but actually in conflict with all the dominant religious and secular moral traditions of our day. Whether one stood in any of the great modern religious traditions or in any of the camps of secular philosophy—the liberal tradition of political philosophy, Marxism, or more recent feminist or communitarian views—the Hippocratic ethic was wrong, both metaethically (epistemologically) and normatively. (344)

Veatch does not just privilege a universalistic philosophical perspective. Instead, Veatch's method attempts to reconcile a social contractarian approach based on the philosopher John Rawls with the conviction that "ethical principles should be seen as preexisting in the fabric of the moral universe" (348–49). As the product of the American 1960s generation, the fabric of Veatch's professional moral universe consists of individual rights and opposition to authority, exemplified in medical authoritarianism and paternalism. Opposed to privileging the medical perspective, Veatch instead emphasizes an "ethic of the lay person in the medical role" (350). More than anything else, Veatch is concerned with removing the main decision-making authority from physicians and placing it into the hands of society.

In summary, Veatch's analysis finds medical-moral intuitions attributed to an ancient Hippocratic ethic devoid of substance and application for contemporary secular and democratic society. He sees no reason why physician intuitions should be privileged over those of patients. He regards the medical principle of beneficence as nothing other than a cloak for medical power. While Veatch emphasizes a patient ethic, he privileges the medical ethicist as the person best trained to determine the preexisting moral universe. Thus, for Veatch the moral universe as a social construct is best observed through an empiricist method by a group of "ideal scientific observers" (348–49). Even though Veatch is a strong advocate for a patient ethic, his popular ethic still requires articulation by an elite class of philosophers and theologians, or other experts trained in the social norms of contemporary American society.

While other philosopher bioethicists are not as extreme in their opposition to physician involvement in medical ethics, a recurrent theme is the notion that philosophers are the best trained to evaluate medical ethics questions. Thus, Baruch Brody's application of moral intuitionism to medical ethics privileges philosophical training in providing the ability to formalize moral intuitions into philosophical theories or principles. The kinds of moral intuitions privileged in Brody's theory are derived through philosophical training and reflection, and not from clinical experience.[34]

Physician turned philosopher Tristram Engelhardt has taken a middle position between medicine and philosophy in defining the nascent discipline of medical ethics. And yet, a close reading of an early article of his, entitled "The Philosophy of Medicine: A New Endeavor" (1973), demonstrates that for Engelhardt philosophy provides the ultimate tools for reflection on the problems associated with medical facts and techniques. Engelhardt argues in this article that the revolutionary advances in medical technology necessitate a "new endeavor" that will see "medical ethical problems within the context of general philosophical issues such as the relationship between values and science, human nature and technology" (444). Moreover, health as the traditional Hippocratic goal of medicine is now to be philosophically reconceptualized:

> In short, deciding what counts as health requires a decision about what counts as an appropriate goal for man. And to be sound, such a decision requires clear logic, breadth of reasoning, and creative sensitivity with respect to ethical issues. *These are philosophical problems as much as they are medical problems.* (446; italics mine.)

While Engelhardt privileges philosophy over medicine in providing the conceptual tools to evaluate medicine, medicine appears here as a neutral application of the biological sciences, rather than as possessing any claims to inherent value.

Stephen Toulmin of all analytic philosophers is unusual in privileging medical experience over philosophy. In an oft cited article entitled "How Medicine Saved the Life of Ethics" (1982), Toulmin provides an uncharacteristic philosophical voice arguing that, in fact, medicine offers the philosopher the opportunity to find its relevance. Toulmin, thus, reverses the traditional dependency of medicine on philosophy. While Toulmin's appeal to medicine for philosophical relevance is uncharacteristic of a philosopher, it does fit in with his larger philosophical project to contextualize philosophy historically and to return philosophical abstraction to commonsense reasoning and concern with day-to-day human affairs.[35]

In their study and revindication of casuistry, Toulmin and Jonsen (1988) argue that medical case-based reasoning provides a good model for moral reasoning. Clinical reasoning about cases using analogy provides for Toulmin an exemplary model for case-based reasoning regarding moral quandaries. Toulmin claims that as with diagnostic reasoning,

> the procedures that casuists have used to resolve moral problems appeal to understood and agreed *paradigms*, or *type cases*, from which they survey their way analogically to less understood, still disputed issues. (44)

While medical ethics provides a convenient contemporary example for Toulmin's proposed revision of moral philosophy, the foundations of his argument are ultimately philosophical and Aristotelian. Thus, Toulmin advocates a reappropriation of Aristotelian practical reasoning, or *phronesis*. In his *Nicomachean Ethics* Aristotle distinguished between *phronesis* and abstract scientific reasoning, or *epistemé*. In a famous paragraph that Toulmin is fond of quoting, Aristotle writes that

> our discussion will be adequate if it has as much clearness as the subject matter admits of, for precision is not to be sought for alike in all discussions, any more than in all the products of the crafts. . . . For it is the mark of an educated man to look for precision in each class of things just so far as the nature of the subject admits; it is evidently equally foolish to accept probable reasoning from a mathematician and to demand from a rhetorician scientific proofs. (*Nich. Ethics*, 1094b, trans. Ross)

This paragraph of Aristotle's encapsulates much of Toulmin's attempt to return moral philosophy to concrete human concerns. Aristotle's point is that it is epistemologically false to attempt to establish certainty in domains of practical reasoning, such as medicine, characterized by contingency and lack of certainty. In these domains, practical knowledge is not only sufficient, but also necessary. As Toulmin writes, in the practical realm, certitude does not depend on a "prior grasp of definitions, general principles and axioms," as in the theoretical realm, but rather on "accumulated experience of particular situations" (1988, 26).

Pierre Bourdieu: Intuitions in Practice

There are two main senses, sociological and philosophical, in which one can understand the discussion between physicians and philosophers over the nature and scope of medical ethics. Firstly, and most obviously, the conflictual relation between physicians and philosophers, exemplified by the positions of Siegler and Veatch, can be understood in sociological terms as a contestation over professional power and authority. The new profession of medical ethics, which applied philosophical reflection to moral problems arising in the context of medicine, offered a fertile terrain for philosophers to expand their professional influence and threatened the traditional hegemony of physicians over bedside decision making. Secondly, the divergent intuitions regarding key ethical principles, as well as the attitude toward intuition, are indicative of an epistemological and ontological divide between physicians and philosophers arising from their respective clinical and reflective practices. Both of these points can be developed through the use of French sociologist Pierre Bourdieu's concept of social *habitus*.

The radical insight derived from Bourdieu, seen from the very beginning of his theory of practice, is that intuitions as prereflexive elements of human cognition are already imprinted with the sociological. Bourdieu's complex concept of *habitus*, outlined in his influential *Outline of a Theory of Practice* ([1977] 1999), presents a materialist reading of intuitive judgment. The centrality of intuition for Bourdieu's critique is evident right at the start of his groundbreaking work, in a paragraph cited approvingly from Marx's *Theses on Feuerbach*:

> The principal defect of all materialism up to now—including that of Feuerbach—is that the external object, reality, the sensible, is grasped in the form of *an object or an intuition*; but not as *concrete human activity*, as *practice* in a subjective way. This is why the active aspect was developed by idealism, in opposition to materialism—but only in an abstract way, since idealism naturally does not know real concrete activity as such.

Implicitly drawing on a philosophical tradition going back to Aristotle's theory of practical wisdom, or *phronesis*, Bourdieu opposes social practice to the reified philosophical intuition developed in German idealism. Instead, for Bourdieu *habitus* is that conceptual element that mediates between the individual and the social. How does *habitus* incorporate individual intuitions into the sociological? Individual intuitions would seem to resist the socio-

Bourdieu claims that the *habitus* is a "subjective but not individual system of internalized structures, schemes of perception, conception, and action common to all members of the same group or class and constituting the precondition for all objectification and apperception" (86).[36] *Habitus* mediates between the individual and the social because it is an actual physiological incorporation of social norms by the biological individual. The *habitus* as a mode of action is only fully revealed in its concrete operation. While the *habitus* informs *all* thought and action, it is not determinable through conscious reflection and prediction. As Bourdieu writes, "Agents are possessed more by their habitus than they possess it" ([1977] 1999, 18). Through the internalization of class norms in the biological individual, the concept of *habitus* allows an observer or practitioner to explain behavior, while recognizing the elusive substance of action and thought resistant to complete explanation. Thus, the internalization of social norms in the *habitus* applies not only at the level of action, but also of thought. Even the private subjective reasoning of individuals, such as intuitions, or especially intuitions, is materialized for Bourdieu through an internalization of group norms.

Through Bourdieu, the epistemological reasons for the conflict between physicians and philosophers over the scope of medical ethics and the question of intuition become more readily explicit. The different understanding and use of intuitions in moral reasoning in medicine arise from the internalization of divergent group norms belonging to physicians and philosophers; these norms emanate from their respective realms of action and reflection. The experience of caring for patients is the foundry of the principle of medical beneficence. Likewise, philosophical reflection in medical ethics tends to support those moral intuitions justified by universal reason, most obviously the principle of autonomy derived from the self-legislating ability of the moral will. Intuitions, and intuitions about intuitions, possessed by physicians and philosophers in the context of medical ethics examined here, present an exemplary confirmation of Bourdieu's theory of practice. In short, the intuitions of physicians and philosophers each represent the subjective reasoning of an elite social group that has internalized a set of professional norms. The heated, if not passionate, nature of the debate is explained both by the certainty of different individuals as to the correctness of their moral intuitions, and also by the feeling of the significance of medical ethical issues for the public.

The moral intuitions of medical ethicists are special in giving rise to principles and norms that appear intrinsically beneficent. Using Bourdieu to analyze the material basis of professional intuitions reveals a more complex structure of social processes. And yet, relating professional intuitions in medical ethics, even those that have become crystallized into fixed principles, to Bourdieu's concept of *habitus*, does not render these intuitions absolutely determinable in practice. The *habitus* in practice can never be ultimately reduced to a set of norms. Rather, Bourdieu compares and contrasts the scientific estimation of probabilities with practical reasoning that "brings into play a whole body of wisdom, sayings, commonplaces," and "ethical precepts" (72). What is remarkable about Bourdieu's theory of practice is that it accounts for these opposing intuitions as the internalization of group norms into *habitus*, yet also allows for the possibility of individual variation or chance. Thus, the sociological analysis of professional intuitions does not exhaust the possibility of action. The theory of *habitus* requires a continual engagement with actual practices.

Bourdieu's analysis of the historical and sociological basis for the divergent intuitions possessed by physicians and philosophers does not obviate the significance of actual intuitions. Despite the determinable pattern of professional intuitions theorized by Bourdieu's *habitus*, the temporal dimension of *habitus* prevents the complete reification of social norms. Likewise, the contingency of human experience prevents medical ethics from being reified into positions represented by philosophical and physician-based reasoning. These intuitions are the crystallization of attitudes that are hardened in the crucible of real human experience.

Conclusion

It is likely that the dichotomies presented by physicians and philosophers in the nature and scope of clinical medical ethics—dichotomies that are revealed through the respective use and understanding of intuition in medical and moral reasoning—cannot be ultimately reconciled. The primary dichotomies are characterized in terms of clinical experience versus theoretical reflection, authority versus reasoned argument, and autonomy versus beneficence. These divergent intuitions and their related dichotomies are the result of an epistemological and ontological divide, which, though dependent on social norms and psychological processes, are not reducible to them. The contemporary debate about the nature and scope of medical ethics demonstrates that the ancient tension between medicine and philosophy continues into the present. It does so, in part, because medicine still requires the conceptual reworking of Aristotelian notions of practice demonstrates how this ancient tension between philosophy and medicine as an ideal form of practice continues in the present. As Bourdieu demonstrates, *habitus* may explain human action, but cannot predict it. Practice then and now deals with what is variable and contingent. Clinical reasoning about individuals provides a model for moral reasoning more generally. Because moral intuitions are not reducible to their social and psychological grounds, moral intuitions present the appearance of moral choice free from the constraints of determinism. This possibility of ethical alterity within moral reasoning indicates that the epistemological divide between physicians and philosophers is not empty, but is filled by an ethical space.[37] This point needs to be unpacked further. A major thesis of this book, to be explored in further chapters, is that the ethical space that arises from the treatment of individuals animates this tension between medicine and philosophy, between theory and practice in medicine, and explains medicine's continual relevance for philosophical reflection.

2

Moral Intuitionism

Clinical reasoning is singular in combining philosophical and practical intuition. By joining these, perhaps antithetical, forms of cognition, clinical reasoning unites direct philosophical intuition as direct perception with commonsense reasoning. The distinction between intuition as philosophical certainty and commonsense knowledge about the sensible world can be traced back to Aristotle. In general, for Aristotle, the *sensus communis* was the primary sense organ, used to make sense of sensible perception. As such, common sense was an aspect of reason, but residing at a more physiological level than that of intuitive judgment.[1] As such, perception provides the link between philosophical intuition and commonsense reasoning. The notion that moral judgments are akin to aesthetic judgments and are derived from sentiment, and not reason, has been developed most famously by the eighteenth-century Scottish Enlightenment philosopher David Hume (1711–76). Hume wrote in this regard that we attain moral knowledge by an "immediate feeling and fine internal sense," and not by a "chain of argument and induction" (Hume 1960, 2). Hume's moral theory has received stimulus from recent neuropsychological research on the neural correlates of emotional and moral reasoning.[2] However, this notion that the faculty of moral reasoning arises through a kind of sense perception goes counter to another famous idea espoused by Hume in an oft-quoted paragraph that has become known as the "is"/"ought" distinction, and relatedly as the "naturalistic fallacy":

> In every system of morality which I have hitherto met with, I have always

usual copulations of propositions, *is*, and *is not*, I meet with no proposition that is not connected with an *ought*, or an *ought not*. This change is imperceptible; but is, however, of the last consequence. For as this *ought* or *ought not*, expresses some new relation or affirmation, 'tis necessary that it should be observ'd and explain'd; and at the same time that a reason should be given, for what seems altogether inconceivable, how this new relation can be a deduction from others, which are entirely different from it. But as authors do not commonly use this precaution, I shall presume to recommend it to the readers; and am persuaded that this small attention wou'd subvert all the vulgar systems of morality, and let us see, that the distinction of vice and virtue is not founded merely on the relations of objects, nor is perceiv'd by reason. (1896, III.i.3)

That Hume posits here the unbridgeable dichotomy between "is" and "ought" is itself generally considered a matter of fact by many analytic philosophers. However, Hume's exact meaning in this paragraph has been a matter of scholarly debate.[3] For example, Alasdair MacIntyre, in supporting a naturalist ethic, claims that Hume was in fact arguing for the correctness of the relation between "is" and "ought."[4] Accepting for the moment the majority opinion that Hume did actually intend to posit the fact/value distinction, the next question is whether he was correct in doing so. The widespread acceptance of the unquestionable separation between "is" and "ought" in regard to moral issues is largely due to the reworking of the Humean fact/value dichotomy by the early twentieth-century British moral philosopher G. E. Moore in his concept of the "naturalistic fallacy." Moore claims that it is a fallacy to attribute any natural properties to the term "goodness." Following Moore, other analytic philosophers—for example, R. M. Hare and C. L. Stevenson—have developed their own nonnaturalistic theories of moral philosophy on the basis of the fact/value distinction. Despite its long currency, Moore's argument against the naturalistic fallacy and the absolute dichotomy between the realms of fact versus value has also been contested by some analytic philosophers. Notably, Philippa Foot has argued for an inseparable connection between moral judgment and human will.[5]

This question of the validity of the fact/value dichotomy is important for an understanding of moral reasoning in medicine and medical ethics. This gap between "is" and "ought" provides, arguably, the crucial ontological factor responsible for the opposition between naturalistic and nonnaturalistic ethics in medicine; bridging this gap is equally important in developing a moral theory of clinical reasoning. For example, as discussed in the previous chapter, the medical privileging of beneficence arises from physician-based experience of caring for actual patients. Beneficence is a naturalistic ethics principle inherent to medicine as a profession. The duty to care for patients arises directly from their factual vulnerability and the power physicians have to harm or to heal. Autonomy, on the other hand, is a nonnaturalistic principle derived from the Kantian philosophical conception of people's duty of moral self-determination. Autonomy might be empirically influenced by the mental capacity of patients, but its moral force arises irrespective of particular empirical concerns. Finding a way of bridging the "is"/"ought" separation provides, therefore, a way of mediating between divergent kinds of moral intuitions in medicine. Mediating between naturalistic and nonnaturalistic moral intuitions parallels the process of clinical reasoning that links intuition as a form of direct perception and commonsense reasoning.[6]

The method I propose in this chapter of analyzing the fact/value distinction in clinical reasoning occurs via an analysis of moral intuitionism, the philosophical theory dealing directly with the question of the validity of relying on our moral intuitions. Because of the close relation between moral intuitionism and the fact/value distinction, this chapter analyzes moral intuitionism in medical ethics in relation to the naturalistic fallacy. Moral intuitionism is also associated with the philosopher G. E. Moore, who is best remembered for his associated critique of the "naturalistic fallacy." As developed by Moore, moral intuitionism is a type of nonnaturalism in that it posits goodness as a nonnatural category. William Frankena has provided the following useful definition of moral intuitionism that emphasizes the distinction between intuitionism and naturalism: "An intuitionist must believe in simple indefinable properties, properties that are of a peculiar non-natural or normative sort, a priori or non empirical concepts, and self-evident or synthetic necessary propositions" (1973, 103).

Frankena's definition establishes a distinction between empirical reasoning from evidence and intuitionism as a form of a priori rationalism. While Moore's moral philosophy espoused a nonnaturalist and intuitionist approach, nonnaturalism and moral intuitionism are not necessarily synonymous. Philosophers indebted to Moore have been nonnaturalist and nonintuitionist, or naturalist and intuitionist. Evaluating the relation between intuitionism and naturalism can lead, therefore, into an intellectual thicket. Examining the relation between naturalism and intuitionism vis-à-vis medical ethics provides a convenient framing structure with which to analyze this relation.

It is important to point out that not all philosophers who rely on intuitions support placing their ethical approach under the rubric of moral intuitionism.

indefeasible and that the theory of moral intuitionism therefore supports an irrationally grounded theory of moral philosophy. This conception, as will be seen, is not necessarily true. On the contrary, theories of moral intuitionism provide methods of comparing and contrasting divergent intuitions. Rather than accepting that because intuitions are pretheoretical they are equally indefeasible, an evaluation of moral intuitionism offers a means of evaluating divergent intuitions and negotiating between apparently incommensurable positions.

This chapter is divided into three sections. In the first half I analyze three theoretical approaches in moral philosophy: naturalism, nonnaturalism, and moral intuitionism. While the main concern is with moral intuitionism, the other two approaches provide useful contextual background for comparison. Following this theoretical discussion I analyze Baruch Brody's application of moral intuitionism to medical ethics. Brody's theoretical method is evaluated in relation to an insightful case that he includes in *Life and Death Decision Making*. In the final section of this chapter, Brody's analytic theory of moral intuitionism is critiqued in relation to the question of the relevance of proximity to death in end-of-life decision making. I argue in conclusion that while moral intuitionism is a valuable resource in medical ethics, the analytic theories of moral intuitionism should incorporate a phenomenological awareness of temporality into their theoretical structure.

G. E. Moore's "Naturalistic Fallacy"

G. E. Moore's (1873–1958) moral philosophy embodies the philosophical approach that is at once intuitionist and nonnaturalist. Much of twentieth-century analytic moral philosophy has taken shape under the influence of G. E. Moore's *Principia Ethica*. In particular, a considerable part of the literature resulting from this work is devoted to contesting or exploring the consequences of Moore's concept of the so-called naturalistic fallacy. In the *Principia Ethica* Moore argues that much of moral philosophy has fallen short in assuming that the philosophical notion of "the good" can be defined through an analysis of the properties belonging to the object described as good. In a famous passage Moore states that

> "good" is a simple notion, just as "yellow" is a simple notion; that, just as you cannot, by any manner of means, explain to any one who does not already know it, what yellow is, so you cannot explain what good is. (1903, 7)

Thus as a simple quality, good can never be reduced to anything simpler, and additionally cannot be understood in terms not related to goodness, such as natural objects. Moore describes the attempt to depict goodness in natural terms as the "naturalistic fallacy," supposedly committed for centuries by moral philosophers.[8]

Moore's naturalistic fallacy is derived from Hume's separation between "is" and "ought." By claiming that goodness is a simple quality and has no relation to the properties of objects, Moore is in essential agreement with those who attribute to Hume the absolute separation between "is" and "ought." The approaches supporting or contesting the fact/value distinction and its offshoot, the naturalistic fallacy, have created a fault line between two significant approaches in analytic moral philosophy—between naturalism and nonnaturalism, respectively.[9] Thus, naturalists can be defined as those who believe that moral terms refer to natural properties that can be observed by the physical senses. Nonnaturalists, of whom Moore is exemplary, believe that moral terms refer to nonnatural properties. Intuitionists fit into the nonnaturalist category, since they generally believe that moral knowledge is derived ultimately neither through deductive reason, nor from the senses.[10] Rather, for them goodness as a nonnatural property is perceived directly through our faculty of intuition. Both strands of Moore's theory of goodness, nonnaturalism and intuitionism, can be traced in regard to medical ethics.

Naturalist-Based Medical Ethics

It is relatively easy to trace the link between naturalism and medicine. As seen in the previous chapter, physicians have a tendency to trace the foundations of medical ethics to a Hippocratic ethic rooted in empirical practice. Defending a naturalist-based virtue ethics, MacIntyre takes Moore to task for the naturalistic fallacy, arguing that statements about the good *do* belong to a type of factual statement. These factual statements about the good cannot be separated from a philosophical anthropology:

> Human beings, like the members of all other species, have a specific nature; and that nature is such that they have certain aims and goals, such that they move by nature towards a specific *telos*. The good is defined in terms of their specific characteristics. Hence Aristotle's ethics, as he expounds it, presupposes his metaphysical biology. Aristotle thus set himself the task of giving an account of the good which is at once local and particular—located in and partially defined by the characteristics of the *polis*—and yet also cosmic and

Naturalists, such as MacIntyre, not only accept but also advocate the essential relation between being and obligation. MacIntyre traces this natu ralistic ethics back to Aristotle's *Ethics*, arguing that for Aristotle there is no ultimate separation between fact and value. Interestingly, MacIntyre draws the connection between Aristotle's ethics and his metaphysical biology. Other commentators on Aristotle, too, have noted the important influence of Aristotle's experience as a biologist on his *Ethics*. For example, Marjorie Grene writes in her *Portrait of Aristotle* that

> what distinguishes Aristotle's "emphasis of attention" from Plato's or Des-
> cartes's or any other philosopher's, I shall argue, is closely related to a certain
> kind of field naturalist's passion for the minute observation of the structures
> and life histories of living things. This is a passion which antedates, and helps
> to determine, the whole of the Corpus as we have it, that is, it bears essentially
> and deeply on Aristotle himself, on the mind of the most neatly and elabo-
> rately systematic of Western thinkers as from his own writings we can and do
> know him. (1963, 33–34)

Grene argues here that Aristotle learned from his work as a biologist not to stray from the concrete realm of observation and experience, but also to value the contingent nature of human knowledge. The influence of medi-cine and biology is evident in the widespread use of medical metaphors and analogies in Aristotle's *Ethics*. Notably, at the beginning of the *Nicomachean Ethics* Aristotle uses a medical analogy to inform us that as there are different types of knowledge, there are different types of goods at which different hu-man actions aim.[11]

Following on from Aristotle, natural philosophers continue the idea that medicine, as the convergence of biology with human values, links the realms of facts and values. In support of this view, William Stempsey has convinc-ingly argued for a value-dependent realism where "all facts in medicine, in-cluding facts about diagnosis, depend on values for their specification" (1999, 49). While medical facts for Stempsey are not free from human values, values in medicine in turn reflect an objective reality as much as hard physiological data. For example, a simple diagnostic blood test to investigate the presence of the HIV virus cannot be separated from the human values associated with the test's results. Stempsey's argument does not need to be interpreted as a refutation of Moore's naturalistic fallacy. Rather, his argument demonstrates the close interaction between facts and values in medical practice. Medicine provides a model for distinguishing fact and value while admitting their close interaction in practical human affairs.

The close relation between fact and value in medicine tends to contradict the fact/value distinction, yet one can hold a position close to the naturalist one without claiming an ultimate link between fact and value. Similarly, an intuitive faculty might be supported in a naturalistic framework, provided its faculty of moral reasoning is grounded in commonsense perception. The situation is, however, different for moral intuitionists who, like Moore, claim that goodness does not possess objective natural properties and is known through a nonperceptual faculty of intuition.

Nonnaturalism

The next branch of moral philosophy coming out of Moore's philosophy is the influential nonnaturalist approach developed by the group of noncognitivist linguistic philosophers. The different approaches taken by these philosophers are unified by their opposition to moral intuitionism and through their focus on the structure of language obtaining in moral statements.[12] Thus, philosophers such as A. J. Ayer, C. L. Stevenson, and R. M. Hare have evaded the problems faced by naturalists and intuitionists by focusing on the meaning of moral language. The noncognitivist perspective has been summarized as follows:

> Theories in which it is denied that ethical statements have truth-values (at least *qua* ethical) will be termed non-cognitivist truth-values. As the non-cognitivists deny any reality to moral properties, they require no moral epistemology, for there are no moral truths to know. (Sterling 1994, xii)

Since according to the noncognitivist approach there is no such thing as moral properties, natural or otherwise, there is no need for a cognitive faculty of intuition. While the noncognitivist approach is nonintuitionist, it affirms the validity of Moore's naturalistic fallacy. Common to noncognitivism is the acceptance that in the commonsensical, everyday world there appears to be a correlation between facts and values; yet in an ultimate philosophical sense there is no intrinsic manner of transmuting natural facts into ethical obligations. Even nonnaturalists admit that natural empirical properties may have importance in moral judgments, but this does not mean that natural facts can be transmuted into ethical obligations.

The allowance by noncognitivists for the importance of facts in everyday moral decisions, while they deny their validity at the level of philosophical "moral supervenience." Hudson provides a useful description of this complicated concept:

> What he [Hare] meant by supervenience has, perhaps, been slightly misrepresented in my account of it this far. The point which he notes about, e.g., "X is good," is not simply that one may ask a reason why and universalize the answer. It is rather that one can always ask, "What is good about it?" and that the answer can never be "Just its goodness." This is where "X is good" differs from e.g., "X is yellow." To "What is yellow about it?" the answer may, though it need not, be "Just its yellowness." Goodness (and, equally, rightness or oughtness) is always necessarily supervenient upon other characteristics as yellowness (or any other non-evaluative characteristic) is not. (1970, 183)

In other words, by moral supervenience, Hare is arguing that while moral values are not properties in the sense construed by naturalists and intuitionists, moral properties can only be determined through recognition of the objective properties on which goodness is dependent.[13] Of course, one should bear in mind that when discussing goodness, Hare means to refer to the words and statements that convey value, rather than holding that such things as value or goodness actually do exist objectively beyond their meaning in language.[14]

This analysis of the relation between fact and value in Hare's approach is enriched through his understanding of the practical syllogism. According to Hare's understanding, the relation between fact and value is maintained in the practical syllogism. The practical syllogism is of particular interest to Hare, since it appears to provide instances where one can derive "is" from "ought." Syllogisms, if one recalls from Aristotle, are comprised of a major premise, a minor premise, and a conclusion. A moral syllogism would repeat the form of the syllogism in general, but would, as Hare argues, contain an "ought" principle in the major premise and an "is" statement in the minor premise. The resulting conclusion would therefore contain a particular "ought" judgment. Thus, the fact/value distinction is apparently overcome through syllogisms that introduce moral evaluations into statements of fact.[15] Hare argues, therefore, that the moral imperatives resulting from the practical syllogism are a function of the language inherent within the structure of the syllogism, rather than the result of an objective fact:

> It has been argued, convincingly in my opinion, that all deductive inference is analytic in character; that is to say, that the function of a deductive inference is not to get from the premisses "something further" not implicit in them [even if that is what Aristotle meant (2.4)], but to make explicit what was implicit

in the conjunction of the premisses. This has been shown to follow from the very nature of language; for to say anything we have, as we have already noticed, to obey some rules, and these rules—especially but not only the rules for the use of so-called logical words—mean, firstly, that to say what is in the premisses of a valid inference is to say, at least, what is in the conclusion, and secondly, that if anything is said in the conclusion which is not said, implicitly or explicitly, in the premisses, the inference is invalid. We cannot be said to understand fully the meaning of premisses and conclusion unless we admit the validity of the inference. Thus, if someone professed to admit that all men were mortal and that Socrates was a man, but refused to admit that Socrates was mortal, the correct thing to do would be not, as has sometimes been suggested, to accuse him of some kind of logical purblindness, but to say "You evidently don't know the meaning of the word 'all'; for if you did you would *eo ipso* know how to make inferences of this sort." (1952, 32–33)[16]

This brief summary of Hare's concept of moral supervenience and his use of the practical syllogism emphasizes the close relation in practice between "is" and "ought," despite the denial at an abstract philosophical level by those philosophers who seek to uphold Moore's naturalistic fallacy. As Nicholas Rescher has pointed out, despite the very real gap between facts and values, the "inferential gap" between them is actually very narrow, often being crossed by no more than a mere truism.[17] It is obvious that while there is a real philosophical difference between those who support the fact/value distinction in theory, in practice there is real commensurability between the two camps in admitting the everyday conflation of fact and value. Yet, the noncognitivist claim that moral concepts are structures of language, rather than resulting from objective moral properties, leads them to deny the validity of our faculty of moral intuitions.

Moral Intuitionism

Moral intuitionism is the second branch of Moore's approach in moral philosophy and the focus of discussion for the remainder of this chapter. Intuitionists generally believe that moral knowledge is derived neither through deductive reason nor from the senses. Thus, intuitionists maintain that intuition provides a separate and independent means of deriving moral knowledge. There are two characteristics which people generally refer to in talking about the classical sense of moral intuition: firstly that it cannot be doubted, and secondly that it cannot be false. Additionally, this type of intuition is cannot stand from a position logically prior to intuition in order to doubt it. Aristotle originally made this point in affirming his notion of *nous* as independent of and in fact grounding processes of logic, the corollary of this being an endless regression.[19] Moral intuitionism in the tradition of analytic philosophy is, however, more rooted in Descartes's notion of direct certainty. Moral intuitionism as a philosophical method in the tradition of analytic philosophy can be traced from Ralph Cudworth in the seventeenth century.[20] Cudworth's notion of intuition most resembles the notion of intuition as a form of infallible certainty. With William Whewell in the nineteenth century, one finds for the first time the notion of a moral intuitionism that is progressive, or dependent on social institutions, particularly in issues of justice. Despite the importance of Whewell's contribution to the progressive notion of intuition, it was not Whewell but Henry Sidgwick who has had the greatest influence on twentieth-century moral intuitionists. In his influential *The Methods of Ethics*, Sidgwick described three forms of intuitionism. He identified firstly an immediate intuitionism that "recognizes simple . . . intuitions alone" (1907, 100). Secondly, he identified an intuitionism which discerns "general rules with really clear and finally valid intuition." This form of intuition is "implicit in the moral reasoning of ordinary men" (101). Finally, Sidgwick identified a form of intuitionism only available to trained philosophers:

> In short, without being disposed to deny that conduct commonly judged to right is so, we may yet require some deeper explanation why it is so. From this demand springs a third species or phase of Intuitionism, which, while accepting the morality of common sense as in the main sound, still attempts to find for it a philosophic basis which it does not itself offer: to get one or more principles more absolutely and undeniably true and evidence, from which the current rules might be deduced, either just as they are commonly received or with slight modifications and rectifications. (101–2)

Accordingly, for Sidgwick, intuitions as ultimate evidence provide the moral data, which are then philosophically understood through philosophical abstraction.

In the twentieth century other philosophers besides Moore who stand out as standard bearers of moral intuitionism include H. A. Prichard, W. D. Ross, and John Rawls. More recently Robert Audi has articulated a comprehensive theory of moral intuitionism, and Baruch Brody has applied a modified theory of moral intuitionism to the field of clinical medical ethics. For the sake of completeness I shall briefly describe the first three, before providing a more detailed review of Audi's and Brody's theories of moral intuitionism in the context of clinical medical ethics.

H.A. PRICHARD

In a well-known article entitled "Does Moral Philosophy Rest on a Mistake?," H. A. Prichard argued for a type of intuitive "moral thinking" akin to mathematical knowledge. Thus Prichard writes that "this apprehension is immediate, in precisely the sense in which a mathematical apprehension is immediate" (1949 [1912], 8). What is most interesting about Prichard's model of intuition is that he argues for a form of intuition both at the levels of presentation of data and the interpretation of that data. There is, therefore, for Prichard a correlation between intuitive apprehension and moral reasoning.

W.D. ROSS

Intuitionism as a moral theory is frequently associated with the deontologist W. D. Ross's appeal to prima facie principles.[21] Ross relies on intuition to discern different principles such as goodness, rightness, and duty in different contexts. Ross's theory is commonly associated with two conceptions of intuitionism: its irreducible pluralism, and the emphasis on the self-evidence of propositions referring to our prima facie duties. Ross refers to the self-evidence of prima facie intuitions in the following paragraph from his classic work, *The Right and the Good*, worth quoting:

> That an act qua fulfilling a promise, or qua effected a just distribution of good . . . is prima facie right, is self-evident; not in the sense that it is evident from the beginning of our lives, or as soon as we attend to the proposition for the first time, but in the sense that when we have reached sufficient mental maturity and have given sufficient attention to the proposition it is evident without any need of proof, or of evidence beyond itself. It is evident just as a mathematical axiom, or the validity of a form of inference, is evident. . . . In our confidence that these propositions are true there is involved the same confidence in our reason that is involved in our confidence in mathematics. . . . In both cases we are dealing with propositions that cannot be proved, but that, just as certainly need no proof. (2002, 8)

JOHN RAWLS

In the latter half of the twentieth century the influential political philosopher John Rawls espoused a form of intuitionism in his theory of justice. Rawls appears to unite the two aspects of intuition developed by Prichards and Ross: intuition as clear moral power, and intuition as the tool for evaluating divergent moral choices. According to Rawls, our moral intuitions provide

the highest-order constructive criteria for determining the competing principles of justice.[22]

Robert Audi, extending Ross's theory, has proposed a sophisticated version
of moral intuitionism deserving of special attention. Audi points out that intuitionism is used mainly to refer either to an "overall kind of ethical theory,"
or else to a "moral epistemology characteristic of such theories" (1997, 33). As
an overall theory, intuitionism possesses three characteristics:

> (1) It is an ethical pluralism, a position affirming an irreducible plurality of ba-
> sic moral principles. (2) Each principle centers on a different kind of ground,
> in the sense of a factor implying a prima facie moral duty, such as making
> a promise or noticing a person who will bleed to death without one's help.
> (3) Each principle is taken to be in some sense intuitively known. (Ibid.)

As a moral epistemology intuition is held to refer to a noninferential faculty
of moral reasoning. It is this stronger claim that accounts for the persistent
criticism of intuitionism as indefeasible, despite the continuation of intuitionist theories up to and including Rawls's. Opponents of intuitionism argue that since intuition does not provide evidence other than an appeal to intuition as that upon which moral knowledge is ultimately founded, intuition
does not in fact increase our moral knowledge at all.

Cognizant of this type of criticism Audi proposes a version of intuitionism that is not indefeasible. His conception of intuitionism possesses four
characteristics:

> (1) An intuition must be non-inferential, in the sense that the intuited prop-
> osition in question is not—at the same time it is intuitively held—held on
> the basis of a premise. (2) An intuition must be a moderately firm cognition.
> (3) Intuitions must be formed in the light of an adequate understanding of
> their propositional objects. In other words, intuitions require a certain level of
> theoretical understanding of the context in which they are formed. (4) Intu-
> itions are pretheoretical: roughly, they are neither evidentially dependent on
> theories nor themselves theoretical hypotheses. (1997, 40–2)

Audi's version of modified intuitionism is original in proposing that intuitions can be both pretheoretical and theoretically justifiable. One manner
in which this can occur is that a pretheoretical intuition can evolve into a
judgment grounded in theory. Audi proposes that pretheoretical intuitions
are noninferential, yet require conscious understanding of their propo-
sitional objects. Furthermore, intuitions can manifest themselves, not only

at the level of an initial apprehension but in the form of a rational conclusion. Stated differently, while intuitions may be expressible in the form of a theoretically grounded premise, rational beliefs are not necessarily arrived at in the form of such premises. Moreover, such intuitions may appear following periods of intense reflection and are not simply spontaneous psychological feelings. Audi claims in this regard that "an intuition may not emerge until reflection proceeds for some time. Such an intuition can be a conclusion of reflection, temporally as well as epistemically; and it may be either empirical or a priori" (44).

Characteristic of such intuitions are their epistemic flexibility. These intuitions are not indefeasible and, like Ross's intuitions regarding prima facie principles, are context-dependent. Since they may be both empirical and a priori, Audi's understanding of moral intuitions resists the division between empiricist naturalism and nonnaturalist rationalism. His is a self-described moral epistemology that is "qualifiedly rationalistic" and "moderately intuitionist," and an ontology of ethics that is "realist, pluralist, and nonreductively naturalistic." Additionally, it is a moral psychology that "countenances unconscious motivation and cognition" (v).

More than a theoretical formulation, Audi's modified version of moral intuitionism describes an introspective process for developing awareness around our intentions vis-à-vis moral objects:

> It is more like a response to viewing a painting or seeing an expressive face than to propositionally represented information. One responds to a pattern: one notices an emotional tone in the otherwise factual listing of deficiencies; one hears him compare her work to some that he once did; and so forth. The conclusion of reflection is a wrapping up of the question, similar to concluding a practical matter with a decision. One has not added up the evidences and formulated their implication; one has obtained a view of the whole and characterized it overall. (43)

In arguing that the process of moral intuitionism is akin to processes of facial interpretation, Audi posits a type of moral physiognomy. His theory fulfills the need described by Putnam of doing moral philosophy having in mind a moral image of the world. It is particularly interesting, therefore, to test Audi's form of intuitionism in the medical context. While, as far as I am aware, there has not yet been such an application, there is one serious attempt to develop a version of modified moral intuitionism in the medical context that has been carried out by the philosopher and medical ethicist,

understand medical ethics using analytic philosophy, but they also provide
test cases to check the validity of this philosophy in the crucible of everyday
medical life. I now wish to turn to analyze Brody's attempt to apply moral
intuitionism in the medical context. Brody's intuitionism, as will be seen,
repeats some of the criteria noted with regard to other intuitionists, especially
those of Ross and Audi, but is also an original version in its own right.

Baruch Brody's Pluralistic Casuistry

Brody first developed his theory of intuitionism in an essay entitled "Intuitions and Objective Moral Truth," published in the philosophical journal
The Monist in 1979. As an active clinical ethicist, Brody applied this approach
in the context of medical ethics. The development of Brody's theory of moral
intuitionism in medical ethics has been most fully developed in his book *Life
and Death Decision Making* (1988). The title of this book reflects the types of
issues that Brody has worked with as the head of an active clinical consult
service. More recently, Brody (2003) has reaffirmed his theory of moral intuitionism in a collection of his essays entitled *Taking Issue: Pluralism and
Casuistry in Bioethics.*[23]

   As the title suggests, Brody considers his philosophical approach to medical or bioethics to be the combination of moral pluralism with casuistry. As a
"normative moral pluralist," Brody believes that "one can draw conclusions
about the rightness or wrongness of actions from premises that attribute several independent properties to the action in question" (2). The existence of
"moral ambiguity"—where there is disagreement as to the correct course of
action even where there is agreement regarding the facts of a case—leads
Brody to propose his theory of moral pluralism. Moral pluralism explains
this moral ambiguity as consequent to the necessary existence of "different
legitimate moral appeals supporting different conclusions about what to do
in the cases in question combined with there being no clear way in those
cases to decide which appeal takes precedence" (3). In contradistinction to
Veatch, Brody argues that there is no "lexical priority" between different moral
appeals. What is an important precedent in one case can become secondary
in another. The contingent nature of particular cases modifies, therefore, the
relevance of particular moral appeals. The importance of the case-based context explains casuistry as the second element within Brody's philosophical
theory of clinical ethics. The second reason why Brody's method is a form
of casuistry is that he bases the knowledge of the legitimacy of moral appeals and their related factors to the generalization from moral intuitions in

particular cases. In other words, moral intuitions provide the ultimate foundation upon which particular moral claims are based. As such, Brody's pluralistic casuistry is dependent on a method of moral intuitionism.

An examination of Brody's understanding of intuitionism reveals the appeal of an intuitionist approach, as well as some of its limitations. In advocating a type of intuitionism in clinical medical ethics, Brody combines the intuitionist approach developed in particular by Sidgwick with Hare's notion of moral supervenience.[24] His is a modified form of intuitionism that affirms the presence of intuitions as the product of a natural cognitive capacity to form moral judgments. At the same time Brody, like Audi, rejects intuitionism as a form of incorrigible knowledge. There are a number of key elements that constitute Brody's approach.

Firstly, Brody claims that his notion of intuition does not imply complete self-evidence or indubitability, as is generally assumed by critics of philosophical intuitionism. Rather, Brody's modified intuitionism claims that intuitions are

> tentative judgments about particular individuals, actions, and social arrangements which are based upon our observations of these particular individuals, actions, or arrangements, but which go beyond what is observed or what can be deductively or inductively inferred from what is observed. (1988, 446)

Furthermore, Brody assumes from previous metaethical discussions that moral properties are supervenient properties. In other words, "while their possession is dependent upon the nonmoral properties of individuals, actions, and social arrangements, their possession is neither deductively nor inductively inferable from the possession of those nonmoral properties" (447). Thus, particular contexts and situations affect the determination of moral judgments, but the moral good cannot be logically inferred from these nonmoral properties. Intuitions, according to Brody's conception, provide the evaluations of experiences rather than simply reports of what has happened. By defining intuitions as a form of moral data collection, Brody attempts to develop a moral intuitionism that is neither a moral sense theory nor a theory of moral reasoning.

Finally, Brody distinguishes between intuitive judgments and moral rules. As previously seen Brody does not allow for moral rule formation at the level of intuitive judgment. Rather, intuitive judgments provide evidence regarding particular cases, while moral rules can be formed at a later stage using the data provided by moral intuitions. Moral rules can, therefore, be flexible tests scientific principles through empirical investigation. The application of moral intuitionism to particular cases or moral actions distinguishes Brody's theory from Ross's intuitionism, where moral intuitions are examined at the more general level of prima facie rules.

With his modified method of casuistic moral intuitionism, Brody attempts to provide a moral theory that is a form of moral realism, yet allows for the complexity of human experience. In summary, Brody's modified intuitionism is a sophisticated version of moral intuitionism and can be defended philosophically, irrespective of its application to medicine. Its philosophical validity has the merits and constraints comparable with other versions of moral intuitionism, such as those provided by Ross and Audi. What is most relevant here, however, is the development of this form of modified intuitionism in the medical context. Since his method emphasizes the particularity of particular cases, it is important to examine Brody's theory in its application.

A Case Study

As a test case for Brody's method I have singled out one particular case for consideration that he considers in *Life and Death Decision Making*:

> Mrs. G is an 83-year-old woman who has suffered from circulation problems in her lower extremities for the past twenty years and who became bedridden and institutionalized in a nursing home seven years ago. Two years ago, she became incontinent; she also began to report that she suffers from constant body pain, the etiology of which is unclear. Recently, she was found in her room in the nursing home having difficulties breathing and was brought to the emergency room. There, her $PaCO_2$ was 70, so that she underwent emergency intubation and was admitted to the ICU. It is difficult to communicate with her, and Psychiatry is not prepared to make a formal assessment of her competency, but she is alert and oriented and writes in response to questions that she is suffering from so many diseases that she just wants to be allowed to die. The trouble is that the etiology of her current problems is unclear. Is her retention of CO_2 caused by drugs? Does it indicate significant obstructive pulmonary disease? No clear answer has emerged, the team is not at all convinced that she is suffering from a terminal illness, and she has no family to consult.
>
> Questions: This case, like several earlier cases of intubated patients, raises a special problem in getting a confident assessment of competency given the difficulties of communicating with the patient. Nevertheless, some members of the team feel that the patient's wishes should be respected, because they are her wishes and/or because of the low quality of her life in recent years and/or because she is going to die in the relatively near future no matter what

is done. Other team members disagree. They find the patient's wishes to be an inadequate reason for stopping the treatment because of the difficulty of assessing her competency, partly because she is intubated and partly because she is heavily medicated in response to her chronic pain problems. Moreover, they claim, we cannot treat her as a terminally ill patient, because the etiology of her problem is unknown. Finally, they suggest, we have no way of assessing the quality-of-life factors influencing some members of the team—the patient is in chronic pain, is bedridden, and is incontinent. A different question has also attracted considerable attention. Should we take as another reason for not treating the patient the fact that she is alone, institutionalized and a burden? Or, as one member of the team strongly argues in response, should we treat this patient precisely because we want to avoid prejudices against the elderly institutionalized patient? (122–23)

The example presented by Brody is a useful demonstration of the complexity of everyday decision making in contemporary clinical medicine. Furthermore, this case demonstrates the theory-rich nature of case-based thinking—a case, like a picture, is worth a thousand words. Brody highlights the moral questions that this case elicits, that is, whether it is permissible in this case to withdraw treatment and allow this elderly woman to die as she requests. Besides Brody's own insights about this case, a number of metaethical observations can be made.

First of all, one sees the importance in the American context of autonomy. If this woman had demonstrated clear mental coherence, there would in all likelihood have been less argument about acquiescing to the patient's wishes to be allowed to die. The problem in this instance is that it is not apparent that she is making a so-called fully informed decision. The ethical dilemma here hinges on the medical situation: whether this woman is able as a result of the mind-altering medical treatment she has received to make a competent decision, and secondly whether she is indeed suffering from a diagnosable terminal illness (other than old age).

In light of the previous discussion regarding the divergent types of medical and philosophical intuitions, one can see the two ethical positions as philosophical approaches grounded in nonnaturalistic and naturalistic ethics, respectively. Thus, those who would grant this woman the right to relinquish her right to life base their decision in part out of a respect for the principle of autonomy. Respect for autonomy is in turn founded upon a moral intuition held by medical ethicists that autonomy is one of the—if not *the*—fundamental bases of moral freedom. The second approach wishes to persist with lence and would fit well with the physicians who argue that clinical ethics is a branch of medicine.[25] Brody came to a similar conclusion in an article he wrote on ethical issues in the management of patients in "persistent vegetative states" (PVS). In this context, he argues that the question of whether to prolong life through medical treatment of people existing in this condition depends on whether one accepts an ethic intrinsic to medicine, and the prolongation of life as a normative medical goal.[26]

Both approaches in this case are dependent on the medical context. The decision to respect the patient's wishes to be allowed to die were motivated by her low quality of life and probable closeness to death; whereas, the decision to continue treatment was motivated by the inadequacy of determining mental competence, as well as the inability to treat the patient as terminally ill because of the undetermined medical etiology of the presenting illness. While the medical context is important for both positions, it is apparent that it carries greater significance for the opinion based on medical beneficence than for that emphasizing patient autonomy. Brody does not evaluate the differences between these two positions, since according to his method of pluralistic casuistry both positions are morally acceptable. What he calls "moral ambiguity" is a necessary consequence of the reality of divergent moral positions. The moral intuitions of the two approaches are the result of divergent moral responses to a single medical context. These intuitions can then become formalized into principles such as autonomy and beneficence as I have done, or else in alternative formulations such as the right to life versus respect for persons as Brody does.[27]

Proximity to Death

Brody's approach of providing rigorous reflection on our intuitions that arise in specific cases can also be described in Audi's terms as a process of introspection leading to increased awareness and intention about moral objects. Yet there is an aporia in Brody's case that reveals his philosophical bias in advocating a moral intuitionism that privileges philosophical reflection. Furthermore, this aporia also reveals the distinction between the pretheoretical intuitions possessed by physicians and philosophers. Despite being sensitive to the medical dimensions of ethical questions, including the issue of diagnostic and prognostic certainty, Brody does not fully explore the significance of the patient's proximity to death in his discussion of the moral intuitions pertaining to this case. One wonders what difference having a terminal illness should make to the question of whether to treat or not? That it *does* make a difference in practice is clear. Literature spanning the spectrum of attitudes toward physician-assisted suicide affirms the permissibility of administering potentially lethal doses of sedating medicine to terminal patients suffering from intractable pain.[28] In other words, proximity to death grants a person suffering from intractable pain the right to pain medication at the risk of inducing death, far more readily than a nonterminal patient suffering from equivalent intensity of pain. This indicates that proximity to death introduces a singular structure into moral reasoning in the medical context. Since the right to terminal sedation is only given to terminally ill patients, the significant factor here is not the entity of pain interfering with quality of life so much as the closing of the temporal finitude of a particular human life, which carries an ethical imperative. In the case brought by Brody, the diagnosis of a terminal illness would have sealed the discussion about granting the woman's wishes to be allowed to die.

Yet, while the fact of terminality appears natural to physicians involved in palliative care, the importance of proximity to death has been philosophically contested. Consider the article by medical ethicist Lynn Jansen (2003) entitled "The Moral Irrelevance of Proximity to Death." In this article Jansen develops an intuitive approach that contests the assumption that proximity to death is a morally important factor in the permissibility of terminal sedation. Here "terminal sedation" is a specific term referring to the procedure whereby doctors induce a state of continuing unconsciousness (such as by a barbiturate coma) wherein the patient is denied nutrition and hydration until the onset of death. More generally, Jansen rejects ascribing any intrinsic moral content to proximity to death in palliative care. She argues that proximity to death has no moral importance once the factors often correlated with it have been isolated. Jansen traces three main reasons traditionally presented in the medical ethics literature that supports ascribing moral significance to proximity of death: (1) the argument that human life has unconditional value, (2) the argument that distance from death is important because of the possibility of recovery, and (3) the argument that when a patient is close to death, his or her death is more "natural" than the deaths of patients who are far from death.

I shall only deal with Jansen's third argument, the naturalistic one, because of all three arguments it has the most philosophical weight, and also because it pertains to the relation between naturalism and nonnaturalism in medicine. Those upholding this position claim that there is an important difference between the terminal sedation of a patient far from death and that of one close to death. In the former instance, the physician's intervention is close to death, terminal sedation should not be considered an act of killing. Jansen argues that this reasoning is fallacious since whether a patient has a terminal diagnosis or not, the procedure of terminal sedation may result in the death of a patient and is therefore the causative event of death, irrespective of the underlying disease. Jansen concludes, therefore, that the naturalistic argument in support of the moral relevance of the proximity to death does not hold water.

In arguing against the relevance of the moral proximity to death Jansen does not articulate any opinion about terminal sedation or physician-assisted suicide. By emphasizing the importance of suffering rather than proximity to death in deliberating about terminal sedation, Jansen's argument could be construed to support physician-assisted suicide. Respect for the relevance of moral proximity to death is associated with the moral intuitions possessed by many physicians derived from a naturalistic ethic intrinsic to medicine, which proscribes physicians from killing patients. The importance of the moral proximity to death for physicians is encapsulated in the law of double effect, whereby actions are permitted even though they lead to unintended though foreseen consequences.[29] For example, in administering high doses of analgesia to patients the unintended consequence of death is not considered killing, since the intention was primarily to relieve intractable suffering. The law of double effect allows physicians to administer adequate palliative care to patients, even leading to death of patients, yet it opposes physician-assisted suicide and euthanasia. The law of double effect developed in Catholic casuistry finds ready applicability in the medical context because it is in general accordance with physicians' intuitions regarding the ethical practice of medicine.[30] Likewise, in the application of the law of double effect to terminal sedation, the proximity to death is also of crucial significance in alleviating the moral conscience of physicians in helping patients to die with dignity.

While not mentioning the law of double effect specifically, Jansen undoubtedly would ascribe the reliance on proximity to death in this instance, too, as a psychological salve to a practitioner's divided conscience and still lacking in any real philosophical moral content. Yet, should this moral intuition of physicians be dismissed so lightly? It is of interest to note that Jansen's paper elicited fierce opposition by the humanist physician Eric Cassell at the medical ethics conference where it was first presented.[31] The intense response can be explained by a clash of intuitions regarding the relevance of the moral proximity to death. These divergent intuitions can be attributed to the different ontological realms of reflection and experience rooted in philosophical and medical practice. More than this, however, one wonders if the failure to explain the deep medical intuition regarding the moral proximity to death is not revealing of an aporia in the structure of analytic reasoning itself, particularly in its application to lived experience intrinsic to the medical context. This would explain Brody's failure to draw out the significance of terminal illness in his case discussion cited earlier, as well as Jansen's inability to account adequately for the moral basis of physicians' intuitions regarding the moral relevance of proximity to death. This aporia can be seen in the case used as a model to describe Brody's application of moral intuitionism, despite his approach providing a method of introspective attention to our intuitions of moral properties in the medical context.

Phenomenological Structure of Temporality

G. C. Sterling has noted that the relevant evidence in support of philosophical intuition is primarily phenomenological in nature.[32] By phenomenological, Sterling ably refers to a descriptive philosophical method that argues a position by revealing the essence of an object or situation. In attempting to flesh out the moral questions associated with Brody's or any ethics case, a phenomenological method is called for, which can reveal as completely as possible the life circumstances of the patient in order to reach the most nuanced and correct ethical decision. In Brody's case, this would have included paying attention to the structure of temporality affected by a terminal diagnosis, which Jansen and Brody's analytic approach are limited in doing.

The analytic structure of time utilized by Jansen in arguing for the irrelevance of the proximity to death in medical ethics decision making is by definition a purely mechanical time unimbued with any human concept of meaningfulness. A phenomenological understanding of time, on the other hand, provides the philosophical resources to expand a theory of moral intuitionism to include sensitivity to the temporal foundation of human experience. In tracing a phenomenology of time, Paul Ricoeur claims that "time becomes human insofar as it is articulated in a narrative manner." "On the other hand," Ricoeur continues, "narrative is significant insofar as it outlines the character of temporal experience" (1983, 17; translation mine). In thinking through ethics cases, there is an imperative to include awareness of the temporal grounds of human narrative experience.[33]

Erwin Straus, a phenomenological philosopher and psychiatrist, has elucidated some important insights regarding the temporality of human life relevant to this discussion. Straus describes the psychological affect of human temporality in terms of a dialectic between subjectivity and finitude. He argues that one senses a distinctive tension in the relation of the single moment of a life to the whole of that life. To justify this claim Straus uses the example of lovers' "readiness or even . . . blissfulness at death," to demonstrate how death can become the "consummation of life." As Straus states, "Life is not surrendered because it no longer carries meaning or because it has become unbearable, but rather because in this one moment the whole seems to be completed" (1982, 80–81). In contrast, Straus mentions the example of how people who were caught in a wartime bombardment felt no fulfillment of temporal experience, despite their proximity of death. Of course, in fact the opposite was the case.

Straus's insights regarding the temporal dimensions of human experience in imbuing our finite existences with existential meaning relates well to the ethical discussion here. In regard to Brody's case, the proximity to death heralded by a definite terminal medical diagnosis would make it possible for the second members of the medical team to acquiesce to the death of the elderly woman. The prognosis related the moment of death to the person's gestalt, including both her medical condition and her temporal life horizon. For the first team, on the other hand, the poor quality of the patient's life and her expressed desire to die was sufficient evidence for them to feel satisfied in their decision not to provide life-sustaining medical treatment. In a sense, this woman's old age and poor physical condition was itself a type of terminal diagnosis; or rather, the actual medical diagnosis was not a significant factor in the first team members' evaluation of the personal whole.

The advantage of framing this analysis in a narrative framework is that it allows for the inclusion of a structure of phenomenological temporality in the analysis of our moral intuitions. Moreover, this analysis emphasizes that the moral intuitions possessed by clinicians often take account of this narrative dimension, even if clinicians lack the philosophical tools to unpack these intuitions in a rigorous and systematic manner. Analytic philosophers, as has been demonstrated, may ignore the temporal aspect of moral intuitions and yet believe that all aspects of our moral intuitions have been analyzed. This study suggests that a respect for the moral intuitions of clinicians, as well as a modified moral intuitionism able to incorporate narrative experience, would provide a strong approach upon which to found a theory of medical ethics.

Conclusion

I wish to conclude this analysis of moral intuitionism with a word about the type of moral reasoning in professional medical ethics. The types of cases that clinical medical ethics deal with fall under the category of what Engelhardt has termed the "ethics of strangers."[34] Thus, Engelhardt distinguishes between the morality of strangers and of friends. In other words, for Engel-hardt a "content-full" morality can only be provided by a moral commu-nity such as one finds amongst different religious communities. An ethics of strangers, on the other hand, is the type of ethics that is practiced by profes-sional medical ethicists and is limited to what is deemed permissible through public agreement. While a morality of strangers is the necessary minimum in a pluralistic society, it is not sufficient to provide an all-encompassing moral vision. As Stuart Hampshire notes, however, in an essay examining public and private morality, that while both types of morality do differ in their so-cial responsibility, they can become compromised through an abstract com-putational morality. For Hampshire, an "intuitive discrimination" that pays attention to tacit forms of moral knowledge is necessary to avoid an abstract moral reasoning inadequate to the complexity of lived experience. Thus, Hampshire claims that

> the model of practical reasoning in difficult and substantial cases over-simplifies the difficulties by over-assimilation to reasoning in theoretical inquiries which demand coherence; it leaves too little place for intuitive dis-crimination alongside abstract general principles and the explicit computa-tion of consequences. (1978, 48–49)

It is possible that a phenomenologically grounded moral intuitionism, while still necessarily an ethics of strangers, is able to compensate for this per-sonal alienation through its content-full methodology sensitive to the moral imperatives that result from ontological structures present in the medical life world.

The Place of Aristotelian *Phronesis* in Clinical Reasoning

A patient arrives in the emergency room cyanotic, acidotic, mentally confused and struggling for breath. Under ordinary circumstances this patient
would automatically be intubated by the emergency physicians. However,
this patient also has a living will or durable power of attorney forbidding
intubation. Should this injunction be respected? This and other similar cases
are mentioned by David Thomasma and Edmund Pellegrino, two influential philosophers of medicine and bioethicists, in their chapter on *phronesis*,
or practical wisdom, described as "medicine's indispensable virtue" in their
analysis of virtues in medical practice.[1] Pellegrino and Thomasma note that
complex clinical decisions like the one mentioned call for "moral insight, for
that combination of intuitive grasp by natural inclination of what is right and
good here," together with prudence, in order to resolve "conflicts in ways no
formula can guarantee" (1993, 89).

While Pellegrino and Thomasma following Thomas Aquinas translate
phronesis as prudence to include the Christian notion of charity, it is more
widely known for its Aristotelian roots. Aristotle, in his *Nicomachean Ethics*, lists *phronesis* (φρονησις) as one of the intellectual virtues together with
philosophic wisdom, or *sophia* (σοφια), and understanding, or *nous* (νους).[2]
Even though Aristotle famously defended practical knowledge by claiming
that different types of knowledge require different methodologies[3], in his
philosophical writings Aristotle did privilege theoretical over practical wisdom.[4] Recently, however, philosophers have attempted to reverse this privileging of *sophia* over *phronesis*. For example, Christopher Long argues that
phronesis emerges as a genuine alternative to *sophia*, "because it points to
the possibility of developing a critically self-reflective model of ontological

knowledge firmly embedded in the finite world" (2002, 36).[5] *Phronesis* has similarly been seen as a resource by contemporary medical epistemologists and philosophers of medicine. Thus, several present-day commentators on the nature of medicine have articulated the idea that clinical reasoning is a form of *phronesis*.[6] However, Pellegrino and Thomasma go further than others in building their philosophy of medicine on *phronesis*. In their study *A Philosophical Basis of Medical Practice*, they define medicine as "simply a habit of *practical understanding* refined and perfected by experience in dealing with patients" (1981, 59; italics mine).

Pellegrino and Thomasma's study of *phronesis* in medicine is an important, influential example of the contemporary return of *phronesis* to medicine. Yet, at the same time, their appropriation of Aristotelian *phronesis* is revealing in its lack of appreciation for the importance Aristotle placed on the existence of *nous*, or intuitive understanding, in practical wisdom. Because of this perceived omission of *nous* from *phronesis*, I take issue with Pellegrino and Thomasma's understanding of medical *phronesis*. I argue that the failure to appreciate the place of *nous* in applying an Aristotelian concept of *phronesis* to medicine has important epistemological, ontological, and ethical implications that need to be accounted for in an adequate philosophy of medicine. Pellegrino and Thomasma's intuitions are correct in turning to Aristotelian *phronesis* to ground their theory of clinical reasoning. Aristotle correctly provides a resource upon which to base a modern synthesis of medicine and humanistic concerns. As Steven Toulmin noted, Aristotelian *phronesis* is of central importance in medicine's saving of philosophical ethics.[7] However, Pellegrino and Thomasma's omission of Aristotelian *nous* from *phronesis* betrays their thoroughly modernist reading of Aristotle and weakens their attempt to rehumanize medicine. As I shall make clear in this chapter, the task of developing a model of clinical reasoning that is equal to the challenge of dealing with lived experience requires a more nuanced reading of Aristotle's classic insights into practical wisdom. Only a reading of Aristotelian *phronesis* as both corporeal and intellectual can provide the firm basis for an ethics of medicine that is able to reflect adequately about the variable and contingent that characterizes the clinical practice of medicine.

In order to ascertain the significance of the omission of *nous* from Pellegrino and Thomasma's resuscitation of *phronesis* in medicine, it is necessary first of all to examine in more detail the relation between *phronesis* and *nous* in Aristotle. The relation has been a much-debated philosophical question.[8] The singular approach followed here is to examine the relation a method to gain important insights into the contemporary application of *phronesis* to medicine, but also a prism to refract the relation between *nous* and *phronesis*.

The approach developed here is somewhat complicated in structure but is intended to be simple in its argument. Firstly, from a close reading of Aristotle and secondary texts on Aristotle, I flesh out a unifying conception of his notion of intellectual *nous* and of *phronesis*. Following this I introduce the medical analogy in Aristotle's depiction of *phronesis*. This discussion provides the backdrop for the subsequent critique of Pellegrino and Thomasma's application of *phronesis* in medicine. I argue that their notion of *phronesis* is deficient since it does not account for Aristotle's notion of intuition, or *nous*, that is present in his theory of practical wisdom. In other words, I make the association between intellectual *nous* and *phronesis* in practical intuition. While Pellegrino and Thomasma's work in the philosophy of medicine attempts to contest a perceived dehumanism in medicine, a true humanization of clinical medicine modeled on Aristotelian *phronesis* requires the incorporation of *nous*.

Aristotelian Phronesis

Most of Aristotle's statements about *phronesis* occur in book 6 of the *Nicomachean Ethics*, which details the intellectual virtues. Here Aristotle famously defines the *phronimos*, or the person endowed with the virtue of practical wisdom:

> Regarding *practical wisdom* we shall get at the truth by considering who are the persons we credit with it. Now it is thought to be the mark of a man of practical wisdom to be able to deliberate well about what is good and expedient for himself, not in some particular respect, e.g. about what sorts of thing conduce to health or to strength, but about what sorts of thing conduce to the good life in general. This is shown by the fact that we credit men with practical wisdom in some particular respect when they have calculated well with a view to some good end which is one of those that are not the object of any art. It follows that in the general sense also the man who is capable of deliberating has practical wisdom. Now no one deliberates about things that are invariable, nor about things that it is impossible for him to do. Therefore, since scientific knowledge involves demonstration, but there is no demonstration of things whose first principles are variable (for all such things might actually be otherwise), and since it is impossible to deliberate about things that are of necessity, practical wisdom cannot be scientific knowledge nor art; not science

because that which can be done is capable of being otherwise, not art because action and making are different kinds of things. The remaining alternative, then, is that it is a true and reasoned state of capacity to act with regard to the things that are good or bad for man. (1140a, trans. Ross)

And a few lines later Aristotle expands on the theme of the *phronimos*:

Practical wisdom on the other hand is concerned with things human and things about which it is possible to deliberate; for we say this above all the work of the man of practical wisdom, to deliberate well, but no one deliberates about things invariable, nor about things which have not an end, and that a good that can be brought about by action. The man who is without qualification good at deliberating is the man who is capable of aiming in accordance with calculation at the best for man of things attainable by action. Nor is practical wisdom concerned with universals only—it must also recognize the particulars; for it is practical, and practice is concerned with particulars. This is why some who do not know, and especially those who have experience, are more practical than others who know; for if a man knew that light meats are digestible and wholesome, but did not know which sorts of meat are light, he would not produce health, but the man who knows that chicken is wholesome is more likely to produce health. (1141b, trans. Ross)

These two paragraphs lay out the main features of *phronesis*, conveniently summarized by Carlo Natali:

(1) *Phronesis* deals with human affairs and the object of deliberation; (2) it deals with things that can be otherwise; (3) it deals with things that have a *telos*, as the practical good of humanity has; (4) for *phronesis* it is more important to know the minor premise, regarding the particular situation, and to reach an individual decision here and now, than to know only the principles in a universal and abstract way. (2001, 22)

As Natali stresses, Aristotle's articulation of *phronesis* is in opposition to his concept of *sophia*, or wisdom. Thus, *phronesis*, unlike *sophia*, deals with the variable elements of human life. *Sophia*, in contrast, deals only with immutable objects. It is not surprising, therefore, that Aristotle claims that *sophia* is knowledge concerned with first principles and intuition:

Therefore wisdom must plainly be the most finished of the forms of knowledge. It follows that the wise man must not only know what follows from the first principles, but must also possess truth about the first principles. Therefore wisdom must be intuitive reason combined with scientific knowledge— scientific knowledge of the highest objects which has received as it were its

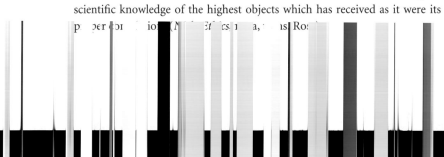

Aristotelian *Nous*

Nous refers to an incorrigible knowledge about the world that does not seek its foundations in reason, but rather provides the foundations upon which reason, such as deduction, and ultimately induction, rests. Besides its role in philosophical wisdom, Aristotle's concept of *nous* has a predominant role in Aristotle's conception of science (*epistemé*). This type of *nous* is exemplified in chapter 19, book 2 of the *Posterior Analytics*, where Aristotle asserts an intuition of first principles upon which scientific knowledge rests:

> Now of the thinking states by which we grasp truth, some are unfailingly true, others admit of error—opinion, for instance, and calculation, whereas scientific knowing and intuition are always true: further, no other kind of thought except intuition is more accurate than scientific knowledge, whereas primary premises are more knowable than demonstrations, and all scientific knowledge is discursive. From these considerations it follows that there will be no scientific knowledge of the primary premises, and since except intuition nothing can be truer than scientific knowledge, it will be intuition that apprehends the primary premises—a result which also follows from the fact that demonstration cannot be the originative source of demonstration, nor consequently, scientific knowledge of scientific knowledge. If, therefore, it is the only other kind of true thinking except scientific knowing, intuition will be the originative source of scientific knowledge. And the originative source of science grasps the original basic premises, while science as a whole is similarly related as originative source to the whole body of fact. (100b, trans. Ross)

It is apparent from this paragraph that Aristotle asserts two different kinds of truth: scientific truth and intuition. Scientific facts are known through a process of induction, whereas intuition is knowledge of first principles. Yet, as Kal notes, Aristotle bases ultimate veracity on an intuitive mind that does not reason.[9] In other words, induction is a discursive reasoning, and intuition, while grounding reason, is not itself reducible to processes of reason. Similarly, Marjorie Grene has highlighted the apparent paradox that Aristotle here resorts to an a priori argument in order to ground a finite, empirical structure of science.[10]

It is logical according to Aristotle's scheme that *sophia* and *epistemé* should be associated since they are both concerned with immutable forms of knowledge. It is more surprising, however, that even while distinguishing *phronesis* from *nous*, Aristotle posits a *nous* of practical wisdom, concerned as *phronesis* is with the particular and everyday.

ARISTOTLE'S *NOUS* OF PRACTICAL REASON

That Aristotle does posit a kind of intuition for practical wisdom is apparent from a difficult passage in the *Nicomachean Ethics*, where Aristotle intimates that there is a type of intuition possessed by both science (*epistemé*) and *phronesis*:

> And intuitive reason is concerned with the ultimates in both directions; for both the first terms and the last are objects of intuitive reason and not of argument, and the intuitive reason, which is presupposed by demonstrations grasps the unchangeable and first terms, while the intuitive reason involved in practical reasonings grasps the last and variable fact, i.e. the minor premiss. For these variables facts are the starting-points for the apprehension of the end, since the universals are reached from the particulars; of these therefore we must have perception, and this perception is intuitive reason. (1143a3b, trans. Ross)[11]

This passage has presented difficulties to interpreters of Aristotle because the notion of there being a *nous* of *phronesis* goes against the grain of Aristotle's other statements regarding their relation. Simply put, *nous* traditionally relates to speculative knowledge, a completely different sphere from practical reasoning. Christopher Rowe, for example, claims that in the *Nicomachean Ethics* the "distinction between the two spheres is complete. Ethics and the theoretical sciences no longer have anything in common, since their subject matters are now established as being totally different in kind" (1971, 70–73, quoted in Kenny 1978, 162). Anthony Kenny, on the other hand, interprets this passage in a literal fashion to argue that there are different types of Aristotelian *nous* for speculative and practical reasoning. Furthermore, Kenny claims that there is a binary division within practical *nous*: a particular practical *nous* and a universal practical *nous*.[12]

The existence of a universal and a practical *nous* renders explicable for Kenny how Aristotelian *phronesis* can be concerned with both ends and means. Moreover, since according to Kenny's understanding, *nous* can be concerned with ends, Kenny claims that

> practical reasoning ends with a judgement about what is to be done, a self-addressed command (1143a9) or a piece of advice to another (1143a15). This too can be called *nous* (1143a27) whether or not it is backed up in a particular case by a statement of reasons (1143b14). (Ibid.)

Ke y's r er et on, h ntest ng m ch f he an cede t n
mer a or tl is ra ap h t h is t e me t c ta din g s iously it it

eral meaning that "(intuitive) reason is concerned with the ultimates in both directions," that is, that there is a practical *nous* concerned with both the ends and the means of a practical decision.[13] While not wanting to decide between the various commentators of Aristotle on this paragraph, it is more than plausible to consider that Aristotle did argue for the presence of *nous* of practical reason.[14] Gabriel Richardson Lear takes a similar position, in arguing that there is a structural similarity between practical and theoretical wisdom.[15] However, rather than attempting to resolve the question I propose instead to take the relation between *nous* and *phronesis* as a given and analyze their relation in the context of medicine.

The Medical Analogy

Medicine lies close at hand to the discussion about *phronesis.* A striking aspect of these two passages regarding the *phronimos* is the importance that Aristotle gives to health as a metaphor. Thus, in the first passage, the metaphor of health is used to demonstrate that *phronesis* is not concerned with particulars. In the second passage Aristotle uses the example of knowledge of the health benefits of eating light meat to explain that practical reasoning is concerned with both ends and means. The obvious connection between medicine and *phronesis* demonstrated in these paragraphs, which motivates Aristotle to draw on the medical analogy, is that both medicine and practical reasoning are inseparable from day-to-day human action. Additionally, they are both concerned with what Aristotle calls knowledge of the "variable" and what "could be otherwise."[16]

Other interpreters of Aristotle have commented on the prevalent use of images of health in his writings. Indeed, the use of metaphors of health was a common trope in ancient philosophy. However, whereas Werner Jaeger emphasizes the importance of medicine for ancient philosophy, another influential classicist, Ludwig Edelstein, argues that philosophy influenced medicine and not the other way round. According to Edelstein medicine was a useful didactic metaphor for ancient philosophers to describe the philosophical effects on the soul.[17] While Edelstein's point might have general validity, it does not seem to apply in regard to *phronesis. Phronesis* as a virtue of practical reasoning bears strong actual resemblance to clinical reasoning. Aristotelian *phronesis* has a much more direct relation with medicine than as an incidental didactic occurrence. For example, there is a strong resemblance between Aristotle's example of the eating of light meats, and a passage in the Hippocratic Corpus *On Ancient Medicine.* In chapter 20 of that book, the Hippocratic author claims:

For this at least about nature I am convinced that a physician must know, and devote himself to knowing, if he is going to do anything of his duty, the nature of man in relation to what he eats and drinks, and in relation to his habits generally, and what will be the effect of each on each individual. He must not be content with the unqualified statement that "cheese is a bad food, for it gives a pain to the man who has eaten his fill of it." We must know what the pain is, the reason for the pain and to what constituent of the man cheese is unsuitable. . . . Cheese, to take the example I used, does not harm all men alike; there are some who eat their fill without being hurt at all, but when cheese agrees with them are even wonderfully strengthened by it . . . (Jones, 1946, 84–5.)

Conceptually it would not change the substance of this passage at all to replace the example of cheese for Aristotle's example of light meat and vice versa. The Hippocratic author had intended to contest the influence of philosophy on medicine.[18] In the tradition of Hippocratic empiricism he argued that a dogmatic theoretical medicine could never understand and effectively treat the individual patient. Disease, in other words, varies too much in individual patients to be able to derive a general theory of disease. Similarly, Aristotle uses the example of eating light meat to explain that the *phronimos* is concerned with particulars. Perhaps Aristotle had the Hippocratic author of *On Ancient Medicine* in mind when he used the metaphor of health to support his argument about *phronesis*.[19] Regarding *phronesis*, what Aristotle might have derived from Hippocratic medicine was the understanding that, firstly, practical knowledge, like medicine, is concerned with the variable, and secondly, the impossibility of deriving a universal theory of knowledge about the individual. Even though for Aristotle, medicine as a productive discipline is an art, or *techné*, the knowledge about its correct application is a form of *phronesis*. It is in its correct application that medicine becomes the most fitting analogy for the moral virtues.

Further support for the cultural association between Aristotle and the Hippocratic physicians and the relation between medicine as *techné*, as well as its correct application as *phronesis*, can be seen from an examination of the word *empeira*.[20] In Hippocratic medicine, the distinction between knowledge of the individual patient and the distillation of this knowledge has been distinguished as *peira* and *empeira*, respectively.[21] *Empeira* is associated with a well-known passage at the beginning of Aristotle's *Metaphysics*, in reference to both medicine and individual knowledge:

And experience seems pretty much like science and art, but really science and art come to men *through* experience; for "experience made art," as Polus says "but inexperie   e   icl   v t aria s when from many notions ain
y experienc one t v s   en it m de about a cla s of objects   pr

duced. *For to have a judgement that when Callias was ill of this disease this did him good, and similarly in the case of Socrates and in many individual cases, is a matter of experience; but to judge that it has done good to all persons' of a certain constitution, marked off in one class, when they were ill of this disease, e.g. to phlegmatic or bilious people when burning with fever—this is a matter of art.* [Italics mine.]

With a view to action experience seems in no respect inferior to art, and men of experience succeed even better than those who have theory without experience. The reason is that experience is knowledge of individuals, art of universals, and actions and productions are all concerned with the individual; for the physician does not cure man, except in an incidental way, but Callias or Socrates or some other called by some such individual name, who happens to be a man. If, then, a man has the theory with the experience, and recognizes the universal but does not know the individual included in this, he will often fail to cure; for it is the individual that is to be cured. (981a1–24, trans. Ross)

In this passage, Aristotle distinguishes between experience of the individual and general medical knowledge, which he terms art (*techné*). As is apparent, Aristotle opines here that the good physician needs to possess both experience and art. Aristotle, therefore, attempts to balance these two types of knowledge, the experiential and the theoretical. This attempt to balance knowledge of the individual with general medical science is the real challenge for medical ethics, both in antiquity and in the present. Pellegrino and Thomasma's concept of *phronesis*, as will be seen in greater detail in the following section, is an attempt to strike such a balance. In his commentary on *phronesis* in Pellegrino's philosophy of medicine, Daniel Davis links Pellegrino's concept of *phronesis* with *empeira*, arguing that that the physician—"as *phronimos*—must give an epistemological and ontological priority to *peira*" (1996, 360). By linking *phronesis* with *empeira*, Davis affirms Pellegrino's claim that the prudential physician must be able to use general medical knowledge in order to make appropriate decisions for particular patients. The link between medicine and *phronesis* is not merely historical, but one present in Pellegrino and Thomasma's contemporary notion of clinical reasoning as a type of *phronesis*. It remains to be seen, however, how faithfully Pellegrino and Thomasma apply Aristotelian *phronesis* to medicine.

Phronesis as Clinical Reasoning: Pellegrino and Thomasma's Philosophy of Medicine

Pellegrino and Thomasma's philosophy of medicine is spelled out in their two major works, *A Philosophical Basis of Medical Practice* (1981) and *The Virtues in Medical Practice* (1993).[22] Whereas in *A Philosophical Basis* they attempt to develop a systematic philosophy of medicine, in *The Virtues* their concern is rather to develop a medical ethics modeled on neo-Aristotelian virtue ethics. In this more recent book, Pellegrino and Thomasma apply the Aristotelian notion of virtue as "habitual disposition to act well" to the person of the physician (5). They define *phronesis*, or prudence, as "establishing right reason in action, *recta ratio agibilium*, as St. Thomas called it" (xii). Despite their debt to Aquinas, it was Aristotle who originally developed the notion of *phronesis*. The inheritance from Aristotle is clear in Pellegrino and Thomasma's further definition of *phronesis* as "both a moral and an intellectual virtue that disposes one habitually to choose the right thing to do in a concrete moral situation" (21). Pellegrino and Thomasma faithfully identify an Aristotelian notion of *phronesis* as the most important virtue of the physician. Like Aristotle they make a distinction between *phronesis*, the intellectual virtue that "disposes us habitually to attain truth for the sake of action," and *sophia*, or "speculative wisdom" (ibid.). Furthermore, for Pellegrino and Thomasma, *phronesis* is a special kind of virtue that links the intellectual virtues, such as science (*epistemé*), art (*techné*), and intuitive wisdom (*nous*), with the moral virtues such as temperance and courage. Finally, *phronesis* provides "a grasp of the end" and "enables us to discern which means are most appropriate to the good in particular circumstances" (ibid.).

The virtues that Pellegrino and Thomasma lay out as central to medical practice include fidelity to trust, compassion, *phronesis*, justice, fortitude, temperance, integrity, and self-effacement. Of these, *phronesis* is described as medicine's "indispensable virtue."[23] In his study of the place of *phronesis* in Pellegrino's philosophy of medicine, Daniel Davis summarizes the reasons for this: Firstly, *phronesis* offers a conceptual link between other contemporary divergent ethical approaches. Secondly, *phronesis* is considered an intrinsic part of the nature of clinical medicine. Thirdly, *phronesis* offers a practical mediation of clinical medicine's "intellectual virtues," such as compassion and temperance (1996, 186–87). Finally, *phronesis* is essential for the application of medicine's "moral virtues in the individual clinical encounter." Moreover, these four points do not stand independently of each other, but are inextricably linked. In other words, *phronesis* as embodied in the clinical encounter means that clinical reasoning is always concerned for the good of the individual patient. Or as Pellegrino and Thomasma write, "the good of the patient provides the architectonic of the relationship" (1993, 53).

Additionally, while different ethical approaches might be mediated through *phronesis*, the patient's good is not reducible to any particular set of ethical principles according to Pellegrino and Thomasma. Thus, the emphasis on a virtue ethic with *phronesis* as the cardinal virtue reverses standard philosophical medical ethics. Different philosophical ethical theories—such as the generally accepted consequentialist, utilitarian, and deontological approaches—become secondary to particular phenomena of the medical context. The important principle of beneficence is itself, Pellegrino and Thomasma argue, part of the nature of medical activity and not a requirement of a system of philosophy applied to medicine. Even the important philosophical principle of respect for autonomy is derived from medicine, because "to violate the patient's values is to violate her person and, therefore, a maleficent act that distorts the healing end of the relationship" (ibid.). Ethical theories are useful to the extent that they allow one to analyze systematically and critically analyze these "human realities" derived from the healing encounter.

Pellegrino and Thomasma's point that *phronesis* reverses the relation between philosophy and experience is of course of especial significance for the claim made in chapter 1 that philosophers and physicians occupy parallel moral universes reflected through their frequently divergent moral intuitions. Pellegrino and Thomasma do not, however, fit squarely into the physician or the philosophy camp in their endeavor to establish a systematic philosophy of medicine. Their discussion of *phronesis* understandably draws on both clinical experience and philosophical argument. Their concept of *phronesis* can be understood as an attempt to validate clinical experience using a neo-Aristotelian philosophical framework. Their modeling of clinical reasoning on *phronesis* is generally convincing, and yet; in positing *phronesis* as the "indispensable" virtue in medicine, an aporia concerning intuition as part of *phronesis* is present in their work. For Pellegrino, medicine's claim to be a rigorous science means precisely that intuition must be discarded. For example, he noted in a chapter in *The Philosophical Basis* on the epistemological nature of clinical reasoning that "to resort to terms such as 'art' or 'intuition' is to impede explication of a socially significant process" (141–42). While one may want to differentiate between intuition as part of a scientific process of diagnosis, and *phronesis* as a moral evaluation, the whole point of Pellegrino's concept of *phronesis* is to join the scientific and moral aspects of clinical reasoning. The discussion of Aristotle earlier in this chapter emphasizes, however, that in practical reasoning *nous* is not separate from *phronesis*. It is important to ask what the epistemological and ethical consequences are for a theory of clinical reasoning that has excluded intuition from *phronesis*.

Pellegrino and Thomasma's conceptual structure of medical reasoning is laid out explicitly by Pellegrino in a paper, "The Anatomy of Clinical Judgments" (1977),[24] as well as in chapter 6 of *A Philosophical Basis*, where the

arguments in the "Anatomy" are repeated. At the beginning of the "Anatomy," Pellegrino states that his aim is to "locate more precisely the several
reasoning modes useful at each of the sequential and simultaneous steps
which eventuate ultimately in a clinical action" (170). In the *Philosophical
Basis*, Pellegrino and Thomasma define medicine as "neither solely an art nor
solely a science in the modern sense of those terms. Instead . . . medicine is a
distinct intermediate discipline, a *tertium quid*, between art and science but
distinct from both of them" (59).

While medicine shares elements with both the sciences and the humanities, the processes of clinical reasoning and action for Pellegrino and Thomasma can be divided into a foundational triad of science, art and prudence.
Prudential reasoning, or *phronesis*, distinguishes clinical action as a special
type of practical activity. Science and art have important, though delimited,
contributions to medicine; and intuition has no, or only a very limited, part
to contribute to the foundations of clinical reasoning. It is worthwhile to
briefly examine these three elements—science, art, and intuition—in comparison with *phronesis*.

For Pellegrino and Thomasma, present-day medicine incorporates a scientific method developed in the seventeenth century. The conception of science that they use is the generally accepted one that consists of "a method,
a body of knowledge built up by that method, and a post facto explanation
of reality based on generalizable laws which relate the facts acquired by the
scientific method to each other" (1981, 146). The rules of inferential logic are
used in medicine just as in any other science. Medicine is a specific discipline
in that the scientific method is used in order to make diagnoses and evaluate treatments. Medicine especially demonstrates its scientific basis when it
"seeks explanations of clinical phenomena in theories and mechanisms of
disease" (ibid.). And yet medicine is not distinguished by being a science.
Since medicine has a timeless concern for the good of the individual patient,
medicine cannot be reduced to a scientific method. Rather, "medicine exists as medicine only when it engages in the full range of activities which
constitute clinical judgment and which lead to decisive action in the interest
of a particular patient" (146). It is in this application of scientific knowledge
for the betterment of individuals that distinguishes medicine as both art and
prudence.

While *phronesis* provides the end of treatment, for Pellegrino and Thomasma the art of medicine refers to medicine as a form of technique, or *techné*,
that merely provides the technical know-how or prowess to achieve a specific
end. *Techné* in this case is also modeled on Aristotle, for whom *techné* applies
to the act of producing or making. Pellegrino and Thomasma do not define

medicine solely in terms of being a *techné* because of the importance they give to *phronesis* in molding clinical reasoning. However, Pellegrino and Thomasma's definition of medical technique as *techné* is in conscious distinction to the popular association of the art of medicine with intuitive reasoning.[25] Pellegrino's distinction between art and intuition can already be seen in an early article of his entitled "Medicine, Science, Art: an Old Controversy Revisited." Here Pellegrino writes that

> art is not synonymous with mysterious intuitive personal endowments peculiar to some and not to others. Though some residuum of the inexplicable will, perhaps, always remain, the art of medicine is not synonymous with that residuum. The better artist of medicine is simply the better craftsman of medicine. (1979, 50)[26]

In summary, intuition as neither art nor science nor prudence has no real place in Pellegrino and Thomasma's architectonic of medicine. On the one hand, intuition does not form part of practical wisdom since intuition is perceived as a form of mysticism, irreducible to reason. Intuition is not reproducible in the same way that *phronesis* is. It provides no link between the emotional and intellectual virtues. On the other hand, because of his modern sensibility, Pellegrino does not affirm intuition in the philosophical sense, either, in the sense that Aristotle uses it—as that form of direct perception or understanding upon which science is founded. Pellegrino and Thomasma also explicitly mention, but only to exclude its applicability to clinical judgment, intuition conceived of as a form of tacit knowledge, modeled on the work of Polanyi and Lonergan:

> There is no reason to suspect that clinical diagnosis is unique in this regard. The phenomena of "insight" and "discovery" are common to both scientific and nonscientific endeavors. Polanyi and Lonergan have attempted to describe the deep epistemological structures and relationships which permit the leap from the obvious and known to the previously unknown. Polanyi holds that scientific knowledge is never wholly explicit but resides in tacit understanding which provides the belief that makes thinking about a truth possible. Lonergan links belief to immanently generated knowledge, Polanyi's "discovery" and Lonergan's "insight" are likened by their authors to the "Eureka" of Archimedes. To what extent these epistemological notions can account for the obscure features of clinical reasoning is problematic. What must be avoided is the easy appeal to some special illumination peculiar to clinicians. Zimmerman's appeal to "genius," . . . is a case in point. To resort to terms such as "art" or "intuition" is to impede explication of a socially significant process. (1981, 141–42)[27]

Michael Polanyi's Theory of Tacit Knowledge

Pellegrino and Thomasma's passing reference to Polanyi provides a key with which to deduce the implications of their elision of intuition from clinical reasoning as a form of *phronesis.* The philosopher of science Michael Polanyi developed his theory of tacit knowledge most explicitly in his book entitled *Personal Knowledge* (1974). Polanyi's work is an important postcritical philosophy, in which he argues for the importance of paying attention to the subjective element within objective scientific knowledge.

Intuition plays an important part in Polanyi's theory of tacit knowledge, since intuition is to some extent synonymous with tacit knowledge. For example, in the following paragraph Polanyi summarizes his theory of personal knowledge by referring directly to intuition, even of mathematical knowledge as a kind of intuition shared with animal life:

> I have shown how all the proofs and theorems of mathematics have been originally discovered by relying on their intuitive anticipation; how the established results of such discoveries are properly taught, understood, remembered in the form of their intuitively grasped outline; how these results are effectively reapplied and developed further by pondering their intuitive content; and that they can therefore gain our legitimate assent only in terms of our intuitive approval. I have indeed shown that all articulation depends on a tacit component of the same kind for conveying a meaning accredited by the person uttering it. And also that this comprehension-cum-affirmation is continuous with the active principal of animal life by which we both shape and accept our knowledge at all its levels, down to that of drives, motoricity and perception, with which as animals we are equipped by nature. (188)

It should be emphasized that Polanyi is not against science but is concerned to demonstrate that "complete objectivity usually attributed to the exact sciences is a delusion and is in fact a false ideal" (18). For Polanyi, so-called objective science falls short due to its positivism. Paying attention to the tacit dimension, the intuitive, or what Polanyi calls "clues,"[28] increases our epistemological horizons to a greater awareness of the whole. Thus, in referring to intuition, Polanyi is not arguing for a philosophical idea of intuition as an incorrigible certainty, but rather as a practical skill.[29] While intuition makes hidden logical associations, this does not preclude but rather requires that we spend time trying to ascertain the tacit elements of scientific reasoning. Polanyi's theory of tacit knowledge goes against modern sentiment in the sense that it posits rationality within the natural universe. Polanyi writes in *Personal Knowledge*:

> For modern man has set up as the ideal of knowledge the conception of natural science as a set of statements which is "objective" in the sense that its substance is entirely determined by observation, even while its presentation may be shaped by convention. This conception, stemming from a craving rooted in the very depths of our culture, would be shattered if the intuition of rationality in nature had to be acknowledged as a justifiable and indeed essential part of scientific theory. (1974, 16)

In this paragraph intuition and rationality in nature are associated. The corollary of this statement is equally true. Not only does the acknowledgement of the intuition of rationality in nature shatter positivistic science, but rationality in nature affirms and is dependent on the validity of intuition. Pellegrino's concept of *phronesis* is thoroughly modernist in its suspicion and elimination of intuition from clinical reasoning.

Marjorie Grene has emphasized Pellegrino's dismissal of Polanyi's theory of tacit knowledge. In a short critique of Pellegrino's model of clinical reasoning in a response to Pellegrino's paper "The Anatomy" (at the conference at which it was originally presented), Grene (1977) had three essential criticisms of Pellegrino's application of *phronesis* to medicine: Firstly, she did not accept that the medical scientific method is distinguishable from the scientific method more generally. Secondly, she argued that Pellegrino's application of ancient science to modern medicine is not valid. Thirdly, she was critical of Pellegrino's dismissal of Polanyi's tacit knowledge, since she was of the opinion that it is precisely this antimodernist conception of science which is the most useful concept to apply to medicine in particular, and to the modern scientific method in general. Specifically, in a reference to Polanyi, Grene remarked that it is the reliance on clues that distinguishes clinical judgment as a model for the sciences. She continues her insightful critique of Pellegrino arguing that

> perception, practical skills (including that of the experienced clinician), the practice of theoretical science and, indeed, of aesthetic judgment, all share, if in significantly different ways, this common structure. If philosophers of science would pay closer heed to the character of clinical medicine, with its massive judgmental component, they might, I believe, learn much that too exclusive an attention to the most abstract and theoretical branches of science has allowed them to overlook. That is not to say that clinical judgment should not be made as "scientific," that is, as precise, as possible, in the sense that it should use whatever objective techniques it can find for its improvement and support. *But what is most important, philosophically, in my view, is the opposite insight: that precision comes to be, and is maintained and increased, only under*

the auspices of judgment, of human-all-too human efforts to make sense of situ-
ations that always outrun our control. (197; italics mine)

While Grene does not link Polanyi's tacit knowledge with Aristotle, this connection is implicit in her criticism of Pellegrino and in her writings on Aristotle more generally.

Pellegrino's "Neo-Hippocratic Fusion"

Further support for Grene's claim that Pellegrino's use of terms derived from
ancient science do not fit well with contemporary science can be found in
what Pellegrino (1974) has termed the "neo-Hippocratic fusion." By this
term, Pellegrino means a "fusion of the neo-Hippocratic spirit with a new
mature Cartesian conviction that human illness can be described in physico-
chemical and quantified terms" (1974, 11). In this statement, Pellegrino attempts to unite the holism and respect for the individual generally associated
with Hippocratic medicine together with the real progress in medicine, since
it incorporated modern scientific principles. But, intuition as the art of medicine has no place in this neo-Hippocratic fusion since for Pellegrino intuition
has dubious scientific validity. Yet intuition, rather than *phronesis*, was part
of Hippocratic *techné*.

The role of intuition in clinical reasoning was argued by the medical historian Arturo Castiglioni in an important article published in 1934. Here Castiglioni highlighted a concept that he referred to as the "Neo-Hippocratic
tendency of contemporary medical thought." By this term, Castiglioni meant
a turn to the study of function by biological scientists, or a rebelling against
the mathematicization and mechanization of biology modeled on the physical sciences. In particular, for Castiglioni the "neo-Hippocratic tendency" referred to the reemphasis on clinical empirical judgment in medicine. And for
Castiglioni critical acumen was constituted by "a keen critical observation, a
logical analysis followed by a rapid synthesis, exact proportion of measures
and moderation in the balance between the various opposite tendencies"
(120). It is this emphasis on empirical clinical judgment in medicine that
Castiglioni regarded as Hippocratic. Castiglioni characterized this type of
empirical judgment as a kind of intuition:[30]

> I only think it possible to state without being much mistaken that intuition
> means that psychological process through which from the swift general judg-
> ment of a question or of a complex fact we reach the appreciation of the detail.

which leads to a general conclusion through analysis. We mean only to say that neither of the two methods of judgment is satisfactory by itself and that intuition, that quick general appreciation of the essence of a phenomenon, or of the importance of one of its details, that, often, inexplicable glimpse of the paramount detail of a complex phenomenon which sometimes escapes the eye of a careful observer, plays an extremely important part in medicine. (Ibid.)

Castiglioni takes an opposing tack to Pellegrino by claiming that an emphasis on clinical intuition is an attempt by modern biologists and physicians to overcome the mathematic reductionism of the physical sciences. The suspicion of intuition by physician-philosophers, such as Pellegrino, who still remain influenced by modern physics, implies that a "neo-Hippocratic fusion" without clinical intuition does not actually succeed in uniting the holistic with the scientific. Castiglioni's paper suggests that a real "neo-Hippocratic fusion" must first take account of the ontological and ethical significance of intuition in medicine.

Conclusion: Hans Jonas's Philosophy of Life

What is the significance of intuition, ontologically and ethically, and its converse, the elision of intuition from clinical medicine? In the final section of this chapter, I wish to utilize some key insights from Hans Jonas's philosophical biology to explicate at least one important issue at stake in the omission of intuition from the modeling of clinical reasoning on *phronesis*.

The abandonment of reliance on intuition following the success of mechanistic science is part of the broader replacement of an understanding of teleology within nature by processes of mechanistic causation alone. Hans Jonas has noted that the struggle against teleology (in Western science) "is a stage in the struggle against anthropomorphism" (1966, 36). In other words, the attempt to free science of teleological causation is an attempt to disassociate the genus Homo sapiens from its hierarchical place in the great chain of being. Science's battle against teleology in nature and its struggle against reliance on intuition in scientific reasoning are to a certain extent synonymous. This is because Aristotelian intuition as a faculty of perception that innately provides the foundations of human rationality is also profoundly anthropocentric. As such, the struggle against intuition can be equated with the struggle against an anthropocentric moral philosophy that claims special ontological or ethical uniqueness for humankind. This point reveals the paradox in the attempt by medical humanists such as Pellegrino and Thomasma to restore a perceived lost humanism within medicine without acknowledging the importance that a reevaluation of intuition might play in this endeavor. As Grene emphasizes, medical reasoning requires a "human, all too human" knowledge—not one stripped of its anthropological foundations. It is ironical that the elimination of intuition from medicine can be associated with the same processes of dehumanization charged against modern medicine, which Pellegrino's and Thomasma's philosophy of medicine attempts to remedy.

The second relevant point that Jonas makes concerns the relation between life and death in the life sciences. Jonas claims that modern thought is held under the "ontological dominance of death" (12, 15). By this Jonas means that biological understanding reduces the mystery of life to laws derived from the intelligibility of the human body dissected and analyzed as a corpse. This is particularly apparent in the history of medicine, since the founding of the modern clinic has been attributed to the anatomo-pathological correlations of disease first demonstrated by Giovanni Battista Morgagni (1682–1771) and Xavier Bichat (1771–1802).[31] Accordingly, Jonas writes, "It is the existence of life within a mechanical universe which now calls for an explanation, and explanation has to be in terms of the lifeless" (1966, 10). Jonas's philosophy of metabolism is an attempt to reinstate the classical respect for life, in which death was the final "limit of all understanding" (12, 15).

Jonas's philosophy of the organism contests the idea that the organism, and most of all the human organism, can simply be understood by reducing its purposeful functioning to the level of mechanistic structure. For Jonas, the living organism is greater than the sum of its parts. Jonas is not trying to reverse the real scientific progress made, especially that of the past three hundred years. He does, however, contest the Cartesian dualistic legacy, which on the one hand made this scientific progress possible, and on the other resulted in a forgetting of the corporeal basis of knowledge. Or as Jonas phrases it, "in the body, the knot of being is tied which dualism does not unravel but cut" (25). As opposed to a simplistic but clear-cut separation between mind and body in dualism, the phrase "knot of being" suggests a complex intertwining of consciousness and embodiment.

These abstract ideas find a practical application in Jonas's opposition to the modern definition of brain death. In his polemical essay entitled "Against the Stream: Comments on the Definition and Redefinition of Death," Jonas examined the ethical implications of a radically dualistic medical culture in its redefinition of human life in the shadow of death. Jonas's article was remarkably prescient. Forty years after the definition of brain death, there is growing unease toward the definition of brain death, particularly in its failure to address the neural mechanisms of brain function that are maintained
despite "whole brain" criteria of brain death. Additionally, Jonas's suspicion

that the public need for harvestable organs was a primary motive for the definition of brain death has become increasingly plain over the years.[32]

Besides its contemporary moral relevance, Jonas's essay is valuable in providing a clue which links his insights into the philosophy of the organism with my own analysis of *phronesis*. This connection is evidenced at the beginning of Jonas's paper, where he responds to the charge of philosophical vagueness by arguing that it is the definition of death that is by necessity unclear and not his argument, which is philosophically "precise" (1974, 134). Jonas cites in support of his argument the well-known passage in the *Nicomachean Ethics*, where Aristotle observes that "it is the mark of a well-educated man not to insist on greater precision in knowledge than the subject admits" (ibid.). Jonas, therefore, applies Aristotle's insight about practical reasoning to the scientific issue of defining death. It is not simply fortuitous that Jonas turns to Aristotelian practical reasoning to give support for his argument about brain death. There is an analogy between Jonas's argument about brain death and the place of *phronesis* in medicine. In other words, the lack of precision in being able to define and unravel the "knot of being" is due to the complexity of the subject matter rather than a lack of philosophical precision. Jonas's "knot of being" refers at the very least to the intimate association between consciousness and metabolism in the human and other organisms. For Jonas, dualism, which separates mind from body, but allows for scientific advancements, does not do justice to the complexity of the human organism.[33] Aristotelian *phronesis* does, however, do justice to this human complexity. As a type of practical knowledge that is concerned with everyday affairs but is also connected with intellectual *nous*, *phronesis* is archetypically a nondualistic form of knowledge. In consequence, the attempt to reclaim the ancient wisdom of Aristotelian *phronesis* for clinical reasoning is arguably an important strategy in contesting the predominance of the static anatomopathological correlate for clinical reasoning. *Phronetic* knowledge, in other words, as opposed to mechanistic dualism, preserves the unity of body and mind captured in the phrase "knot of being." Likewise, the incorporation of *nous* into *phronesis* reties this knot by acknowledging a *telos* in nature in which human reasoning partakes.

There is evidence to suggest that David Thomasma would have been sympathetic to this critique. In an article entitled "The Comatose Patient, the Ontology of Death, and the Decision to Stop Treatment," Thomasma describes the problem of a so-called ontology of death in modern society. Thomasma argues for an "ontology of death" that "is described through a relationship with life, rather than as an absence of life." Thomasma's argument for a definition of brain death and his critique of an "ontology of death" appears quite close, if not identical to Jonas's position on brain death and argument against the "ontological dominance of death." Thomasma might even have agreed with my analysis of *phronesis* as reversing this negative ontology through its association with Aristotelian *nous*. However, the omission of *nous* in Pellegrino and Thomasma's model of clinical reasoning on *phronesis* remains associated with a Cartesian dualism that repeats the error they attempt to address.

Aristotle's Practical Syllogism: Accounting for the Individual through a Theory of Action and Cognition

> Why, in forging our metaphysics, should we not begin by acknowledging the integral living forms we experience, whether firs, roses, bees, beetles, macaques, or finches—in the manner precisely of Aristotle, not to say of Darwin? Why, indeed, should we not have a metaphysics that is first of all consonant with living things as they are in the changing realities of their lives—in their movement and rest, in their generation, growth and decay? Why should we have a metaphysics that commences with the inanimate rather than the animate, especially since that metaphysics typically either fails to do justice to, or ignores altogether, a natural history? Moreover why should the mind/body problem in particular be a problem solved only at the level of a 20th-century conception of matter? Why should it not be a problem solvable at the level of mindbodies themselves, at the level of the "manifestation of persistent wholes," of Darwinian bodies, of intact living beings—of individuals like Descartes himself, in the flesh?
>
> MAXINE SHEETS-JOHNSTONE, *The Primacy of Movement*

In the previous analysis of Aristotelian *phronesis* I argued that Edmund Pellegrino's and David Thomasma's attempt to model clinical reasoning on *phronesis* was deficient in not accounting for the presence of intellectual *nous*. This account suggested that Aristotelian *nous* is an essential component of human practical wisdom. Yet, this analysis only tentatively sketched out the relation between *phronesis* and *nous*. It did not address, for example, the question of how Aristotelian *nous* becomes modified through its participation in practical wisdom. A common strategy among Aristotle scholars is to analyze the relation between *nous* and *phronesis* through the practical syllogism, an important element in Aristotle's theory of action.[1] In this chapter I continue, therefore, the analysis of *phronesis* and *nous* by examining Aristotle's practical syllogism in relation to medicine. This is an important exercise, since the practical syllogism provides the means to examine the manner of deepening the investigation of the problem of the individual. The line of my argument here is that *nous* of *phronesis* as it occurs in the practical syllogism connects the individual with the cognitive process of practical reasoning.[2] Traditionally associated with noninferential intuition, it can take account of individual variability because it is not merely conceptual but has a corporeal basis, and is, therefore, itself a product of the variable and particular. Analyzing the practical syllogism adds, therefore, another piece in the Aristotelian conceptual apparatus of accounting for individual variability, the central ethical concern of both medicine and *phronesis*.[3]

The Practical Syllogism in Aristotle

Aristotle's concept of the practical syllogism refers to the implied syllogistic structure in practical reasoning. In Aristotle's logic a syllogism is a piece of reasoning that consists of a major premise, a minor premise, and a conclusion. The particular conclusions follow necessarily from the two premises. Some interpreters of Aristotle accord to him an analogous mental process occurring in action.[4] W. F. R. Hardie, for example, refers to Aristotle's practical syllogism as the analogy between syllogistic proofs in demonstrative science and the application of practical rules to particular situations.[5] D. J. Allan (1955) writes similarly that "Aristotle makes use of an analogy between the demonstrative syllogism and the performance of actions from established dispositions of character. This is the so-called theory of the practical syllogism" (1955, 325). What is common to these two exemplary definitions is the application of the general syllogistic structure to practical decision making. Thus, the practical syllogism uses the syllogistic structure to demonstrate the causal association between deliberation and action.

The structure and application of the practical syllogism has generated much debate among interpreters of Aristotle. One reason for this is that Aristotle does not actually use the term "practical syllogism." The passage in the *Nicomachean Ethics* in which he comes nearest to doing so is in book 6, chapter 12: "For the syllogisms which deal with acts to be done (*ton prakton*) are things which involve a starting point, viz. since the end."[6] Yet very different interpreters of Aristotle have accepted the fact that Aristotle does refer to the practical syllogism in his theory of practical reasoning.[7] Moreover, since discussion of the nature of the practical syllogism is part and parcel of the literature dealing with the problem of the meaning of *nous* in *phronesis*, an analysis of the practical syllogism helps to clarify the manner in which they relate to each other. Well-known examples of the practical syllogism have been attributed to Aristotle in books 6 and 7 of the *Nicomachean Ethics*, as well as passages in the *De Anima* and the *De Motu Animalium*. Analysis of a few selected examples of the practical syllogism helps to clarify its meaning.

Hardie claims that the following passage in the *De Anima* provides the formula for the practical syllogism[8]:

the first tells us that such and such a mind of man should do such and such a kind of act, and the second that this is an act of the mind meant, and I a person of the type intended), it is the latter opinion that originates movement, not the universal; or rather it is both, but the one does so while it remains in a state more like rest, while the other partakes in movement. (434 a16–21, trans. Smith)

Hardie elicits the structure of the practical syllogism from this passage as consisting of a major and minor premise:

> Where the major premiss is "such and such a kind of man should do such and such a kind of act" and the minor premiss "this is an act, and I am a person, of the kind meant." (1968, 228–29)

In other words, for Hardie the major premise supplies the general rule or motive for action, while the minor premise provides the particular instance in which this action occurs. Hardie's theory can be seen to occupy the middle ground in the debate about the practical syllogism. On the one hand, he argues against John Cooper that the practical syllogism is part of the process of deliberation.[9] On the other hand, while agreeing with Allan that the practical syllogism does participate in the process of deliberation, Hardie has a more modest position than Allan, who claims that the major premise of the practical syllogism provides both the means to an end and the true understanding of that end.[10] For Hardie it is sufficient that the major premise in a practical syllogism recommending the means already encompasses the "thought of the end." Thus, Hardie criticizes those interpreters of Aristotle who make the major premise state the end of an action. For Hardie, the major premise specifies effective means for the attainment of an end, but does not refer to the understanding of that end (1968, 228–29).

These respective positions can be clarified by focusing on the example of the practical syllogism that occurs in one of the paragraphs cited in the previous chapter referring to the *phronimos* in Aristotle's *Nicomachean Ethics*. This passage is further evidence that the practical syllogism provides a concrete instance of *phronetic* reasoning:

> The man who is without qualification good at deliberating is the man who is capable of aiming in accordance with calculation at the best for man of things attainable by action. Nor is practical wisdom concerned with universals only—it must also recognize the particulars; for it is practical, and practice is concerned with particulars. *This is why some who do not know, and especially those who have experience, are more practical than others who know; for if a man knew that light meats are digestible and wholesome, but did not know which sorts of meat are light, he would not produce health, but the man*

who knows that chicken is wholesome is more likely to produce health. (VI.vii.7, 1141b, trans. Ross; italics mine)

According to Hardie's definition of the practical syllogism, this example is typical in that knowledge that "light meats are digestible and wholesome" is an example of the major premise specifying effective means to an end (health). Cooper, however, in this case, emphasizes the role of the minor premise. He defines the practical syllogism as consisting of a

> major and a minor premiss in which the major specifies a type of action to be done and the minor records by means of demonstratives and personal pronouns the fact that persons or objects of types specified in the major are present; and the performance of the action follows immediately, as the syllogism's outcome. (1975, 26)

Cooper's definition bears resemblance to Hardie's, except that according to Cooper, knowledge of the chicken species is achieved through intuitive understanding. The knowledge that this particular piece of meat is indeed chicken is provided through the minor premises of the practical syllogism. The healthful benefit of eating this form of light meat is an immediate consequence of intuition (*nous*) and the minor premise of the practical syllogism, leading to the action of eating.[11]

One issue at stake in this apparent hair-splitting over the nature of the practical syllogism is the fate of the fact/value distinction in Aristotle. For, if deliberation about the good end is part of a process of deliberation as Allan claims, then Aristotle would, it seems, conflate reason with value, and therefore be a proponent or victim of the naturalistic fallacy, depending on which side of the debate one stood. Hardie makes this clear when he writes that "in Aristotle's scheme the minor premiss does not recognize a value; it merely states a fact." The result of this is that "the practical syllogism has to be inflated in order to do the work expected by commentators, and its shape gets distorted in the process" (1968, 249–50). Cooper, for his part, by placing the practical syllogism outside of deliberation, implies that the practical syllogism is associated with values originating from perception, and that deliberation and values are separate realms.

Aristotle's position on the fact/value distinction is not at all clear. In his analysis of normativity in Aristotle, Oates argues that Aristotle, unlike Plato, did emphasize being over value and, therefore, did ultimately separate fact from value. Yet Oates also makes clear that there are passages in which Aristotle appears to affirm the relation of being and value.[12] *Phronesis* is exemplary in this regard. Aristotle at the beginning of book 6 distinguishes between two parts of the intellectual soul which grasp invariable causes and variable things. The intellectual categories, as stated earlier, include: art, scientific knowledge, practical wisdom, philosophic wisdom, and intuitive reason. *Phronesis* is distinguished from scientific knowledge and philosophic wisdom by being able to address that which is variable. The difficulty is to explain how, as a type of intuitive knowledge of first principles, *phronesis* can be concerned with variable knowledge. The answer suggested from this review of the practical syllogism is that *phronesis* contains elements of both the intellectual and emotional psyche. To put it differently, *phronesis*, in addition to incorporating a type of intellectual *nous*, is also akin to the appetitive soul. Aristotle points to this corporeal aspect in describing *phronesis* as a type of perception, even though as he makes clear it is "not the perception of qualities peculiar to one sense but a perception akin to that by which we perceive that the particular figure before us is a triangle" (*Nic. Ethics*, 1142a). As a unique type of perception, it is not surprising that Aristotle, at the end of chapter 6, claims that *phronesis* requires both intellectual and moral virtues.[13]

In summary, *phronesis* is a type of understanding associated with the intellectual, the appetitive and the moral parts of the human psyche. It is understandable that there should be a close association in *phronesis* between being and value. The various possible combinations of intellect, emotions, and morals explain the different interpretations of the practical syllogism. Furthermore, the tension between the moral and the intellectual, the appetitive, and the rational all contained under the aegis of *phronesis* explains the difficulty in defining the nature of the relation between *nous* and *phronesis*.

From the above it can be seen why *phronesis* is representative of a type of essential ontological knowledge that refers to what Jonas has termed the "knot of being." It is not surprising that for Aristotle, this knowledge, while exemplified in human beings, is not specific to them but exists in other animals, too.[14] This sharing of *phronesis* with other animals indicates that *phronesis* is a corporeal or visceral type of knowledge associated with animal drives and perception.[15] One Aristotle commentator, Takatsura Andō, claims justifiably that practical wisdom is a form of *sensus communis* that is "accompanied by physiological phenomena, especially those of the heart" ([1958] 1971, 209). Additionally, as a type of intellect, it "is not a mere function of the body, but bears some transcendent character" (ibid.).

The Corporeal Foundation of *Phronesis* and *Nous*

This argument for the corporeal relation between *phronesis* and *nous* vis-à-vis the practical syllogism finds support in the classicist Richard Braxton Onians's philological analysis of the origins of European thought. Thus, Onians argues that for Homer, the Greek word *phronein* (φρονείν) generally understood as an intellectual sense "to think" or to "have understanding" had a more comprehensive sense referring to "undifferentiated psychic activity, the activity of the *phrenes* (φρένες), involving 'emotion' and 'conation' also" (1951, 14). Likewise, for Homer the word *phrenes* from which *phronein* and *phronesis* are derived, should not mean merely "wits," but the "physical organ which is also the seat of intelligence" (35). Similarly, *nous* (νόος), which functioned in Greek philosophy as the "dynamic ordering factor in the universe" has a corporeal association, being located in the chest and identified with the heart (83). However, Onians claims that in its origin, *nous* did not refer to a permanent organ of the body. Rather, he suggests it is a formation:

> (From νέομαι 'I go,' νέω 'I move in liquid, swim') like πνόος a 'blowing' or a 'wind' from πνέω, ρόος a 'flowing' or a 'river' from ρέω. It expresses either the particular movement, purpose, or, relatively permanent, that which moves, the purposing consciousness. It darts (άίξη), rushes (όρνυται), is restrained (ίσχανε), turned (τρέπεται, cf. έπιγνάμπτει). . . . It makes the difference between uncontrolled and intelligent, purposive, conscious (e.g. μή χαλέπαινε παρέκ νόον) as in a different way the defining frame of the θρένες did. Thus, like θρένες, it gets something of the value of 'intelligence' or 'intellect' but, unlike θρένες, it is not obviously material, tangible, pierced by weapons, etc. It is not mere intellect; it is dynamic, as we have seen, and emotional . . . as the case may be. (82–83)

Besides providing support linking *phronesis* with *nous*, Onians's philological analysis helps explain Aristotle's related theory of action. Thus, according to Onians, in the weltanschauung of classical Greece, perception or cognition was invariably followed by or associated with a tendency to action and an emotion varying in degree and kind according to the nature of the object perceived.[16] It is logical, therefore, that Aristotelian *phronesis* developed as part of a larger weltanschauung that related bodily parts and functions to abstract thought, and formed the foundations of Aristotle's theory of action in his practical syllogism.

Onians's insight regarding the close relation between intellect and perception in Greek culture is supported by another example of the practical syllogism from the *De Motu Animalium*. Thus, in the *De Motu Animalium*, Aristotle uses the structure of the practical syllogism to describe how the thought of movement becomes movement:

> But how does it happen that thinking is sometimes accompanied by action and sometimes not, sometimes by motion and sometimes not? It looks as

if almost the same thing happens as in the case of reasoning and making inferences about unchanging objects. But in that case the end is a speculative
proposition (for whenever one thinks the two premises, one thinks and puts
together the conclusion), whereas here the conclusion which results from the
two premises is the action. For example, whenever someone thinks that every
man should take walks, and that he is a man, at once he takes a walk. . . .

But just as questioners in dialectical contests sometimes do, so here too
thought does not stop and consider at all the second premiss, the obvious
one. For example, if walking is good for a man it doesn't spend any time over
the fact that one is a man oneself. Hence in actions that we perform without
calculation we act quickly. For when one is actually using his power of perception in connection with an end in view, or his "imagination" or intellect,
he does at once that which he desires: for the active desire takes the place
of inquiry or thinking, "I ought to drink," says appetite; "This is a drink,"
perception or "imagination" or intellect says—he drinks at once. (701a10–36,
trans. Nussbaum)

Two important points for the present discussion can be derived from
this passage: Firstly is the importance of the appetitive element of desire in
motivating human action. Secondly, as Cooper explains about this example,
Aristotle does not mean that the minor premise simply disappears or is unimportant, but that as something obvious, it is not explicitly formulated in
the mind. In this passage, the minor premise refers to the fact of being a man:
"If walking is good for a man it doesn't spend any time over the fact that one
is a man oneself" (1975, 52–53).

Extending this reading further, the fact of being a human is not merely
coincidental as the content of the minor premise in this example of the practical syllogism. The practical syllogism, as has been shown, is that form of
practical understanding that unites reason, emotion and the virtues. It is exemplary in humans. Hence, the anthropological and ethical implications of
this example should not be underestimated. The fact of being a human is
glossed over in this practical syllogism, and yet this is due to its obviousness,
and not to its insignificance. The centrality of the human being is essential for
the practical syllogism, as it is for *phronesis* more generally. Practical *nous*, as
the intellectual element of *phronesis*, cannot be separated as well from *phronesis's* implicit anthropocentrism, whereby the human image represents the
overarching structure upon which human practical reasoning is modeled.

The anthropocentrism implicit in this example of the practical syllogism
is not an isolated phenomenon in Aristotle. Consider the following passage
in Aristotle's *De Anima:*

The so-called abstract objects the mind thinks just as, if one had thought of the snub-nosed not as snub-nosed but as hollow, one would have thought of an actuality without the flesh in which it is embodied: it is thus that the mind when it is thinking of the objects of Mathematics thinks as separate, elements which do not exist separate. (431b, trans. Smith)

Here one finds Aristotle presenting a critique of the type of thinking exemplified by the later Cartesian method that reduces living forms to mathematical formulae. One can, Aristotle claims, understand the snub of a nose as simply a geometrical form, that is, as concave. Yet, this would not do justice to the embodied flesh of the nose, and presumably to the human face to which the nose is attached. Again the human form is so central for human reasoning that one is likely to ignore it.

Conclusion

In summary, this review of Aristotle's practical syllogism suggests that the *nous* of *phronesis* is a particular kind of intellectual intuition that not only deals with the variable in human experience, but also arises from a corporeal substrate. Practical reasoning is both physiological and rational. The examples of the practical syllogism demonstrate the intrinsically anthropocentric nature of Aristotelian practical reasoning. Bringing this discussion to bear on the relation between *phronesis* and medicine, it can be said that medicine, like *phronesis*, faces the ontological, epistemological and ethical conundrum of how to reconcile universal understanding with the individual particular. I wholeheartedly agree with Natali that practical *nous* is very like the practical *empeiria* used by Aristotle at the beginning of the *Metaphysics*.[17]

In the light of this analysis of the relation between *nous* and *phronesis* in the practical syllogism it is worthwhile again to read this passage that I cited in the previous chapter:

And experience seems pretty much like science and art, but really science and art come to men *through* experience; for "experience made art," as Polus says, "but inexperience luck." Now art arises when from many notions gained by experience once universal judgement made about a class of objects is produced. *For to have a judgement that when Callias was ill of this disease this did him good, and similarly in the case of Socrates and in many individual cases, is a matter of experience; but to judge that it has done good to all persons' of a certain constitution, marked off in one class, when they were ill of this disease, e.g. to phlegmatic or bilious people when burning with fever—this is a matter of art* (italics mine).

> With a view to action experience seems in no respect inferior to art, and
> men of experience succeed even better than those who have theory without
> experience. (The reason is that experience is knowledge of individuals, art of
> universals, and actions and productions are all concerned with the individual;
> for the physician does not cure man, except in an incidental way, but Callias
> or Socrates or some other called by some such individual name, who happens
> to be a man. If, then, a man has the theory with the experience, and recognizes
> the universal but does not know the individual included in this, he will often
> fail to cure; for it is the individual that is to be cured. (981a1–24, trans. Ross)

Empeira, like *phronesis*, draws its rationality from its association with intellectual *nous*. While practical wisdom makes sense of the variability of individual events and situations, *empeira* refers to the variability of individuals
themselves. Both receive their rational force from their association with Aristotelian intuition, which is not ultimately separate from practical reasoning.
Their applicability for clinical reasoning derives from the ability of *empeira*
and *phronesis* to reason rationally about an individual without subsuming
her into a category of universal reason. As Marjorie Grene (1963, 24) claims,
individuals are the only "fully real" entities in Aristotle's *Metaphysics*: "Callias ruddy, turning pale; Socrates young, growing old—of such as these the
catalogue of realities is made" (Grene 1963, 24). Analysis of Aristotle's practical syllogism shows that the fully real entity of the individual is not simply
derived from explicit conscious awareness, but has a prereflexive dimension
that is constituted through the human corporeal schema and human action.

Individual and Statistical Physiognomy:
The Art and Science of Making the Invisible Visible

In tracing *The Evolution of Modern Medicine* Sir William Osler (1921) describes how modern medicine based on inductive science finally freed itself from the hold of astrology. Osler praises Rabelais's satirical critique of astrology in chapter twenty-five of the third book of *Pantagruel*:

> Panurge goes to consult Her Trippa—the famous Cornelius Agrippa, whose opinion of astrology has already been quoted, but who nevertheless, as court astrologer to Louise of Savoy, has a great contemporary reputation. After looking Panurge in the face and making conclusions by metoscopy and physiognomy, he casts his horoscope *secundum artem*, then taking a branch of tamarisk, a favorite tree from which to get the divining rod, he names some twenty-nine or thirty mantic arts, from pyromancy to necromancy, by which he offers to predict his future. While full of rare humor, this chapter throws an interesting light on the extraordinary number of modes of divination that have been employed. Small wonder that Panurge repented of his visit! (122)

In decrying the premodern association of medicine with the mantic arts Osler makes an automatic link between astrology, metoscopy—the art of reading the signification of lines on the forehead—and physiognomy. Physiognomy refers to the arcane discipline of diagnosing character through facial expression. In making this association Osler in all likelihood had in mind the seventeenth-century book on physiognomy by Richard Saunders entitled *Physiognomie, Chiromancie, Metoscopie*, first published in 1653. Yet Osler's immediate inclusion of physiognomy as an aspect of purely premodern medicine is premature. For one thing, Osler immediately continues his analysis of astrology with a critical quote from the *Pseudodoxia Epidemica* by Sir Thomas Browne, the seventeenth-century English author and physician. Yet Browne himself was a fervent believer in physiognomy, writing in another work, *Religio Medici,* that "certain characters which carry in them the motto of our Soules, wherein he that cannot read A.B.C. may read our natures. . . . The finger of God hath left an inscription upon all his works" (1909, 2.2.1.3.8). A more important reason to distinguish physiognomy from astrology is the historical role of physiognomy as form of classification that directly informed diagnostic procedures and treatment.[1] Osler's skepticism toward physiognomy was shared by many seventeenth- and eighteenth-century authors on the subject.[2] Despite this universal skepticism, physiognomy returned in its modern formulation through J. C. Lavater in the eighteenth century. Particularly through the statistical physiognomy of Francis Galton in the nineteenth century, physiognomy became an important element in the development of modern physiology and psychology. Yet that this skepticism was maintained and physiognomy not completely ultimately overcome, or that the attempt was made to free physiognomy from its association with astrology, indicates the convincing power of physiognomical inference for clinicians, even as medical nosology transformed toward modern classifications of disease. The incorporation of the term *pathophysiognomy* in the medical lexicon, describing the "conditioning exercised by the structure, position, and function of an organ on the characteristic configuration of a pathological process" (Giampalmo and Quaglia 1990) indicates the incorporation of a scientifically transformed physiognomy into our modern clinico-pathological vocabulary and epistemology. This reluctance for medicine to completely jettison physiognomy arises, perhaps, from physiognomy's other historical role as a moral science, "a science of man."[3]

In providing a conceptual apparatus for clinical reasoning, physiognomy is similar to *phronesis,* especially since both rely on intuitive inferences. The intuitive analogy between physiognomy and *phronesis* suggests the need for a more sustained philosophical analysis of these two modes of reasoning in relation to medicine. As a form of cognition related in Aristotle's understanding to a faculty of the soul, *phronesis* is obviously difficult or impossible to visualize. Physiognomy provides an allied medical structure of human reasoning that claims to provide a method of visualizing invisible human characteristics. An analysis of physiognomical discourses provides, therefore, a means of rendering more explicit the prereflexive corporeal basis of practical reasoning. This strategy is not a new one. Physiognomy provides a visual metaphor for practical wisdom, analogous to the role that medicine played in classical antiquity of providing a metaphor for the soul.

In this chapter I provide a hermeneutic reading of the body, which compares the physiological substrate of practical reasoning with that of physiognomy. Physiognomy in the ancient Greek world, particularly as described by Aristotle, shares the corporeal foundations of practical reasoning. I use this corporeal analogy between *phronesis* and ancient physiognomy to examine more modern variants of physiognomy, from J. C. Lavater in the eighteenth century, to the statistical physiognomies of Adolphe Quetelet and Francis Galton in the nineteenth and twentieth centuries, respectively. These examples demonstrate the manner in which modern forms of physiognomy strive to reveal the inner anthropological essence of human reasoning, highlighted in the previous analysis of Aristotle's practical syllogism, but invert its classical form by reducing its inner corporeal substrate to mathematical abstraction to form a "science" of the contingent.[4] This inversion occurs most prominently in Francis Galton's statistical experiments, particularly his photographic composite images of individuals and families. Finally, in the concluding section of this chapter, I contrast Galton's inversion of the anthropological structure in Aristotelian practical reasoning with the German theorist Walter Benjamin's insightful ideas about photographic montage and social physiognomy. Benjamin's social critique provides an important resource with which to develop a microethics in the clinical context.

Before beginning this analysis, a word needs to be said about the, perhaps, strange interest shown here in the pseudoscience of physiognomy and in Galton, who was after all the father of modern eugenics, with all its sinister connotations. In his *Inquiries Into the Human Faculty and Its Development*, Galton defined the word *eugenics*, claiming that it is

> equally applicable to men, brutes, and plants. We greatly want a brief word
> to express the science of improving stock, which is by no means confined to
> questions of judicious mating, but which, especially in the case of man, takes
> cognisance of all influences that tend in however a remote a degree to give
> to the more suitable races or strains of blood a better chance of prevailing
> speedily over the less suitable than they otherwise would have had. ([1883]
> 1951, 24–25n1)

Carlo Ginzburg has noted that even though it is absurd to consider Galton a forerunner of Nazism, his "composite portraits of criminals, individuals affected by phthisis, and Jews cannot be dissociated from his strong campaign for 'stern compulsion'—that is, sterilization—of 'less suitable' races and strains of blood" (2004, 545). Despite this controversial science, Galton's work on heredity led him to discover the concept of statistical correlation, which occupies a rightful place in the pantheon of scientific discoveries.

From this analysis of Galton I argue that one cannot separate this discovery of correlation from an anthropomorphic substrate, and that this insight can be used against a statistical positivism in medicine that has developed in the wake of Galton's discovery. In other words, this analysis presents the basis for an evaluation of the application of statistics in clinical reasoning—one that is intended to undermine a particularly influential and pervasive form of medical positivism. This methodology of using Galton "against himself" in order to make explicit the association between intuition and statistics and to emphasize the anthropomorphic element associated with Aristotelian intuition within medical reasoning—including medical statistics—presents an argument for a moral image within medical epistemology. In this sense, Galton's work may in fact be used against a dehumanizing eugenics program in a revised medico-moral epistemology.

Ancient Physiognomy

As mentioned, physiognomy in its scientific sense refers to the ancient art of reading character through facial expression. Its earliest origins have been traced to ancient Mesopotamia, where according to Jean Bottero it was associated with practices of divination and prognostication. Bottero argues that Mesopotamian physiognomy, in developing a kind of deductive reasoning, provided an early step in the history of the scientific method.[5] Physiognomy's medical associations became more explicit once it was incorporated into the Hippocratic Corpus. For example, in one of the first examples of physiognomy in the Hippocratic Corpus, the *Epidemics* state that "those with a large head, large black eyes and a wide, snub nose are honest."[6]

Aristotle was also familiar with physiognomy.[7] In his *Generation of Animals*, he describes a physiognomist who used to demonstrate how people's faces could be reduced to those of two or three animals (769b). In Aristotle's[8] wide writings on logic, the connection between syllogistic reasoning and physiognomy occurs not with the practical syllogism, but rather with the rhetorical syllogism, or enthymeme.[9] In his *Prior Analytics*, Aristotle uses an example from physiognomy to elucidate his concept of the rhetorical syllogism. For Aristotle an enthymeme is a rhetorical, as opposed to a dialectical or demonstrative, mode of reasoning. It does not, therefore, have the same truth value as proofs provided by other types of reasoning.[10] Since an enthymeme works only from probable propositions, the conjectural science of physiognomy provides a convenient example used by Aristotle to elucidate probabilistic inference from signs. The centrality of Aristotle's description of physiognomy merits its full citation:

It is possible to infer character from features, if it is granted that the body and the soul are changed together by the natural affections: I say "natural," for though perhaps by learning music a man has made some change in his soul, this is not one of those affections which are natural to us; rather I refer to passions and desires when I speak of natural motions. If this then were granted and also that for each change there is a corresponding sign, and we could state the affection and sign proper to each kind of animal, we shall be able to infer character from features. For if there is an affection which belongs properly to an individual kind, e.g. courage to lions, it is necessary that there should be a sign for it: *ex hypothesi* body and soul are affected together. Suppose this sign is the possession of large extremities: this may belong to other kinds also though not universally. For the sign is proper in the sense stated, because the affection is proper to the whole kind, though not proper to it alone, according to our usual manner of speaking. The same thing then will be found in another kind, and man may be brave, and some other kinds of animal as well. They will then have the sign: for *ex hypothesi* there is one sign corresponding to each affection. If this is so, and we can collect signs of this sort in these animals which have only one affection proper to them—but each affection has its sign, since it is necessary that it should have a single sign—we shall then be able to infer character from features. But if the kind as a whole has two properties, e.g. if the lion is both brave and generous, how shall we know which of the signs which are its proper concomitants is the sign of a particular affection? Perhaps if both belong to some other kind though not to the whole of it, and if, in those kinds in which each is found though not in the whole of their members, some members possess one of the affections and not the other: e.g. if a man is brave but not generous, but possesses, of the two signs, large extremities, it is clear that this is the sign of courage in the lion also. (70b, Ross translation)

In this paragraph Aristotle claims that a sign demonstrates the existence of the thing that it signifies. Thus, largeness of extremities in a lion indicates courage, provided that lions as a class are characterized by being large, and not by another quality, such as generosity. This physiognomic knowledge of the character of lions can be applied to judge the more complicated human features, provided that "body and soul change together in all natural affections."

The analogous structure between lion-ness and humanness, allowing both to be accessible to physiognomic evaluation, presents further evidence for the relation between *phronesis* and physiognomy. As is made clear by Marcel Detienne and Jean-Pierre Vernant, *phronesis* can be possessed by animals and is akin to the Greek concept of animal cunning, or *metis*. Likewise, the importance of animals in the structure of physiognomy is not incidental. Tamsyn Barton in her study of physiognomy in the ancient world claims that physiognomical methods are designed to diagnose any divergence toward the incorporation of Monstrous Others: "The physiognomist will sniff out any hint of monstrosity in the subject's body, ever alert for signs of the woman in the man, the foreigner in the Greek, or the animal in the human" (1994, 118). As with *metis*, the attitude of high culture toward the animal aspect of physiognomic rationality is characterized by ambivalence, as the beastly is associated with monstrosity.[12] Despite its animal links, *phronesis*, as an intellectual capacity derived from its element of *nous*, is considered to belong to a higher order of intellectual reason than mere animal reasoning. Nonetheless, the close link between corporeality and animality in physiognomy and *phronesis* presents a clue indicating that they both possess an underground or "radical" association, established on the basis of analogous corporeal foundations.

Physiognomy differs most obviously from *phronesis* in claiming that a particular physical sign denotes the existence of a particular underlying trait, or character of the soul, rather than a process of human reasoning. It is associated with the rhetorical syllogism, because it is a probabilistic mode of reasoning. The lion's extremity, that is, its body, presents a mode of rhetorical proof. Yet, as the previous analysis of Aristotle's practical syllogism shows, the human body presents a similar type of corporeal proof with regard to the practical syllogism. In other words, the human body provides the same type of evidentiary proof in the practical syllogism that the animal body does in physiognomy. While practical reasoning, because of its transcendental qualities as a type of intellectual *nous*, remains conceptual and therefore invisible, physiognomic reasoning is premised on the existence of visible bodily signs. This interpretation of the close relation between *phronesis* and physiognomy suggests that a similar inner corporeal or physiological substrate that physiognomists claim to read from external bodily signs also exists in regard to Aristotelian practical reasoning. The importance of this insight for my analysis of contemporary medical epistemology becomes evident through a comparison of ancient and modern forms of physiognomy.

Modern Forms of Physiognomy

Physiognomy has never disappeared since antiquity, perhaps because we are all physiognomists in our daily affairs. A more or less unbroken tradition of physiognomy was passed down from ancient Greece, via Rome, through Arab physicians in the Middle Ages and into the Renaissance.[13]

GIAMBATTISTA DELLA PORTA (1535?–1615) AND
CHARLES LE BRUN (1619–1690)

Toward the end of the sixteenth century, a natural physiognomy emerged, different from its premodern predecessors in distancing itself from astrology and divination.[14] Giambattista della Porta's *De humana physiognomia*, published in 1586, was probably the most important Renaissance treatise on physiognomy. In it della Porta presented and reinterpreted classical and medieval texts on physiognomy and medicine.[15] Della Porta's work is remembered mostly for its engravings that compare animal and human heads, some of which were reprinted in J. C. Lavater's popular works on physiognomy in the eighteenth century. The physiognomic resemblance between human and animal heads for della Porta is encapsulated in his syllogism: "All parrots are talkers, all men with such noses are like parrots, therefore all such men are talkers" (quoted in Wechsler, 179f12).[16] Della Porta's syllogism was a fundamental rhetorical underpinning of classical physiognomy. While della Porta was important in the transmission from ancient to modern forms of physiognomy, the structure of his physiognomic syllogism is still embedded in that of its ancient precursors.

After della Porta, Charles Le Brun's manual for painters, *Conférence sur l'expression générale et particuliére*, published in 1698, is the best remembered contribution to the European literature of physiognomy during the Renaissance. Le Brun, probably under della Porta's influence, also articulated a similar physiognomical syllogism:

> Courage is discernible from the shape of the nose: the courageous have aquiline noses, but if the whole nose is aquiline, it denotes a talker like a parrot, and if the bump is too low, a mere croaker like a crow. (Quoted in Wechsler 1982, 179n12)

While continuing the classical syllogistic structure, Le Brun's work can be distinguished from della Porta's and traditional physiognomy for a number of reasons. Firstly, as Judith Wechsler has noted, as a manual for painters Le Brun's study reads the same physiognomic code from the opposite direction:

> Where physiognomics, from pseudo-Aristotle through Lavater, starts from the outward sign and teaches how to interpret it in terms of inward character, the treatises for painters start from an emotion or disposition and teach the signs which will express it; and in this they are paralleled by guides to gestures for actors and orators. (Ibid., 16)

Additionally, as it is concerned with emotions rather than character, Le Brun's work develops the allied tradition of pathognomy, or the study of hu-

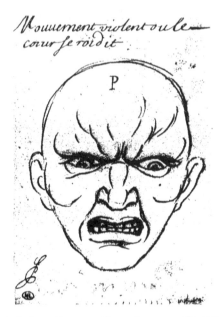

FIGURE 1. From Charles Le Brun, *Movement violent ou le coeur se roidit*, G.M. 6509; Jules Guiffrey and Pierre Marcel, *Inventaire general des dessins du Musée du Louvre et du Musée de Versailles, école française*, vols. 7 and 8 (1912–13).

man passions, rather than just the reading of character in traditional physiognomy. Le Brun's concern with the fluidity of passions has been interpreted as a Cartesian move in breaking with the physiognomical syllogism, and as a vital step toward modern physiology.[17]

The fusing of physiognomy and pathognomy under the modern medical disciplines of physiology and psychology continued in various guises throughout the eighteenth century, flourished through the prolific writing of J. C. Lavater, and reached its statistical climax in the figures of Adophe Quetelet and Francis Galton in the nineteenth century. As will become apparent, Galton figures centrally in this analysis of the manner in which modern physiognomy inverts its classical form. Reviewing these three modern physiognomic discourses helps contrast and highlight Galton's radical statistical discoveries, which emerged from his amateur experiments in statistical physiognomy.

J. C. LAVATER (1741–1801)

Physiognomy as a medical theory was most famously resuscitated in the eighteenth century by the Swiss theologian Johann Caspar Lavater in his popular

Essays on Physiognomy (1789).[18] Lavater's physiognomy can be considered as both a regression toward earlier physiognomic tropes, and an important link in the development of modern physiology. Because of his method of rendering visible the inner elements of physiognomic reasoning and because of his influence on the statisticians Adolphe Quetelet and Francis Galton, Lavater was important in the transition from classical to modern versions of physiognomic reasoning.

As Lucy Hartley points out, Lavater was an essentialist in believing that a person's essence could be known as long as his or her actions, gestures, and expressions could be observed.[19] Lavater defined physiognomy as the "science or knowledge of the correspondence between the external and internal man, the visible superficies and the invisible contents" (1804, 11). Lavater considered his theory of physiognomy to be scientific. Thus Lavater explained that

> physiognomy is as capable of being a science as any one of the sciences, mathematics excepted. As capable as experimental philosophy; as capable as physic, for it is a part of the physical art; as capable as theology, for it is theology; as capable as *belles lettres*, for it appertains to the *belles lettres*. Like all these, it may, to a certain extent be reduced to rule, and acquire an appropriate character, by which it may be taught. As in every other science, so in this, much must be left to sensibility and genius. (37)

Lavater's theory of physiognomy played an important part in nineteenth-century debates about the nature of science. Its theoretical importance lay in mediating aspects of instinct as an important part of everyday life and as part of scientific theorizing.[20]

The instinctual element in Lavater is associated with the vestiges of bestiality in the human countenance and in human rationality. This presence of animality in Lavater's physiognomy indicates both continuity and rupture with its more ancient avatars. Lavater was both aware and critical of his physiognomical predecessors. For example, Lavater, continuing the classical obsession with the physiognomic significance of the nose, writes that "the ancients rightly named the nose *honestamentum faceï*" (1804, 390). Harking back to Hippocratic physiognomy, Lavater, in his plates referring to the nose, mouth, and chin, presents the snub nose as denoting folly. For Lavater, its modern physiognomic importance arises from its "foundation, or abutment of the brain" (ibid.).

Lavater reserves much of his appreciation and criticism for Aristotle as the best exemplar of ancient physiognomy. He paraphrases with approval a number of passages from Aristotle relating human and animal characteristics to their facial and facial expressions (96). Yet, as he describes in his meeting with Emperor Joseph II, Lavater considered his own modern physiognomy distinguishable from its predecessors because of its scientific nature. "I merely observe; and assert nothing but from my own observation," he writes, adding that "I have certainly affirmed much less than the old writers on the subject; but what I have said has been much more precise and defined; and in this science, accuracy and precision are of infinite importance" (lxxxii).

This conception of scienticity does separate Lavater from his classical premodern forebears. Lavater's concern for bestiality within the human visage appears to parallel that of ancient physiognomy. For example, his fusion of moral values with facial expression is epitomized in plates 77 and 79 from his *Essays*; these plates compare the progression of the countenance of a frog's head to the Apollo. For Lavater, the frog's head is the "swollen representative of disgusting bestiality," as opposed to the head of Apollo, representing the "penetrating divinity." Additionally, the comparison between humans and animals, serving to contrast and relate the human and animal countenance, is clearly depicted in Lavater's plates 29 and 30, comparing the human face with that of the monkey, the ox, and the lion.

Despite the important presence of animals in Lavater's physiognomic schema, the apparent similarity between ancient physiognomy's concern to detect animality and monstrosity is deceptive. Lavater's concern with animality can be understood not simply as an attempt to classify the natural order or else to detect the presence of bestiality in the human, but rather, to develop a "science" of the contingent. As Barbara Stafford claims, Lavater's *Essays* "dominated a reductive image of the body inexorably trapped or imprisoned in a geometrical grid" (1991, 103). Lavater was not alone in his endeavors but was associated with the increasing quantification of all branches of knowledge, particularly statistics, during the European Enlightenment. His *Essays* are associated with a neoclassical mentality that promoted "summarization, codification" and "schematicization" (ibid.). In summary, Lavater's physiognomical oeuvre formed part of a larger cultural landscape in which "optical meagerness was anatomy pushed to geometrical anorexia" (ibid.).

Lavater's geometrical physiognomy works counter to Aristotle's criticism in the *De Anima* of the attempt to reduce human contingency to mathematical certainty. By providing a thin description of physiognomy, Lavater's abstractions go against the corporeal basis of practical reasoning in Aristotelian and ancient Greek thought more generally. Lavater's contribution to the eighteenth century's passion to systematize the irrevocable antinomies of "soul and body," "physiognomy and pathognomy," and "certitude and ambiguity,"[21] provides a revealing inversion of Aristotelian thought by stripping practical and physiognomic reasoning of its anthropomorphic bodily essence, and replacing it with an abstract mathematical grid. Moreover, his abstractions demonstrate the modern attempt to visualize or incarnate the invisible, to "seize the liquid inner and outer of things . . . to gain visual knowledge and come to imaginatively possess all that cannot be consumed, or subsumed by words" (45).

This corporeal transmutation of classical structures of practical reasoning becomes most visually obvious with the amateur statisticians Adolphe Quetelet and Francis Galton, both influenced by Lavater's theory of physiognomy. Quetelet was a type of physiognomist in positing an ideal human form that could be discovered through social statistics, while Francis Galton most comprehensively brought together the invisible threads of physiognomy and statistics in his work on heredity. Their respective applications of physiognomy to statistics projected and transformed the anthropomorphic element within practical reasoning to the field of statistics and population studies.

ADOLPHE QUETELET (1796–1874)

Following a visit to Paris in 1823, where he was initiated into the study of mathematical probability and learned about the statistical measurement of errors or observation, it occurred to the Belgian astronomer Adolphe Quetelet that the law of large numbers might apply equally to people and to moral laws as it did to astronomical observations. Quetelet expressed this in his 1835 treatise, *Sur l'homme et le developement de ses facultes*:

> The greater the number of individuals observed, the more do individual peculiarities, whether physical or moral, become effaced, and allow the general facts to predominate by which society exists and is preserved. (1842, 6)

This is the restatement in social terms of Jacques Bernoulli's law of large numbers.[22] It was, in fact, Laplace's central limit theorem that derived the asymptotic normality of the distribution of the mean that captivated Quetelet's attention most fully.[23] If Laplace's theorem could explain how order arises in astronomical observation out of the apparent randomness of individual acts, then why should not this be equally the case with regard to human anthropological data, such as height and birth rate? As a nonmathematician, Quetelet applied Laplace's theorem in a rather simplistic fashion. Yet, more significant than the content of Quetelet's actual mathematical model was its application of mathematical statistics to human data. Thus, this application provided a crucial step in the application of statistics to the social sciences.[24]

Height (inches)	Number of men with chest circumference (inches) of —																Total no. of men in height class
---	33	34	35	36	37	38	39	40	41	42	43	44	45	46	47	48	---
64–65	1	7	31	69	108	154	142	118	66	17	6	3	0	0	0	0	722
66–67	1	9	30	78	170	343	442	337	231	124	34	12	3	1	0	0	1,815
68–69	1	2	16	34	91	187	341	436	367	292	126	70	13	3	2	0	1,981
70–71	0	1	4	7	31	62	117	153	209	148	102	40	16	7	0	0	897
72–73	0	0	0	1	9	7	20	38	62	65	45	43	18	7	1	1	317
Total no. of men in chest-size class	3	19	81	189	409	753	1,062	1,082	935	646	313	168	50	18	3	1	5,732

FIGURE 2. Table of distribution of heights and chest circumference of 5,732 Scottish militia men. From *Edinburgh Medical and Surgical Journal* (1817, 260–64).

Measures of the Chest (Inches)	Number of Men	Proportional Number	Probability according to the Observation	Rank in the Table	Rank according to Calculation	Probability according to the Table	Number of Observations Calculated
33	3	5	0.5000			0.5000	7
34	18	31	0.4995	52	50	0.4993	29
35	81	141	0.4964	42.5	42.5	0.4964	110
36	185	322	0.4823	33.5	34.5	0.4854	323
37	420	732	0.4501	26.0	26.5	0.4531	732
38	749	1305	0.3769	18.0	18.5	0.3799	1333
39	1073	1867	0.2464	10.5	10.5	0.2466	1838
			0.0597	2.5	2.5	0.0628	
40	1079	1882	0.1285	5.5	5.5	0.1359	1987
41	934	1628	0.2913	13	13.5	0.3034	1675
42	658	1148	0.4061	21	21.5	0.4130	1096
43	370	645	0.4706	30	29.5	0.4690	560
44	92	160	0.4866	35	37.5	0.4911	221
45	50	87	0.4953	41	45.5	0.4980	69
46	21	38	0.4991	49.5	53.5	0.4996	16
47	4	7	0.4998	56	61.8	0.4999	3
48	1	2	0.5000			0.5000	1
	5738	1.0000					1.0000

FIGURE 3. Quetelet's analysis of the distribution of the chest circumference of 5,738 Scottish soldiers (1849, 276).

Quetelet's first major example was the statistical evaluation of the chest measurements of 5,738 Scottish soldiers, adapted from an 1817 edition of the *Edinburgh Medical and Surgical Journal*.[25] He proceeded to fit the chest sizes of these tables to the normal curve. In his famous table of this study, Quetelet set out the frequency distributions of these chest measurements.[26]

According to Quetelet, his plotting of the statistical average of the measurement of chest sizes of the population of Scottish soldiers provided the ideal chest size of the individual soldier, as well as the essential chest size of a population. Quetelet summarized this by claiming that the determined distribution was "as if the chests measured had been modeled on the same type, on the same individual, an ideal if you wish, but one whose proportions we can learn from sufficiently prolonged study" (Quetelet 1846, 137, cited in Stigler 1986, 214). The result for Quetelet was that anthropological data corresponded to the normal distribution of the bell-shaped curve derived by Gauss in 1809.[27]

This conflation of the individual with the average essence of a population led Quetelet to develop his second famous concept, the "average man" or *l'homme moyen*. The "average man" represented the central area of a bell-shaped curve where there was the greatest clustering of anthropometrical data. For Quetelet the center of the bell curve represented the ideal essence of human form where deviations from the average were cancelled out. Individual deviation from this central area represented monstrosity and biosocial pathology. The average man, on the other hand, represented for Quetelet all that which is "grand, beautiful, and excellent" in an individual (Quetelet [1842] 1969, 100).[28]

Quetelet's mathematics has been shown to be inaccurate[29] and his conception of the average man maligned. His importance was in providing the bridge between statistics and the social sciences. By successfully converting individual anthropometric data into statistical form, Quetelet showed that all human data could be mathematically determined in compliance with the statistical law of large numbers. Quetelet's concept of the average man was not limited to physical anthropometric data, such as chest sizes, but included moral norms, too. Quetelet hoped that his measurement of physical anthropometrical data, such as chest sizes, could be applied to measure moral

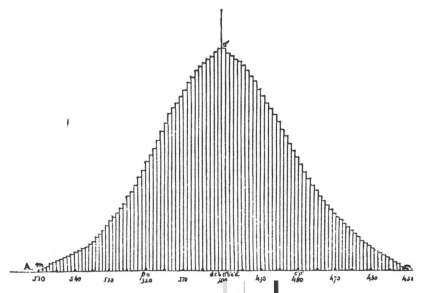

FIGURE 4. Quetelet's repr duction of a symmetric b nc al distr ution with 999 trials, based on the table in figure 9 (1846, 396).

GROUPES DE	RANG des GROUPES.	ÉCHELLE de possibilité. — PROBABILITÉ du tirage de chaque GROUPE. Table A.	ÉCHELLE de précision. — SOMMES des probabilités à partir du groupe le plus probable. Table B.	ÉCHELLE de possibilité. — PROBABILITÉ relative du tir. de chaque GROUPE. Table C.
499 boules blanches et 500 noires. .	1	0.025225	0.025225	1.000000
498 id. 501 id. . .	2	0.025124	0.050349	0.996008
497 id. 502 id. . .	3	0.024924	0.075273	0.988072
496 id. 503 id. . .	4	0.024627	0.099900	0.976285
495 id. 504 id. . .	5	0.024236	0.124136	0.960789
494 id. 505 id. . .	6	0.023756	0.147892	0.941764
493 id. 506 id. . .	7	0.023193	0.171085	0.919429
492 id. 507 id. . .	8	9.022552	0.195657	0.894040
491 id. 508 id. . .	9	0.021842	0.215479	0.865882
490 id. 509 id. . .	10	0.021069	0.236548	0.835261
489 id. 510 id. . .	11	0.020243.	0.256791	0.802506
488 id. 511 id. . .	12	0.019372	0.276163	0.767956
487 id. 512 id. . .	13	0.018464	0.294627	0.731958
486 id. 513 id. . .	14	0.017528	0.312155	0.694860
485 id. 514 id. . .	15	0.016573	0.338728	0.657008
484 id. 515 id. . .	16	0.015608	0.344335	0.618736
483 id. 516 id. . .	17	0.014640	0.358975	0.580364
482 id. 517 id. . .	18	0.013677	0.372652	0.542197
481 id. 518 id. . .	19	0.012726	0.385378	0.504516
480 id. 519 id. . .	20	0.011794	0.397172	0.467576
479 id. 520 id. . .	21	0.010887	0.408060	0.431609
478 id. 521 id. . .	22	0.010008	0.418070	0.396815
477 id. 522 id. . .	23	0.009166	0.427236	0.365366
476 id. 523 id. . .	24	0.008360	0.435595	0.331407

FIGURE 5. A portion of Quetelet's table of a symmetric binomial distribution for 999 trials: "The table lists outcomes ranked by distance from the center, for one side only. The first column gives the outcomes (499 white balls and 500 black, etc.), the second column gives the rank, the last column (Table C) gives the relative probabilities (as a ratio to the central term), the third column (Table A) gives the probabilities themselves, and the next-to-last column (Table B) gives the one-sided cumulative probabilities $P\{500 = X < 500 + r\}$, with X = number of black balls, r = rank." From Quetelet (1846, 374); text from Stigler (1986, 210).

data, such as the penchant of an individual for criminality.[30] The most recalcitrant aspects of individual human behavior and character could, according to Quetelet's conception, be predetermined through statistical analysis.

In reducing the basis of human action to statistical probabilism, Quetelet, like Lavater, inverted the physical anthropomorphic substrate present in Aristotelian physiognomic and practical reasoning. While physiognomy for Aristotle was associated with the probabilistic reasoning of the rhetorical syllogism, for Quetelet it became part of the statistical evaluation of statistical probabilism. Likewise, the anthropomorphic basis of the practical syllogism associated with individual action becomes transmuted into the anthropomorphic data belonging to populations. The inner essence of individuals becomes visible at the population level in the form of the bell-shaped curve. In summary, Quetelet's average man hypostatizes the inner essence of individuals into statistical graphs. This tendency within social statistics becomes most apparent, however, in the statistical studies of Frances Galton.

FRANCIS GALTON (1822–1911)

Frances Galton is remembered for his statistical innovations as well as, somewhat infamously, being the father of eugenics, the scientific movement of social selection based on breeding. His prolific career may be divided into five distinguishable periods, the first three of which are of importance for the present discussion.[31] Between 1869 and 1890 Galton analyzed "the hereditary doctrine" and its utility in the reformation of society.[32] During this period Galton analyzed sets of data demonstrating the relation between characteristics for different generations. Galton's unfolding ideas on the relation between heredity, physiognomy, and statistics are displayed in his book *Hereditary Genius.* Galton introduced this work by claiming that

> the theory of hereditary genius, though usually scouted, has been advocated by a few writers in past as in modern times. But I may claim to be the first to treat the subject in a statistical manner, to arrive at numerical results, and to introduce the 'law of deviation from an average' into discussions on heredity. (vi)

The content of *Hereditary Genius* is filled mainly by listing a number of eminent European men and their families, such as the Bachs and the Bernoullis, in which there was a preponderance of very talented individuals. As Pearson describes, Galton's method, replicating his earlier 1865 paper, "Hereditary Talent and Character," was to take high grades of ability represented by certain eminent people and to measure the frequency of their appearance in relation to a limited population of kinsmen.[33] Finding the appearance of talent amongst eminent families to be in much greater proportion than that in the general population, Galton argued that this result was due to the special talent that was passed down in families.

During the second period, from 1869 to 1876, Galton turned his attention to physiological theories of heredity, attempting together with his cousin Charles Darwin to establish experimental evidence for pangenesis.[34] Between

1874 and 1877 Galton expended most of his effort in analyzing the pattern of inheritance within families. Besides human beings Galton studied sweet peas, pedigreed moths, and hounds.

From 1876 to 1889, the third period of his research, following lack of success in his physiological theorizing, Galton turned his attention to the processes of statistical and anthropometric techniques. His major achievements during this period were the two books *Inquiries into Human Faculty* (Galton [1883] 1951) and *Natural Inheritance* (Galton 1889).[35] As part of his attempt to map and statistically represent the inheritance of genius, Galton turned to Quetelet's application of the Gaussian distribution to anthropometric data.[36] Galton perceived Quetelet's work as useful for his own primary interest in utilizing statistics as a tool to understand the laws of heredity. He first encountered the Gaussian Law of distribution through the biographical memoir of the geographer William Spottiswoode.[37] In turn Galton's understanding of Quetelet's application of this law to analyze anthropometric data was through the influence of the influential scientist John Herschel, who reviewed Quetelet's 1846 work on the social applications of probability.[38] In an early allusion to his later explicit concept of statistical regression toward the mean, Galton noted that there is a tendency for eminence to steadily decrease the further removed one became from the most eminent person in a family.[39] This hereditary truth applied equally to all forms of organic life. Already in *Hereditary Genius*, Galton wrote,

> If a man breeds from strong, well shaped dogs, but of mixed pedigree, the puppies will be sometimes, but rarely, the equal of their parents. They will commonly be of a mongrel, nondescript type, because ancestral peculiarities are apt to crop out in the offspring. (1869, 64)

This statement expresses the statistical concept of regression toward the mean in terms of patterns of inheritance. Galton's studies of talent and mediocrity in families led him to conclude that reversion toward mediocrity in successive generations was a mathematical consequence of the normal curve.

While Galton attempted to visually demonstrate his findings using the statistical physiognomy of Quetelet, he was more interested in distributions and deviations from the mean than in average values. In his early studies, Galton set out to relate mental abilities to facial characteristics. Two representative paragraphs of Galton's physiognomy from his 1883 *Inquiries into Human Faculty* are frequently quoted:

> The difference in human features must be reckoned great, inasmuch as they enable us to distinguish a single face among those of thousands of strangers,

though they are mostly too minute for measurement. At the same time, they are exceedingly numerous. The general expression of a face is a multitude of small details, which are viewed in such rapid succession that we seem to perceive them all at a single glance. If any one of them disagrees with the recollected traits of a known face, the eye is quick at observing it, and it dwells upon the difference. (3)

And:

The physiognomical difference between different men being so numerous and small, it is impossible to measure and compare them each to each, and to discover by ordinary statistical methods the true physiognomy of a race. The usual way is to select individuals who are judged to be representative of the prevalent type, and to photograph them; but this method is not trustworthy, because the judgment itself is fallacious. It is swayed by exceptional and grotesque features more than by ordinary ones, and the portraits supposed to be typical are likely to be caricatures. (4)

Statistical Regression and Correlation

As part of his studies on heredity Galton innovated new statistical methods, most importantly what has come to be known as the statistical laws of regression and correlation. He observed that the regression lines of two variables, when expressed in standardized units, had the same slope; and he suggested that this slope could be used to measure the strength of their relationship.[40] His discovery of correlation demonstrated for the first time a means to statistically evaluate the effect of independent variables in causation, for example, tracing the association between smoking and cancer. The importance of this discovery of correlation was to provide the missing link in the transmission of statistics to the social sciences initiated in the previous century by Quetelet.[41] Galton's initial discovery of regression came about through his work on hereditary transmission in peas. By comparing the marks of parental seed size with filial size on a graph, Galton realized that the marks when connected formed a straight line with a measurable slope. He referred to this slope as the "coefficient of reversion." After a while Galton realized that this coefficient was the result of statistical manipulation and not of heredity, and he replaced reversion with regression.[42] In 1888 he made the conceptual breakthrough that this correlation coefficient could be used to determine the strength of the relation between independent variables.

It is important to note, as other commentators on Galton have done, the centrality of Galton's interest in heredity and eugenics for his discovery of

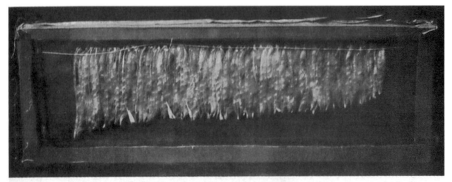

Galton's "Ogive Curve" as exhibited by a marshalled series of Bean Pods. Unfortunately in the many years since Galton built up this illustration several tips have been broken off and in other cases some of the pods have burst open and the shell has curled round.

FIGURE 6. Galton's "Ogive Curve." From Pearson, vol. 3 (1924, plate 2).

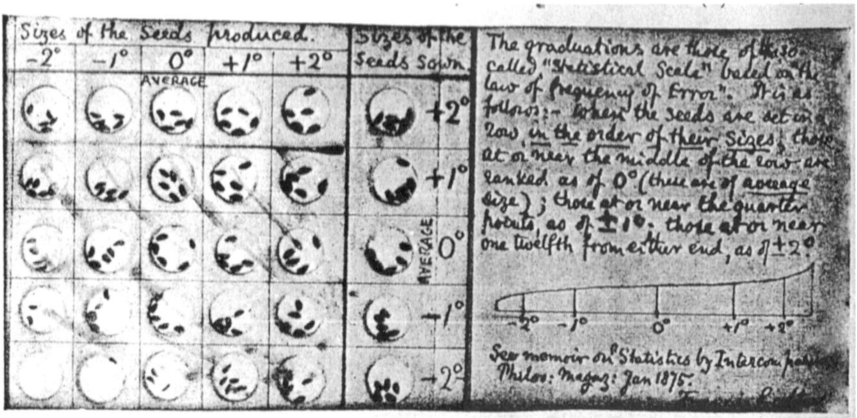

Galton's first illustration of Correlation, *circa* 1875. From the *Galtoniana.*

FIGURE 7. Galton's first illustration of correlation. From Pearson (1924, 2:392)

correlation.[43] As evinced by this brief review, the discovery of correlation resulted from the statistical generalization of concepts originally relating to specific hereditary and anthropometric characteristics. The discovery of correlation resulted from the attempt by Galton to reconcile anthropometric observations with the central limit theorem.[44] Ruth Cowan observes that the term "correlation" "has two roots: first as 'co-relation,' a measure of the coincidence of two variables, and second as 'correlation,' the biological principle which relates the growth of one part of the body to the growth of another" (1972, 527). Summarizing this insight into Galton, Karl Pearson, Galton's friend, biographer and most ardent advocate, writes,

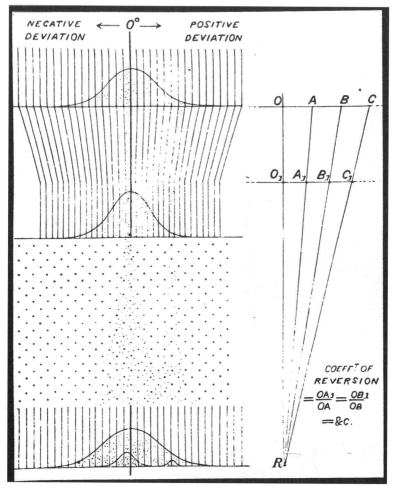

FIGURE 8. Galton's illustration of reversion. Originally published in "Typical Laws of Heredity," *Proceedings of the Royal Institution* (Feb. 9, 1877).

The reader will now grasp how necessary it is to appreciate that the inheritance of mental and moral characters in man was the fundamental concept in Galton's life and work. It led him to all his later quantitative investigations on heredity; it led him to his conception of the "stirp,"[45] or as it was later termed the principle of the continuity of the germ plasm, but it led him also to his rejection of the doctrine of an implanted "soul"—"*talent* and *character* are exhaustive; they include the whole of man's spiritual nature so far as we are able to understand it." Galton's free thought was the product of his views on heredity, and Darwin's *Origin of Species* had led Galton directly to the study of heredity in man. (1924, vol. 2, 82)

In summary, Galton's drive to statistically represent the transmission of hereditary characteristics resulted in his working out the method of correlation. Galton's concern with the inner anthropomorphic essence of heredity, termed the "stirp," connects his work in statistics with Lavater and Quetelet's science of physiognomy. Like them, Galton attempted to render scientific and mathematically precise the intuitive/instinctual element present within physiognomic reasoning. The monstrous element within physiognomy is represented for Galton by the "grotesque features" of individuals at the extremes of statistical variation. Galton's strength, however, lay not in mathematical deduction, but in empirical investigation. In emphasizing the centrality of Galton's eugenic concerns for his discovery of regression and correlation, Cowan writes that "Galton's flair for visual representation of data lies at the heart of his ability to discover these techniques [of regression

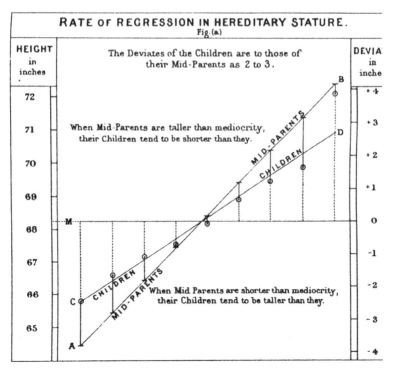

FIGURE 9. Galton's illustration of regression: the circles give the average heights for groups of children whose midparental heights can be read from the line *AB*. The difference between the line *CD* (drawn by the eye to approximate the circles) and *AB* represents regression toward mediocrity. From Galton, "Regression Toward Mediocrity in Hereditary Stature," *Journal of the Anthropological Institute* (1886); text from Stigler (1986, 295).

and correlation], not his success at abstract reasoning" (1977, 185). Besides his charts, Galton was a master in developing practical tools used to test his statistical concepts. His famed quincunx served as an analogue to graphically demonstrate the statistical processes of heredity.[46] Besides their obvious epistemological value, Galton's visual techniques, and in particular his experiments with photography in dealing directly with the human image, provide the most visually compelling examples of his statistical physiognomy. An analysis of Galton's methods of photographic reproduction provides the clearest example of the manner in which modern physiognomy transmutes the anthropomorphic element that is present in Aristotle's structure of practical reasoning.

Galton's Composite and Analytic Photography

Galton developed his method of composite photography in order to provide a "pictorial statistics" of Quetelet's average man. In an 1879 article entitled "Generic Images," Galton described the purpose of his composites:

> The process . . . of pictorial statistics [is] suitable to give us generic pictures of man, such as Quetelet obtained in outline by the ordinary numerical methods of statistics, as described in his work on *Anthropometrie*. . . . By the process of composites we obtain a picture and not a mere outline. (162, cited in Sekula 1986, 48)

Galton achieved his composite images by taking serial photos of faces and exposing them upon a single plate through fractional exposures. Thus, each image was exposed for an inverse amount of time, depending on the total number of images in a series.[47] The result of this process was that distinctive individual features disappeared through underexposure, while common shared features became accentuated. Or as Galton noted,

> Those of its outlines are sharpest and darkest that are common to the largest number of the components; the purely individual peculiarities leave little or no visible trace. The latter being necessarily disposed on both sides of the average, the outline of the composite is the average of all the components. (1878, 134)

Through this method Galton fabricated the ideal image of Quetelet's average man. As for Quetelet, Galton's composite images represented "an ideal composition," because they made manifest specific inherited traits:

> Th eff ct f composite portraitur ? is to bring into evidence all the traits in wh h er is agreement, and to eave but a ghost of a trace of individual

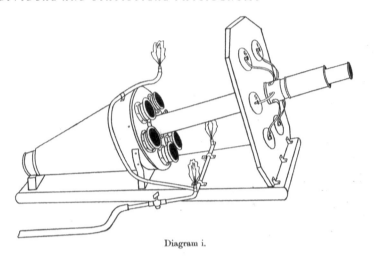

Diagram i.

¹ "Composite Portraits," made by combining those of many different persons into a single resultant figure. *Journal of the Anthropological Institute*, Vol. VIII, pp. 132–42, 1878.

FIGURE 10. Galton's composite maker. From Pearson (1924, 2:285).

particularities. There are so many traits in common in all faces that the composite picture when made from many components is far from being a blur; it has altogether the look of an ideal composition. (Galton 1883, 7)

The effect, as Alan Sekula notes, was to give the symmetrical bell curve a human face.[48] Galton differed from Quetelet, however, in that he was not interested in mapping averages of whole populations, but rather in tracing traits belonging to a group of exceptional individuals.[49] Moreover, Galton came to realize that the early composite was an aggregation rather than an average.[50] Galton was from the start more interested in comparing different variables, than with Quetelet's concept of the statistical average. It was this interest in tracing independent variables that led Galton to discover the statistical law of correlation.

Galton's interest in comparing variables becomes obvious through his advance upon the composite image in the next tool he developed, the "transformer." Galton called the study and production of transformers analytical photography.[51] Whereas composite images allowed Galton to compare between individuals and types, he proposed the idea of the transformer to compare between individuals and individuals, as well as between individuals and types. Like the method of composites, the transformer relied on the superimposition of photographic images to emphasize or eliminate physiognomic characteristics. In a letter published in *Nature* in 1900, Galton provided a concrete example of his method of analytical photography. Here Galton described

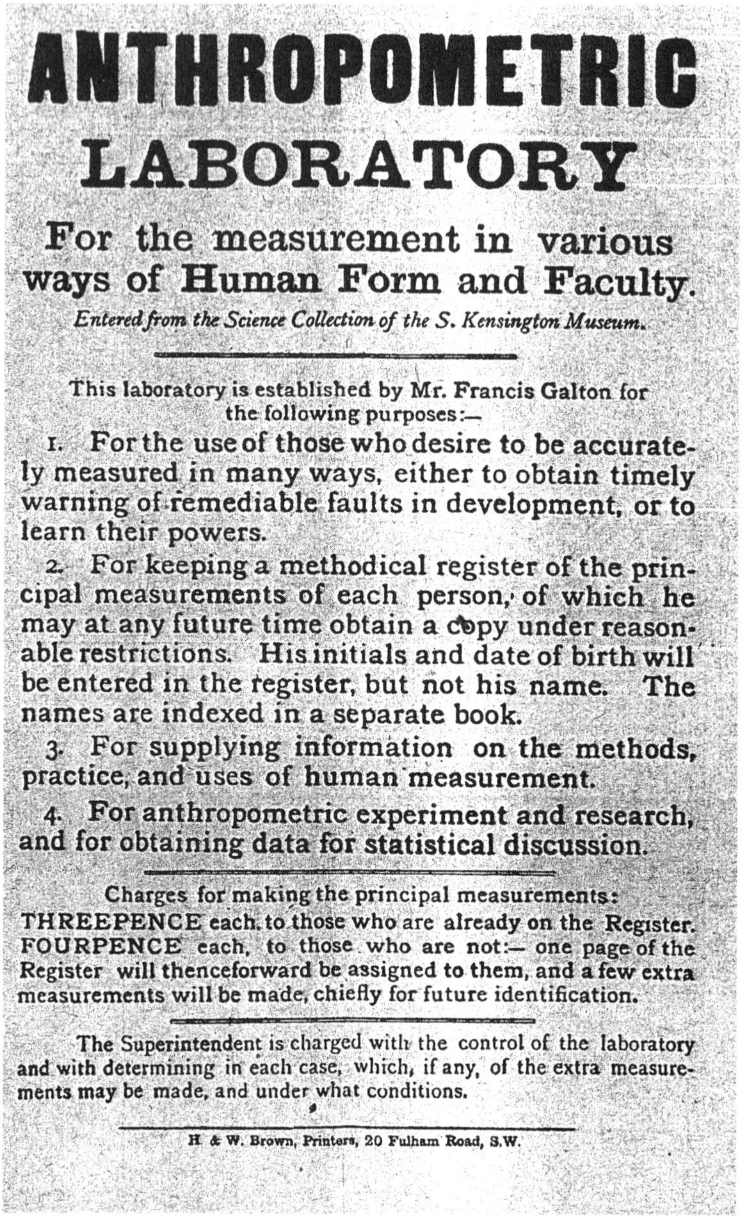

ANTHROPOMETRIC
LABORATORY

For the measurement in various ways of Human Form and Faculty.

Entered from the Science Collection of the S. Kensington Museum.

This laboratory is established by Mr. Francis Galton for the following purposes:—

1. For the use of those who desire to be accurately measured in many ways, either to obtain timely warning of remediable faults in development, or to learn their powers.

2. For keeping a methodical register of the principal measurements of each person, of which he may at any future time obtain a copy under reasonable restrictions. His initials and date of birth will be entered in the register, but not his name. The names are indexed in a separate book.

3. For supplying information on the methods, practice, and uses of human measurement.

4. For anthropometric experiment and research, and for obtaining data for statistical discussion.

Charges for making the principal measurements:
THREEPENCE each, to those who are already on the Register.
FOURPENCE each, to those who are not:— one page of the Register will thenceforward be assigned to them, and a few extra measurements will be made, chiefly for future identification.

The Superintendent is charged with the control of the laboratory and with determining in each case, which, if any, of the extra measurements may be made, and under what conditions.

H. & W. Brown, Printers, 20 Fulham Road, S.W.

FIGURE 11. Commercial poster for Galton's anthropometric laboratory. From Pearson, vol. 2 (1924).

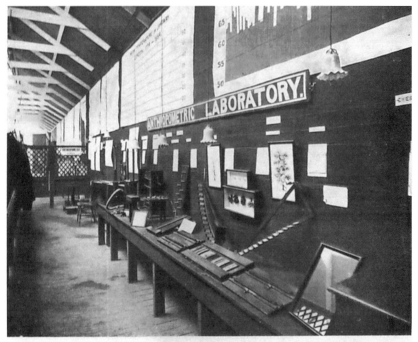

Francis Galton's First Anthropometric Laboratory at the International Health Exhibition, South Kensington, 1884–5.

FIGURE 12. From Pearson, vol. 2 (1924, plate 50).

how he photographed two faces, each in two expressions—the first was glum, and the second was smiling broadly. Galton continued, "I could turn the glum face into the smiling one, or *vice versa*, by means of the suitable transformer; but the transformers were ghastly to look at, and did not at all give the impression of a detached smile or of a detached glumness" (1881, 383).

Pearson summarizes the counterintuitive reasoning behind Galton's analytical photography in the following paragraph:

> A subject *A* and a subject *B*, taken in similar positions and of similar size, have faint transparent positives and faint transparent negatives taken of each. If now positive *A* and negative *A* be thrown accurately adjusted on the same screen, they will antagonise each other and give a uniform grey background. If further positive *A* and negative *B* be thrown on the same screen, they will only antagonise each other where the originals are identical; where they are different, they will only in part antagonise each other. Thus the combination of positive *A* and negative *B* gives a representation of their difference on a grey ground. This Galton calls the "transformer." If the transformer be thrown on the screen with positive *B*, it converts positive *B* into positive *A*. Similarly negative *A* and positive *B* is the transformer, which superimposed

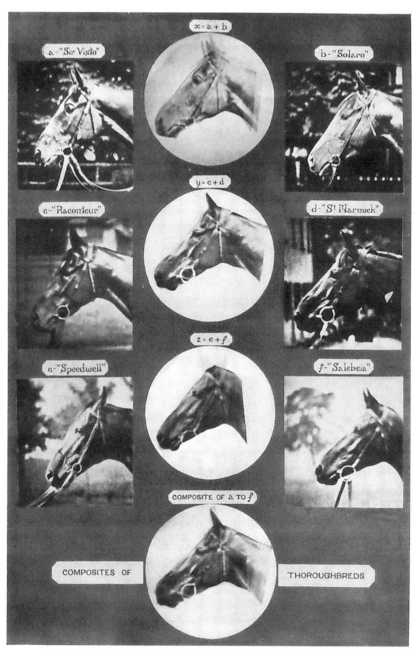

FIGURE 13. Composite of thoroughbreds. From Pearson, vol. 2 (1924, plate 30).

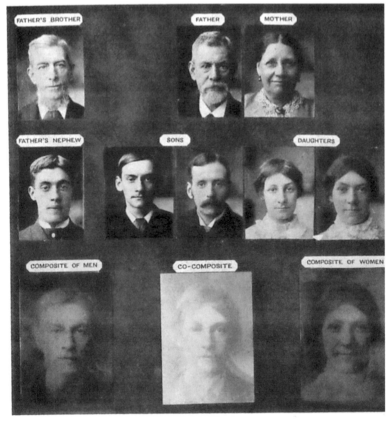

Composites of the Members of a Family.

FIGURE 14. Composite of the members of a family. From Pearson, vol. 2 (1924, plate 31).

on positive *A*, converts it into *B*. The two transformers are in fact positive and negative of the same difference. In both cases the transformed portrait is that of a darkened subject. The fact that our combination of faint positive and faint negative gives a uniform grey or half tone is very important; because it follows that where our transformer adds nothing in the way of difference to *A* to make *B*, it will still add everywhere this grey or half tone. The transformed *B* will therefore be a *darkened* picture of *A*. (1924, vol. 2, 313)

In the photographic image captured by the transformer, or what Galton calls the "example of analytical photography," *A* is the normal subject and *B* the smiling subject, while *C* and *D* are the transformers. *C* is the photograph of a smile, and *D* is the glumness. Pearson claims that Galton realized the transformers were a kind of hieroglyphics requiring a key to their interpretation. Thus, the photograph of a smile is the photograph of their "facial modifications

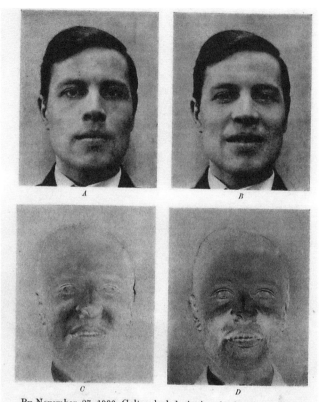

By November 27, 1900, Galton had devised a simple small apparatus[1]

[1] This is now in the Galton Laboratory. It consists essentially of a triple camera; one object is thrown directly on to the focal plane; the other two by aid of two reflecting prisms are also thrown on to the same plane. The three objects thrown on to the plane are positive a, negative a and positive b. By throwing out one or two of the three we can throw on to the screen (i) positive a, (ii) negative a, (iii) positive b, (iv) positive a + negative a to show the uniform grey, (v) negative a + positive b, the transformer, or (vi) positive a + the transformer, giving the darkened b.

FIGURE 15. Example of analytical photography. From Pearson (1924, 2:312).

which failing the stable basis of the face we do not recognize as a smile at all"
(311).

Galton's inversion of Aristotle

Galton's analytical photography provides a clear demonstration of how Galton's statistical physiognomy reverses Aristotle's anthropomorphic image in the *De Anima*, where the concave shape of the snub nose is nothing without the face. Here, in contrast, the smile becomes transformed into an independent variable, free from the particularistic individuality of the human face. Rather tha receiv in me u ing from the h olistic image of the human fa e, th mo tl in ialton'; t ans o mer smile be omes reduced to a fleshless nath ematical abstraction called "glumness." Galton's inversion of Aristotelian physiognomic and practical reasoning not only occurs at the level of images but also, and perhaps most importantly, with regard to Aristotle's theory of action posited through the practical syllogism. Hartley has highlighted the centrality of a theory of action in Galton's statistical physiognomy. She notes that by emphasizing human action, Galton's system of judgment allows the practical application of physiognomic ideas to assume a central role in regulating society.[52]

Galton's interest in mental heredity has been traced to his early 1865 essay published in *MacMillan's* magazine.[53] Here, Galton wrote that it was his intention to demonstrate that mental qualities are controllable in the same way that animal life is controllable by the power breeders. Pearson attributes the earliest evidence for Galton's turning from physical to psychical anthropometry a little later to his 1877 "Address to the Anthropological Department of the British Association." In this paper Galton proposed that "all anthropologists should turn for a time from physical anthropology to study prevalent types of human character and temperament" (Pearson 1924, vol. 2, 228–29). Even Galton's photographic research, as Pearson emphasizes, had its greatest significance for Galton in its psychological implications. The development of Galton's interest in psychology in his different photographic techniques moved from composite images to the transformer to his later work on the Weber-Fechner law, which demonstrated that relative perceptual sensitivity decreased as the level of stimulus increased. Galton's aim in developing his composite photography and analytical photography was to provide a method of overcoming the innate errors of idiosyncratic observation and mental cognition, but also to provide a pictorial statistics of the processes of the mind. Galton referred to this in his paper entitled "Generic Images":

> Our mental generic composites are rarely defined; they have that blur in excess which photographic composites have in a small degree, and their background is crowded with faint and incongruous imagery. The exceptional effects are not overmastered, as they are in the photographic composites, by the large bulk of ordinary effects. Hence in our general impressions far too great weight is attached to what is strange and marvellous, and experience shows that the minds of children, savages and uneducated persons have always had that tendency. Experience warns us against it, and the scientific man takes care to base his conclusions upon actual numbers.
>
> The human mind is therefore a most imperfect apparatus for the elaboration of general ideas. Compared with those of brutes its powers are marvellous, but for all that they fall vastly short of perfection. The criterion of a perfect mind would lie in its capacity of always creating images of a truly

generic kind, deduced from the whole range of its past experiences. General impressions are never to be trusted, Unfortunately when they are of long standing they become fixed rules of life, and assume a prescriptive right not to be questioned. Consequently, those who are not accustomed to original inquiry entertain a hatred and a horror of statistics. They cannot endure the idea of submitting their sacred impressions to cold-blooded verification. But it is the triumph of scientific men to rise superior to such superstitions, to devise tests by which the value of beliefs may be ascertained, and to feel sufficiently masters of themselves to discard contemporaneously whatever may be found untrue. (1879, 168–70.)

Galton's shift from physical to psychometric anthropometry led him toward the end of his life to have less and less faith in any superficial bodily measurements having any real psychological importance.[54] The importance of Galton's research in the history of science, besides his discovery of statistical correlation, lies in marking the shift from a physiognomic theory of expression to a physiological one. The idea of the mind as a spiritual essence became replaced with a physicalist conception of mental states.[55] The irony here, as Hartley observes, is that this naturalized conception of human nature requires the anchor of physiognomy while, at the same time, leads to its dissolution as an acceptable scientific theory.[56]

What social or philosophical sense can one make out of Galton's extraordinarily strange experiments in statistical physiognomy? And what bearing does this review of Galton have on the former comparison of *phronetic* and physiognomic reasoning for an epistemology of clinical reasoning? Carlo Ginzburg celebrates Galton's composite photography as illustrative of a cognitive metaphor using family resemblances that provides a "potentially rewarding research strategy being based on 'blurred edges, mistakes, and anomalies.'" (2004, 556) Yet, this present reading of Galton indicates that the eugenic motivation behind Galton's statistical physiognomy is important in abstracting an Aristotelian structure of practical reasoning. In this sense, Galton's methods of composites may be associated with a research strategy that attempts to ignore or explain away the inherent variability of practice. It will be seen in the final section of this chapter that Galton's discovery of correlation has had important positive and negative influences for clinical reasoning.

Walter Benjamin's Social Physiognomy

In concluding this examination of physiognomy's influence on clinical reasoning I wish to compare Ga ton's method of composites with he theory of montage put forward by the twentieth-century German theorist Walter Benjamin (1892–1940). Benjamin was also absorbed by the subject of physiognomy, however, as a social critic and not as a scientist. For him, montage was a key element in his attempt to construct philosophy out of historical material, especially in his unfinished life project, the *Passagen-Werk*.[57] Benjamin's montage is part of his Marxist dialectical method, which brings archaic images together in order to identify the historically new in the "nature" of commodities.[58] It is, in short, a practical method of analyzing the commodity fetish. The method of montage "counteracts illusion" by "interrupting the context into which it is inserted" (Benjamin 1972, 697–98, cited in Buck-Morss 1999, 67).

Benjamin's concept of montage must be seen in the context of his interest in photography as a modern technique of mimetic reproduction. Photography, in its ability to capture images unavailable to the naked eye, provides an invaluable technique for Benjamin as a social theorist. This sense is captured by a sentence in his remarkable essay "The Work of Art as Mechanical Reproduction," where Benjamin writes, "The camera introduces us to unconscious optics as does psychoanalysis to unconscious impulses" ([1955] 1968, 237).

The photographic technique of montage for Benjamin, like composites for Galton, forms part of a tradition of physiognomic knowledge. This is alluded to in another Benjamin essay, providing a "Small History of Photography":

> At the same time photography reveals in this material the physiognomic aspects of visual worlds which dwell in the smallest things, meaningful yet covert enough to find a hiding place in waking dreams, but which, enlarged and capable of formulation, make the difference between technology and magic visible as a thoroughly historical variable. (1979, pp. 243–34)

There are important differences, however, between Benjamin and Galton's physiognomic knowledge. Firstly, Benjamin's interest in physiognomy was part of his attempt to create philosophy out of history. His physiognomy was not so much of individuals, but rather a social physiognomy culminating in the unfinished project of his *Passagen-Werk* that attempted to reveal through material objects the conditions of nineteenth-century Paris. In this regard Benjamin's social physiognomy bears strong resemblances with the nineteenth-century literary physiognomy exemplified by Balzac (1799–1850), himself strongly influenced by J. C. Lavater.

Balzac's literary theory of physiognomy found expression in the genre that he claimed as his own under the title of *physiologies*, and refers to a series of semicomic pieces he wrote during the 1830s for various Parisian periodicals.

These texts, such as *Physiologie de l'employé* and *Physiologie du rentier,* use overt physical characteristics to describe different sociological types.[59] As Rivers notes, Balzac intended the term *physiologie* to denote the tools of physiognomy in the service of sociology.[60] Judith Wechsler, in her illuminating study of physiognomy and caricature in nineteenth-century Paris, emphasizes the social sense of Balzac's *physiologie.* She notes that "the term *physiologie* suggested objective observation of a type rather than of an individual." As such, "the series dealt with the broad range of middle-class life according to the profession, trade and avocation, diagnosed by habits, customs and manners" (1982, 34).

Another significant shift in Balzac from traditional physiognomy of the individual, expressed in his *Theorie de la demarche,* was to move from concern with facial expression to a "physiognomy of the body," expressed through one's walk and bearing (30).[61] Wechsler has culled the following axioms from Balzac's physiognomy of the body in the following paragraph worth citing:

> The walk announces the man; gesture is thought in action, by which one can decipher vice, remorse, sickness; the look, the voice and walk are equal means by which you can know the entire man; all our body participates in movement, but no part should predominate; when the body is in movement, the face is immobile; economy of movement is the means to render a noble and gracious walk; all jerky movement betrays a vice or bad education; grave favours rounded forms; rest is the silence of the body; work has its effects on our bearing, scholars, for instance, incline their heads; courtesans, actors, spouses and spies, the ambitious and vindictive betray their disingenousness in their walk and bearing. (30–31)

Similarly, with Benjamin one finds a concern for a flourishing analysis of microscopic elements of the human gait. The full paragraph in which Benjamin refers to an "optical unconscious" reads as follows:

> Evidently a different nature opens itself to the camera than opens to the naked eye—if only because an unconsciously penetrated space is substituted for a space consciously explored by man. Even if one has a general knowledge of the way people walk, one knows nothing of a person's posture during the fractional second of a stride. The act of reaching for a lighter or a spoon is familiar routine, yet we hardly know what really goes on between hand and metal, not to mention how this fluctuates with our mood. Here the camera intervenes with the resources of its lowerings and liftings, its interruptions and isolations, its extensions and accelerations, its enlargements and reductions. The camera introduces us to unconscious optics as does psychoanalysis to unconscious impulses. ([1955] 1968, 236–37)

In penetrating below the skin of society the camera adheres, albeit in an attenuated form, to the divinatory powers of the magician or shaman, out of which ancient physiognomy developed. Benjamin uses the analogy of the surgical operation to make this metaphor explicit:

> Even more revealing is the comparison of these circumstances, which differ so much from those of the theater, with the situation in painting. Here the question is: How does the cameraman compare with the painter? To answer this we take recourse to the analogy with a surgical operation. The surgeon represents the polar opposite of the magician. The magician heals a sick person by the laying on of hands; the surgeon cuts into the patient's body. The magician maintains the natural distance between the patient and himself; though he reduces it very slightly by the laying on of hands, he greatly increases it by virtue of his authority. The surgeon does exactly the reverse; he greatly diminishes the distance between himself and the patient by penetrating into the patient's body, and increases it but little by the caution with which his hand moves among the organs. In short, in contrast to the magician—who is still hidden in the medical practitioner—the surgeon at the decisive moment abstains from facing the patient man to man; rather, it is through the operation that he penetrates into him. (233)

In this paragraph one sees that for Benjamin the optical unconscious of the camera is analogous to the surgeon's tinkering inside the human body. Yet, Benjamin's distinction between the shamanistic physician, who maintains a natural distance from the patient, and the surgeon penetrating the living flesh does not simply privilege the camera as an instrument of mathematical precision, a trope of mid-nineteenth century physiognomic literature. By referring to a shamanistic residue within the technology of mechanical reproduction, this paragraph affirms Michael Taussig's observation that Benjamin's favorable regard for the camera is "anything but a straightforward displacement of 'magic' in favor of 'science'" (1993, 24). Applied to the present analysis, Benjamin's emphasis on experience in the flesh provides an important point for a critique of Galton. Thus, for Benjamin the camera provided the optical technology able to capture a social physiognomy, because it substitutes an "unconsciously penetrated space for a space consciously explored by man." Benjamin's use of montage was intended to explode dangerous social ideologies, such as eugenics and scientific racism. Galton, however, assumed that photography could reveal the hidden processes of heredity. Additionally, the use of montage can be used as a critical tool to examine Galton's composites as a type of reactionary montage. Benjamin claims that montage, too, can become illusory when the elements become so artfully fused that "all evidence of incompatibility and contradiction, indeed all evidence of artifice is eliminated—as in the falsified photographic documents, as old as photography itself" (Buck-Morss 1999, 67). Galton's composites are a type of montage intended to reveal the hidden physiological essence of heredity in families. Yet, as "ideal images" they also demonstrate an illusory form of montage where the fusion of faces becomes so artful as to construct an apparently seamless image of a single individual. This single individual presents an idealized version of a physiological essence, and yet one that is stripped of its living flesh through statistical and mathematical abstraction. Benjamin's physiognomy, on the other hand, is characterized precisely through its attempt to render a kind of tactile knowledge of the flesh. Even while the camera renders possible a kind of optical unconscious, the effect of film is to eliminate the human physical presence of the on-stage actor—termed "aura" by Benjamin. For this reason, Benjamin concludes that "the tasks which face the human apparatus of perception at the turning points of history cannot be solved by optical means, that is, by contemplation, alone." Rather, "they are mastered gradually by habit, under the guidance of tactile appropriation" ([1955] 1968, 240).

While Benjamin's social physiognomy bears most obvious resemblance to Balzac's *physiologies* and physiognomy of the moving, walking body, it can also be constructively compared with Aristotle's structure of practical reasoning and action. Benjamin's description of the active body as a fertile field for a theory of tactile or affective reasoning has a strong resonance with Aristotle's practical syllogism in the *De Motu Animalium*. Where Benjamin pleads for knowledge of a "person's posture during the fractional second of a stride," Aristotle writes that "whenever someone thinks that every man should take walks, and that he is a man, at once he takes a walk" (236–37). In both cases, the anthropological substrate is essential for a theory of human action.

This association is more than incidental. Maxine Sheets-Johnstone argues convincingly that for Aristotle, particularly in the *De Anima*, the act of perception is fundamentally a dynamic process, tied with movement:

> He [Aristotle] states there that "sensation depends . . . on a process of movement or affection from without, for it is held to be some sort of change of quality" (*De Anima* 416b34–35). Accordingly, Aristotle appears to be claiming that whatever might constitute a change of quality in specific material terms, change is dependent upon movement and perceiving is thus fundamentally a dynamic process. In other words, that a particular organ of sense is "being affected" or "acted upon" is fundamentally a matter of movement and not a matter of matter. If this is so, then given that the object of sense, via movement, affects the medium, and the medium, via movement, affects the organ of sense, perception is fundamentally and in all cases precisely the kinetic process Aristotle declares it to be. (1999, 99)

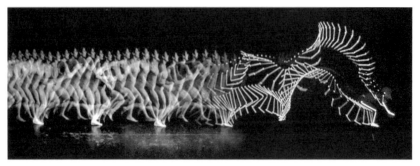

FIGURE 16. Chronophotography of walking. Image by Butch Rovan. Still from interactive installation *Let Us Imagine a Straight Line.* Ami Shulman, dance (© Butch Rovan, rovan@brown.edu, http://www .soundidea.org).

For Aristotle, perception, and consequently all human reasoning derived from perception, is a kinetic process. The previous analysis of the practical syllogism shows how the practical reasoning for Aristotle contains a foundation in perception, which in turn is inseparable from a philosophical anthropology that relies on a moral image to guide practical reasoning. It is perhaps uncanny that Benjamin's theory of tactile reasoning should render Aristotle's practical syllogism so faithfully in a critique of twentieth-century technical reproduction. Yet, the tacit tactile structure of practical reasoning within physiognomic knowledge is traceable, as has been shown through ancient versions of physiognomy, and is retained, though in an inverted form, in its modern forms proposed by Quetelet, Lavater, and especially Francis Galton.

It is possible from this somewhat tortuous comparison of physiognomy with *phronesis* to reach some conclusions relevant for an epistemology of clinical reasoning. The relation between *phronesis* and *nous* in Aristotle's structure of practical reasoning can best be understood as a combination of a physiological and transcendental cognitive process. The anthropological visceral substrate of practical reasoning is made explicit by relating practical reasoning with its medical counterpart, physiognomy, that claims to be able to visualize invisible human essences. While modern versions of physiognomy, epitomized by Lavater, Quetelet, and Galton, are useful for this exercise in attempting to render the inner body visible, they are characterized by a rupture with classical practical reasoning, inverting its structure with the attempt to render the fleshiness of the body into abstract mathematical constructs. This is especially the case with Galton's studies on heredity and statistics. Finally, these insights are of importance for the development of a moral epistemology of clinical reasoning. While Galton's hereditary research was essential for his discovery of the statistical law of correlation, his work has been blemished by its association with the reactionary theories of scientific eugenics.[62] It is likely that these two associations are not incidental. The comparison between Galton's method of composite photography and Walter Benjamin's montage demonstrates, however, the difference between Galton's eugenics that sought to relate social difference to hereditary traits, and Benjamin's social physiognomy that attempted to describe how biology itself is socially mediated. Benjamin's anthropological theory appears to resuscitate the Aristotelian insight that practical reasoning must be molded on a human image in order to be humane. Likewise, a theory of clinical reasoning that is aware of human details within the clinical encounter—details that resist abstraction but are intrinsic to clinical reasoning nonetheless—is required. For Benjamin's social physiognomy these details include the microdetails of what occurs when a hand reaches for a spoon. In the medical context it might be a grimace of pain as a needle is inserted in a vein, or the effect on a moribund patient of the smoothing of a pillow. Moreover, these microdetails cannot be separated from the social context in which disease occurs. These microdetails of human action arise from the human predicament of being embodied individuals gifted with self-awareness. Clinical reasoning modeled on the awareness of microdetails such as these would itself provide a model of human reasoning that is reasonable in being fashioned for its social and human context.

Clinical Intuition versus Statistical Reasoning

Time was, not so long ago, when the standard unit of clinical information was the individual patient, captured in the detail of the case report, often elegantly and precisely at that. But increasing realization of the power of probabilistic reasoning has now shifted from an older anecdotal to a new epidemiologic standard, thus "raising the bar" for the acceptable level of etiologic and diagnostic evidence.

> DAVIDOFF, *"Evidence-Based Medicine: Why All the Fuss?"*

However, the idea of achieving a standardization of professional practice through automatic appeal to mathematical data is immediately simplistic and dangerously naive. Nevertheless, in simplistic and dogmatic fashion, the advocates of "evidence-based medicine" reject medical determinism and personal clinical experience, but glorify probabilism based on mathematical logic, synthesizing a certainty based on what is statistically probable, which—in the clinical setting—does not represent certainty at all.

> POLYCHRONIS ET AL., *"Evidence-Based Medicine: Reference? Dogma?*
> *Neologism? New Orthodoxy?"*

Introduction

During the last few decades of the twentieth century a statistical turn occurred in the epistemology of clinical reasoning.[1] During this period theories of the cognitive processes involved in clinical reasoning became increasingly modeled on the techniques and methods of modern statistics. In particular, the evidence-based medicine movement, which emerged on the medical scene in the early 1990s, represents the most tangible examples of this "trust in numbers" regarding clinical medicine.[2] Proponents of evidence-based medicine argued that medical clinicians needed to incorporate the findings of statistical knowledge into their everyday practice. David Sackett, the movement's founder, defined it in a widely quoted statement as the "conscientious, explicit and judicious use of current best evidence in making decisions about the care of individual patients." And he continued, "the practice of evidence-based medicine means integrating individual clinical experience with the best available external clinical evidence from systematic research" (1997, 4–5). For Sackett, the best external evidence included, but was not limited to, the epidemiological tools of metaanalyses, cross-sectional studies, and randomized trials, the "gold standard" of epidemiological judgment.

Evidence-based medicine emphasizes a model of clinical reasoning by applying statistical data from population studies. In its application of statistics to clinical reasoning, evidence-based medicine relies straightforwardly on the insights of modern statistics. The epistemological basis of evidence-based medicine's application of statistics to clinical medicine mirrors that of modern statistics more generally. Despite the great variety of different statistical theories, contemporary historians of statistics have identified a common epistemological basis of modern statistics. For example, Theodore Porter has defined modern statistics as the "recognition of a distinct and widely applicable set of procedures based on mathematical probability for studying mass phenomena" (Porter 1986, 3). Additionally, Porter argues that statistics has been considered to be especially valuable in eliciting causal relationships where the individual events are difficult to discern or are subject to divergent influences. Its great discovery was that the law of large numbers revealed causes regarding individuals which were previously unknowable, owing to their small size or their exceedingly large number.[3] Another historian, Stephen Stigler, has emphasized the methodological component of modern statistics. For Stigler, modern statistics provided the "logic and methodology for the measurement of uncertainty and for an examination of the consequences of that uncertainty in the planning and interpretation of experimentation and observation" (Stigler 1986, 1). In summary, evidence-based medicine utilizes the insights and methods of modern statistics in order to increase certainty and eliminate error in everyday clinical decision making.

At first glance it does not seem unusual that there should have been attempts to model clinical reasoning on statistics. Medicine is singular of all professions in dealing most directly with the fragile contingency of human biological existence. Why then should modern statistics, which has succeeded in quantifying probability in all aspects of inanimate and biological life, not be easily applicable to the domain of clinical medicine? Stated differently, if modern theories of probability have succeeded in quantifying risk, or in "taming chance,"[4] should this know-how not be important in reducing or even eliminating error in medicine? Yet, despite the success of statistics in measuring probability, the attempt to apply statistics to clinical reasoning presents epistemological difficulties internal to the structure of clinical reasoning. The difficulty, simply stated, is that of reconciling subjective clinical reasoning pertaining to individuals with precise mathematical statistical data, most often derived from population studies.[5]

By providing cogent critiques of expert clinical opinion, evidence-based medicine has deepened the tension between clinical and statistical reasoning. For example, in summarizing the findings of evidence-based medicine and

its counterpart, clinical decision analysis,[6] Arthur Elstein has stated that decades of psychological research on decision making has shown that

> expert clinical judgment was not as expert as we had believed it to be, that
> knowledge transfer was more limited than we had hoped it would be, and that
> judgmental errors were neither limited to medical students nor eradicated by
> experience. (2000, S135)

This statement is significant in indicating that cognitive errors inherent in
clinical reasoning are not eradicated, but may in fact be aggravated, by reliance on so-called expert opinion.[7] In turn, some clinicians have opposed the
encroachment of statistics in clinical medicine, from the conviction of the
necessary place of experience in clinical reasoning.

Intuition is central to understanding the conflict between proponents and
opponents of statistical medicine. The binary opposition between intuitive
and statistical reasoning was detailed in an early pioneering psychological
study by Paul Meehl (1954), entitled *Clinical Intuition Versus Statistical Prediction.* Meehl noted that supporters of the statistical method often referred
to it in positive terms as objective, reliable, rigorous, scientific, and precise.
Others referred to the statistical method in pejorative terms, such as mechanical, atomistic, arbitrary, rigid, and sterile. Proponents of the clinical method
in psychology called it dynamic, global, holistic, rich, deep, and genuine;
while its critics viewed it as mystical, transcendent, metaphysical, unscientific, muddleheaded, and intuitive.[8] Meehl's study was influential in opening
up a new academic field that examined the efficacy of clinical reasoning using
statistical techniques. While Meehl distinguished between the two different
epistemological structures entailed by statistical and intuitive reasoning, he
did not justify, either. Rather, Meehl argued for a division of intellectual la-
bor and application between intuition and statistics in the clinical context.
Yet, the tension between intuition and statistics has proven too great to contain through a superficial epistemological ecumenicalism.

In the decades following Meehl's research, that tension has raged into
the open, particularly in the controversial literature around evidence-based
medicine. It appears from this conflict that clinical reasoning, considered as
a form of practical intuitive reasoning and as the application of techniques
founded on statistical mathematics, is quite different, if not an antithetical
mode of reasoning. The epistemological bases of statistical and clinical intuitive reasoning seem to be founded on contrary presuppositions. In short,
the statistical critique of intuition ruptures the reliance on intuitive reasoning dating back to Hippocratic medicine. Revalorizing the role of intuition
provides a means of reintegrating Hippocratic concern for the whole person

with the modern scientific method. Instead of there being a polar dichotomy between clinical intuition and statistical inference, the analysis of intuition in this and other chapters proves that intuitive and statistical inference represent opposite positions on a single spectrum of human reasoning.

An adequate theory of medical knowledge needs to account for the kinds of processes that physicians use in their actual practice. These processes are accounted for by a theory of tacit knowing,[9] as developed by the philosopher Michael Polanyi. Tacit knowing, according to Polanyi, is analogous to practical intuition.[10] Philosopher Tim Thornton has noted that through the formulation of explicit guidelines and codifications based on evidence gleaned from statistical studies proponents of evidence-based medicine ignore the body of tacit or implicit skill that is ineliminable from clinical practice.[11] However, Thornton claims that by incorporating tacit knowledge into its epistemology, evidence-based medicine would find the unifying factor in its model of clinical judgment. In other words, Thornton suggests that the persistent clinical critique against evidence-based medicine could be attenuated by combining the method of evidence-based medicine with the insights derived from tacit knowing,[12] and that the incorporation of tacit knowledge into its paradigm would undermine the view of evidence-based medicine as algorithmic, or more pejoratively, as a form of "cookbook medicine." Through an appeal to tacit knowledge Thornton intends to unify the tripartite division of evidence-based medicine, that is, to integrate research evidence with clinical expertise and patient values. Yet, as attractive as this argument sounds, because of the dichotomy established between intuitive and statistical reasoning, tacit knowing and evidence-based medicine are diametrically opposed in their epistemological foundations. Primarily because of evidence-based medicine's emphasis on the randomized controlled trial, the epistemology of evidence-based medicine is premised precisely on the dismissal of tacit knowing pertaining to the individual, and therefore cannot incorporate a theory of tacit knowing into its epistemology without transforming into another theory of clinical reasoning. This improved theory already exists in clinical epidemiology, the historical precursor discipline to evidence-based medicine that also advocated the incorporation of public health methods, especially epidemiology, into medical practice. By equally privileging clinical data derived from individual clinical encounters and validating clinical experience, including clinical intuition, together with statistical epidemiology, clinical epidemiology presents an alternative model for the application of statistics to clinical reasoning without sacrificing the fluidity of the clinical context, and thereby retaining the flexibility to account for tacit knowing. In this chap

I evaluate the epistemological basis of evidence-based medicine in relation to clinical reasoning, and demonstrate the dichotomy that evidence-based medicine posits between randomization and clinical intuition. I compare evidence-based medicine with its precursor discipline clinical epidemiology, particularly as developed by the physician Alvan Feinstein. Finally, in the concluding section I reflect on how Polanyi's theory of tacit knowing may take better account than evidence-based medicine of the relation between statistical and clinical intuition.

Evidence-Based Medicine

The term "evidence-based medicine" was first introduced in an article published in the influential *Journal of the American Medical Association* (*JAMA*) in 1992, where its proponents argued that clinicians needed to incorporate the findings of statistical knowledge into their everyday practice. They proposed the founding of a truly scientific medicine through the reevaluation of clinical knowledge by using epidemiological methods. In the *Users' Guide to the Medical Literature*, its authors set out a hierarchy of the evidence-based method used to evaluate new treatments:

- N—of—1 randomized controlled trials;
- systematic reviews of randomized trials;
- a single, randomized trial;
- a systematic review of observational studies addressing patient-important outcomes;
- a single observational study addressing patient-important outcomes;
- physiological studies; and
- unsystematic clinical observations (Guyatt 2002, 7)

As opposed to randomized controlled trials, unsystematic clinical observations are practically synonymous with clinical intuition, associated with the nonscientific error-prone art of clinical medicine. The notion of science established by reliance on the randomized controlled trial as the gold standard for clinical judgment is premised on the dichotomy between scientific, epidemiological expertise and nonscientific, nonepidemiological clinical expertise. In the preface of his 1991 book, *Clinical Epidemiology: A Basic Science for Clinical Medicine*, Sackett traces his understanding of the existence of the dichotomy between the science of epidemiological reasoning versus the art of intuitive judgments to his earliest discovery of epidemiology. Sackett confesses that "it dawned on him that applying these epidemiologic principles (plus a few more from biostatistics) to the beliefs, judgments, and intuitions that comprise the art of medicine might substantially improve the accuracy and efficiency of diagnosis and prognosis" (ix).

In *Clinical Epidemiology* Sackett distinguishes between the "expert" who by publishing treatment recommendations without supporting evidence is on a par with the barefoot doctor and the real experts who cite proper evidence to back their claims from randomized clinical trials (195). This perceived dichotomy between scientific clinical reasoning based on application of data from randomized clinical trials and nonscientific clinical intuition is based on another distinction between inductive and probabilistic reasoning. Categories like intuition and clinical expertise are for Sackett inherently flawed because they are associated with inductive reasoning. For Sackett, the problem with the inductive method is that it is often incapable of exposing false conclusions about treatment efficacy, even when the observations upon which the process of inductive reasoning is based are totally accurate. "The crucial advantage" of the hypothetico-deductive approach,[13] Sackett concludes, "is that it provides, in the randomized controlled trial, the scientifically rigorous opportunity to demonstrate that therapeutic claims are rubbish" (194).

In the almost two decades since its inception, evidence-based medicine has been largely accepted as part of the medical mainstream and has succeeded in reconfiguring the language of academic medicine in its statistical image. It has been difficult for orthodox medicine, priding itself on its scientific foundations, to contend with the argument for mathematical precision and objectivity in medicine, articulated by evidence-based medicine. External signs of the movement's success include the establishment of departmental chairs in evidence-based medicine as well as the medical journal *Evidence-Based Medicine*, first published in 1995.[14]

Clinical Opposition to Evidence-Based Medicine

Despite the movement's success, it has met with persistent opposition by clinicians. The debate between the two sides, if it can be called a debate, has often been heated and defamatory.[15] Arguments against evidence-based medicine can be traced through a series of articles published in the *Journal of Evaluation in Clinical Practice*, also established in 1995. Over time these articles demonstrate a greater confidence in critiquing the theories and methods of evidence-based medicine, particularly since there has been no study demonstrating any greater efficacy using its epidemiological methods of evaluation.[16] Common to all of these articles is an attempt to put into explicit language a tacit anxiety about the claims of evidence-based medicine—an anxiety derived from clinical experience.

The first argument against evidence-based medicine can be framed in terms of the movement's questioning of medical authority. Early in the debate, an editorial in the influential medical journal *The Lancet* (1995) depicted the strident proponents of evidence-based medicine as revolutionaries who demanded that it be hallowed as the "new orthodoxy."[17] This strong backlash from the medical establishment stemmed from the perceived hubris of the founders of evidence-based medicine and their perceived assault on medical authority. What made *The Lancet* bristle was not the movement's emphasis on statistics as much as the tacit implication that it and other nonevidence-based medicine medical journals were less than scientific. In a conciliatory tone, however, the journal editorial offered a place for the "evolving ideas" of evidence-based medicine, provided that its advocates would "lower their profile."[18]

Closely related to the sociological analysis of evidence-based medicine's contestation of authority is the critique of its use of the term "evidence." Eyal Shahar (1997) accuses the protagonists of evidence-based medicine of "throwing sand in the eyes of their critics" by adopting a persistently anti-authoritarian stance that conceals their attempt to set themselves up as new authority figures with the right to define and interpret evidence. Also critiquing the evidentiary basis of evidence-based medicine, Kirsti Malterud (2002) argues that subjective elements, such as "intuition and invisible algorithms," are irreducible from diagnostic reasoning and clinical knowledge and are not presently accounted for by the practitioners of evidence-based medicine. Malterud argues that in giving preeminence to statistical knowledge, evidence-based medicine is guilty of a form of scientific objectivism that is not adequately scientific in neglecting clinical knowledge arising from the realm of "valid evidence," that is, subjective clinical experience.

Similarly, Polychronis and his colleagues (1996) criticize the proponents of evidence-based medicine for implying that the increased power of probabilistic reasoning will render clinical judgment obsolete:

> However, the idea of achieving a standardization of professional practice through automatic appeal to mathematical data is immediately simplistic and dangerously naive. Nevertheless, in simplistic and dogmatic fashion, the advocates of "evidence-based medicine" reject medical determinism and personal clinical experience, but glorify probabilism based on mathematical logic, synthesizing a certainty based on what is statistically probable, which—in the clinical setting—does not represent certainty at all. (2)

Polychronis's critique gets to the heart of the clinicians' opposition to evidence-based medicine. He finds difficulty with the attempt of evidence-based medicine to replace clinical experience with probabilistic reasoning and thereby introduce a false sense of certainty into the clinical medical domain. The problem, then, is not that evidence-based medicine uses statistics, but that it introduces a definition of certainty that is antithetical to clinical reasoning. It does so because it mistakenly replaces clinical reasoning pertaining to individuals with statistical evidence derived from population studies. According to Polychronis's critique, evidence-based medicine is not simply an application of statistics to medicine, but a revolutionary attempt to rewrite clinical medicine.[19]

The Randomized Controlled Trial

Evidence-based medicine's positivistic application of statistics derived from populations to individuals is evidenced from its use of the randomized controlled trial. Randomized controlled trials have been recognized as the "gold standard" method in evidence-based medicine for eliminating clinical bias. Yet, this reliance and usage is not entirely warranted epistemologically. This is evidenced by examining the work of the British statistician R. A. Fisher (1890–1962) and the epidemiologist Austin Bradford Hill (1897–1991).

The insight that randomization of experimental units renders it possible to evaluate whether the difference in outcome between treatment groups is related to chance or to a specific and identifiable cause was first demonstrated by R. A. Fisher. As part of agricultural experiments during the late 1920s and 1930s, he showed that randomization provided the theoretical foundation for tests of statistical significance. In his landmark 1926 article, entitled "The Arrangement of Field Experiments," Fisher noted that

> one way of making sure that a valid estimate of error will be obtained is to arrange the plots deliberately at random, so that no distinction can creep in between pairs of plots treated alike and pairs treated differently; in such a case an estimate of error, derived in the usual way from variation of sets of plots treated alike, may be applied to test the significance of the observed difference between the averages of plots treated differently (506–7).

In his well-known work *The Design of Experiments*, Fisher added that "the purpose of randomisation . . . is to guarantee the validity of the test of significance, this test being based on an estimate of error made possible by replication" ([1935] 1951, 26). Fisher's discovery of randomization was an extension of Galton's discovery of correlation, which was refined by Karl Pearson. Thus, randomization provided the methodological means to implement the conceptual breakthrough that correlation supplied in evaluating the strength of independent variables.

Randomization was subsequently introduced into medical research by the British epidemiologist Austin Bradford Hill. In the 1940s Bradford Hill introduced randomization into his design of research studies for the Medical Research Council (MRC). His intention in so doing was to eliminate selection bias resulting from personal idiosyncrasies that he had observed in medical trials during the 1930s.[20] In the intervening decades since it has been introduced, the randomized controlled trial has generally been accepted as providing the best means of verifying the statistical significance of variations between two compared groups.[21] Randomized controlled trials reduce the risk of bias in statistical comparison between two groups and increase the probability of proving the efficacy of particular treatments. In contrast to individual observations that carry the inevitable error-prone biases of individual clinicians, randomized controlled trials present the best statistical method of eradicating biases from experimental studies.

Proponents of evidence-based medicine perceive this quality of randomized controlled trials as a revolutionary tool for the reevaluation of clinical reasoning. By subjecting clinical questions to the evaluation of statistical studies—particularly randomized controlled trials—and in building up a readily accessible literature of studies that had passed strict evidentiary reviews, the proponents of evidence-based medicine intend to set clinical reasoning upon, what they considered for the first time, solid scientific foundations. However, it is of more than incidental interest that the two people most important in the introduction of randomization in medical research did not conceive of the randomized controlled trial in the manner that it has been prevalently used, that is, as a statistical weapon against clinical experience and the contingent in medical knowledge.

Bradford Hill conceived of his work in medical statistics as a valuable adjunct to assist medical clinicians in their practice of medicine and research. He was severely critical of statisticians who were out of touch with practical realities and who published material not readily intelligible to nonstatisticians.[22] Bradford Hill came to conceive of statistical analyses as having secondary importance to the internal validity of studies and the actual data acquired from such studies.[23] He wrote about the randomized controlled trial in the 9th edition of his bestseller *Principles of Medical Statistics*, intended for a clinical audience: "It should be designed to promote rather than hinder the traditional method of medicine of acute observation of disease by the clinician at the bedside" (1971, 273). In the 11th edition (1984) of this book Bradford Hill expanded his critique of the randomized controlled trial:

> At its best such a trial shows what can be accomplished with a medicine under careful observation and certain restricted conditions. The same results will not invariably or necessarily be observed when the medicine passes into general use; but the trial has at the least provided background knowledge which the physician can adapt to the individual patient. (Quoted in Horton 2000, 3152)

Richard Horton (2000) points out that Bradford Hill was not only moving from an emphasis on internal validity of statistical tests depending on their clinical context, but also positing the importance of external validity of inferences as they pertain to the generality of future patients. In other words, in direct contrast to Sackett, Bradford Hill emphasized the importance and the problem of inductive clinical reasoning in the application of statistics in general, and the randomized trial in particular, to the clinical context.[24]

With Fisher it is possible to discern a similar presumptive criticism of the unreflective use of the randomized controlled trial. While Fisher's statistical experiments were primarily agricultural, he did have an interest in the application of statistics to medical research.[25] Fisher's advocacy of randomization was related to the search for valid interpretation of statistical significance, and was associated with his lifelong obsession of rigorously specifying uncertainty. In discussing this aspect of Fisher's personality, Harry Marks (2003) notes that

> for Fisher, any statistical inference should indicate "two things: (1) wherein our factual knowledge differs from complete ignorance and (2) wherein it differs from perfect knowledge." Such inferences could be made from either observational or experimental data, but the data from randomized experiments allowed experimenters to make "statements of uncertainty" of the strongest [most rigorous] possible type. (933)

Fisher was, therefore, skeptical that we could ever reach absolute certainty about empirical facts.[26] Instead, his method of "rigorously specified uncertainty," epitomized by randomization, provided the foundations with which to make sense of a probabilistic world. This is quite different, however, from the way in which the randomized controlled trial has often been used as a tool to eliminate uncertainty from clinical medicine altogether. Thus both Bradford Hill and Fischer, the two important founding fathers of randomization in medical research, would likely have opposed the use of the randomized controlled trial to undermine clinical experience and to eliminate the necessary uncertainty of clinical practice.

Alvan Feinstein provides a similar critique of evidence-based medicine's use of randomization, which ignores the dimension of tacit knowledge, or what he refers to as "clinical nuances":

> Derived almost exclusively from randomized trials and meta-analyses, the data do not include many types of treatments or patients seen in clinical practice; and the results show comparative efficacy of treatment for an "average" randomized patient, not for pertinent subgroups formed by such cogent clinical features as severity of symptoms, illness, comorbidity, and other clinical nuances. The intention-to-treat analyses do not reflect important post-randomization events leading to altered treatment; and the results seldom provide suitable background data when therapy is given prophylactically rather than remedially, or when suitable therapeutic advances are equivocal. Randomized trial information is also seldom available for issues in etiology, diagnosis and prognosis, and for clinical decisions that depend on pathophysiological changes, psychosocial factors and support, personal preferences of patients, and strategies for giving comfort and reassurance. (1997, 529)

The gist of Feinstein's critique against evidence-based medicine is that the information hierarchy proposed by it, and in particular that obtained from randomized control trials, does not include soft data that is distinctive to individual patients and particular clinical details that may be crucial for therapeutic decisions. These soft data form the stuff of the clinical encounter, and are inalienable from the processes of clinical reasoning.[27]

Despite this evidence that randomization was never meant to replace but to complement the intuitive basis of clinical reasoning, this is precisely what has often been attempted in evidence-based medicine's application of statistics to clinical reasoning. It would be a mistake to ascribe this phenomenon merely to intellectual laziness; rather, it reflects a tension between the two poles of intuitive and statistical reasoning. While clinical medicine invariably handles the micro-level of phenomena pertaining to individuals, statistical epidemiology in its end formation analyzes and integrates already formalized distributions. What is lacking in the uncritical reliance on randomized controlled trials is the connection between the micro- and macro-levels of emergent statistical phenomena. The emphasis on statistical certainty at the expense of clinical experience is a logical trap that arises when one pole of the intuition-statistics divide is unduly weighted. The use of the randomized controlled trial by proponents of evidence-based medicine provides a pre-eminent example where the temptation to achieve absolute certainty in the contingent realm of the clinic leads to the undermining of the cognitive processes of clinical reasoning, embedded as they are in embodied knowledge. This analysis suggests that instead of a polar dichotomy between statistical and intuitive reasoning, the application of statistics to medicine needs to take account of the intuitive foundations of clinical experience. Mediation between clinical and statistical reasoning requires more than simply superficial acknowledgment of the importance of clinical expertise in clinical reasoning. Moreover, the successful restructuring of the epistemology of clinical reasoning in the image of statistics would require more than just the reliance on randomized control trials and other forms of metaanalyses; rather, it would require the reconceptualization of the cognition of clinical reasoning itself.

Response to Criticism

It is useful to assess how the proponents of evidence-based medicine have responded to some of the cogent critiques directed against it. As detailed in the introduction to this chapter, opponents of evidence-based medicine criticize it for failing to take account of the subjective, tacit element of clinical reasoning. Brian Haynes, one of the early proponents of evidence-based medicine, remarked in light of this kind of criticism of the term "evidence" that it might have been better to have called this approach "evidence in support of practice," which admits a certain hubris in the initial founding of the evidence-based medicine movement.[28] Perhaps the best example of the evidence-based medicine movement's recognition of the criticism directed against it comes from Gordon Guyatt, who has proposed the development of the "N of one" or single patient trial. Conscious of the problem in applying epidemiological data derived from population studies to individuals, Guyatt adapted from psychological research the idea of giving a single patient a random sequence of alternative treatments and comparing the outcomes.[29] The most effective outcome of these various treatments signaled the best treatment option for that particular patient. Sackett himself has admitted that

> good doctors use both individual clinical expertise and the best available external evidence and neither alone is enough. Without clinical expertise, practice risks becoming tyrannized by external evidence, for even excellent external evidence may be inapplicable to or inappropriate for an individual patient. (Sackett et al. 1997, 2)

This statement of Sackett's implies a kind of admission for the necessity of including tacit knowledge in evidence-based medicine's epistemology. And yet this admission does not really change the hierarchy of evidence by giving more validity to clinical intuition and other modes of embodied reasoning, without which this admission is nothing more than lip service to an ideal.

For this reason, Thornton's aim of undermining the view of evidence-based medicine as algorithmic through appealing to tacit knowledge cannot be carried out practically, because evidence-based medicine's epistemological theory is premised precisely on the elimination of clinical tacit knowledge as unreliable. For this reason, Stephen Henry writes that "EBM threatens good medical practice not because it merely fails to recognize that tacit knowledge is an essential part of medical knowledge, but because it actively suppresses tacit knowledge as unreliable and biased" (2006, 205). For evidence-based medicine to extract tacit knowledge from the clinical context and incorporate it into its theoretical structure, a completely different epistemological theory of medicine would be rendered.

Clinical Epidemiology

Historically, evidence-based medicine has had a precursor epistemological movement, i.e., clinical epidemiology, that did incorporate tacit skill as foundational for its theory. This term was first used in 1938 by John Paul, professor of Preventive Medicine at Yale University, who advocated the incorporation of public health methods, especially epidemiology, into medical practice.[30] A number of the leading proponents of evidence-based medicine, such as Sackett, include members who had promoted clinical epidemiology in North America—Canada and the United States—in the late 1960s. Clinical epidemiology applied quantitative methods to the empirical study of clinical practice. Its main proponent was Alvan Feinstein, who aimed to develop an explicit and comprehensive science of bedside medicine.

Sackett was influenced by Feinstein to involve himself in clinical epidemiology at the start of his medical career.[31] In 1985, Sackett's department of clinical epidemiology at McMaster University published *Clinical Epidemiology: A Basic Science for Clinical Medicine*, which aimed to set out the scientific principles of clinical medicine. According to Feinstein, clinical epidemiology was characterized by its use of epidemiological and statistical analytical methods to enhance clinical reasoning. Feinstein has made this point repeatedly. It is well summarized in an article published in 1973, one of three analyzing the structure of diagnostic reasoning:

> This rejection of statistics is probably warranted if we assume that statistics will continue to be used in the unscientific manner portrayed in the previous examples. On the other hand, if suitable specificity can be brought into both the statistical data and the clinical reasoning, a scientific clinician of the future can use statistics as a source of enormous illumination and assistance.

To achieve this goal, however, requires a more effective recognition than has hitherto been given to the different types of decisions made by clinicians, and to the types of statistics needed for the decisions. (280)

By 1992, however, Sackett and his colleagues decided to replace the term "clinical epidemiology" with "evidence-based medicine." In an implicit reference to the earlier discipline of clinical epidemiology, the 1992 announcement of evidence-based medicine argued that "all medical action of diagnosis, prognosis, and therapy should rely on solid quantitative evidence based on the best of *clinical epidemiological* research" (italics mine). The evidence-based medicine movement continued the task initiated by clinical epidemiology of applying statistics to clinical medicine; it also maintained its rationale of determining the scientific basis of scientific medicine. Yet, while Sackett absorbed the statistical techniques advocated by Feinstein's model of clinical epidemiology, he arguably betrayed its epistemic essence by ignoring the subtlety of the clinical context. The newly named movement of evidence-based medicine heralded a shift away from the fluid clinical context and toward the emphasis on fixed definitions of evidence determined by statistics.

In an interview with the sociologist Jeanne Daly, Feinstein clarifies his sense of betrayal by the shift away from the real principles of clinical epidemiology:

> My main trouble with the McMaster gang, whom I love dearly, is that they have, in my opinion, assembled under one roof more brainpower under the title of clinical epidemiology than anywhere in captivity, and I just think they have totally blown it. All the fundamental challenges they have evaded. Instead of taking on the challenges of developing a clinical taxonomy, they have just promulgated randomized trials. And when you couldn't do randomized trials on the big scale, you did N-of-one randomized trials. And when randomized trials couldn't give you the answer, you then did meta-analysis. I mean it just shocks me. (2005, 104)

The epistemological significance of this move away from clinical epidemiology to evidence-based medicine becomes more apparent when evaluated in the light of Feinstein's well-developed epistemology of clinical reasoning. As emphasized, Feinstein argued consistently for a scientific theory of clinical reasoning that is adequate for the clinical context. From 1963 till his death in 2001, he developed a sophisticated theory of clinical reasoning, ranging from his early interest in devising a modern clinical taxonomy pertaining to individuals to the development of clinical epidemiology, clinical biostatistics, and to clinimetrics, a method enabling doctors to remain consistent in evaluating a patient's qualitative conditions, such as pain, distress, and disability, through the use of clinical indexes and rating scales.[32] Feinstein's critique of evidence-based medicine is derived, then, from his well-developed epistemology of clinical reasoning; itself largely influenced by his early background in mathematics, and should be considered the negative corollary of his positive epistemology of clinical reasoning.

The key insights of this theory of clinical reasoning were already laid out in Feinstein's classic study, *Clinical Judgment*. Clinical judgment is distinguished by the fact that it revolves around individuals. Clinical experience is the accumulation of clinical wisdom or knowledge through the experience gathered over time of treating individual patients. Feinstein differentiates between clinical judgment, which depends "not on a knowledge of causes, mechanisms, or names for disease, but on a knowledge of patients," and deductive logic, which is "employed to establish diagnosis, etiology, or pathogenesis of a patient's disease" (1967, 12). In other words, there is a particular kind of clinical experience that cannot be gathered from rote learning, simple investigative procedures, or statistical computations, but is the accumulation of all of these and more in the treatment of individuals.

For Feinstein, the individual physician is the central apparatus of clinical appraisal:

> Yet his human sensory organs give a clinician the power to make many observations of which no inanimate instrument is capable, and his human mind enables him to make constant scientific improvements in the way he performs his observations and interpretations. The clinician cannot begin to improve these functions, however, until he recognizes himself as a unique and powerful piece of scientific equipment. He can then contemplate and, if necessary, revise the fundamental aspects of what he does and how he thinks when he collects the human data for which he is the main and often the only, perceptual apparatus. (53)

Statistical techniques are mere adjuncts to the huge range of data that the good clinician should use in forming clinical judgments. The fundamental task of the clinical method remains acquiring and classifying "the elemental data of the bedside: symptoms, signs, and other personal features of sick people" (53).

Besides clinical observation, Feinstein proposes a revision of clinical reasoning through analyzing the use of mathematics and language in the clinical context. The logic and symbols of mathematics, and in particular Boolean algebra and Venn diagrams, Feinstein claims, provide a "sublime intellectual mechanism for describing the procedures of clinical reasoning" (159). In particular, the problem of overlap of clinical data provided by unbiased

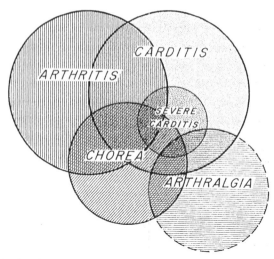

FIGURE 17. The clinical spectrum of acute rheumatic fever. From Feinstein (1967, 184).

clinical observation can be resolved through the mathematics of Boolean algebra and Venn diagrams in which objects or elements have some common defined property. They are also an ideal way to "distinguish multiple properties that could be present or absent, alone or in combination" (10). Thus, applied to human disease, these mathematical concepts provide an explanatory model that could account for the many clinical specificities distinctive to each individual disease.

It is important to emphasize that while Feinstein was concerned with quantitative analysis, the contents of the clinical encounter included nonexplicit epistemological elements associated with tacit knowing. In addition to clinical observation and algebraic formulations, Feinstein's revised nosology requires renewed attention to clinical language. This is because the problem of classification becomes exponential when clinicians advance from first-order observational to subsequent inferential classifications. Feinstein decries the fact that "with uncommon exception," there are "no consistent, generally accepted, and generally used clinical criteria exist today for *any* of the reasoning used in the sequence of second-, third-, and fourth-, or higher-order inferential classifications that lead from clinical observation to anatomic diagnosis" (83). For this reason, the infinite variability of clinical data needs to be matched with a precise clinical language derived from observation and not deductive inference. An adequate clinical epistemology must develop a richly descriptive language that is both scientifically reproducible and thick enough to match the passion-filled domain of clinical medicine.

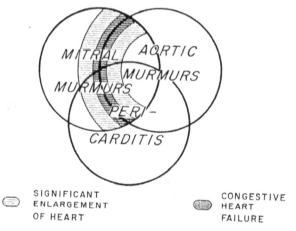

FIGURE 18. The clinical spectrum of acute rheumatic carditis. From Feinstein (1967, 185).

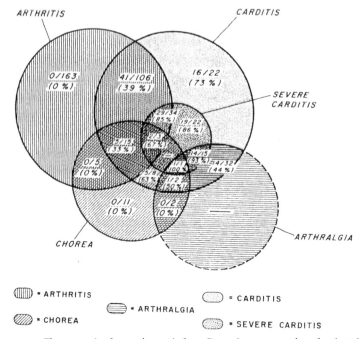

FIGURE 19. The prognosis of acute rheumatic fever. Denominators = number of patients in each subset; numerators = number of patients with clinical evidence of rheumatic heart disease eight years later. From Feinstein (1967, 187).

For example, Feinstein claims that

> there is no ordinary method, for example, of dimensionally measuring the
> difference in physical appearance between a man and a woman. Yet a child
> can give a precise description of most of the distinctions. There is no ordinary
> method of dimensionally measuring the firmness of a carcinoma, the fluctua-
> tion of an abscess, the croak of a rhonchus, or the rasp of a murmur. Yet each
> of these distinctions can be described precisely. There is no ordinary method
> of dimensionally measuring the locations, qualities, and other characteris-
> tics of the different types of pain produced by toothache, migraine, pleurisy,
> abdominal cramps, or angina pectoris. Yet each pain can be differentiated
> distinctly and precisely by verbal description. A dimensional measurement of
> duration can be made for a pain that begins insidiously at a specific moment,
> but not for a pain that starts insidiously. The dimensional duration of the two
> pains may not be needed, however, to determine their origin and significance.
> The descriptive properties of acute onset or of insidious onset are precise fea-
> tures of the two types of pain and can often be used to distinguish between
> them with scientific exactness. (63–64)

Feinstein betrays a utopian desire for a clinical language that can effectively
synthesize the need for qualitative variability with scientific precision.[33] Yet,
despite this desire, Feinstein does not allow himself to become seduced by the
allure of pure statistical mathematics detached from the clinical context.

Intuition

It is enlightening to compare Feinstein's position on intuition that he ar-
ticulates in *Clinical Judgment*. Because he was seeking to develop an explicit
theory of clinical reasoning, Feinstein was critical of clinical intuitions consisting of what he referred to as "hunches" or "nebulously defined" clinical experience (1967, 26). Used in this irrational sense, intuition becomes a
catchall term used to refer to the complex process of clinical reasoning, and
thereby evades the necessary task of scientific explanation:

> Lacking a taxonomy of his own, he [the clinician] *must* be uncertain of where
> and how he got, put or retrieved the data stored in those interstices. When
> asked how he does it, he cannot identify the process because it *had* to be done
> without a conscious order, so he regards it as an unscientific intuition, hunch,
> or mystique, and he calls it *clinical judgment*. (126–27)

It would be a mistake, however, to assume from this paragraph that Feinstein scompletely opposed intuition as part of the process of clinical judgment. Rather, the inclusion ability of an intuitive element within clinical rea-

soning necessitates the attempt to render this subjective, personal, and tacit dimension of clinical reasoning explicit. Echoing, somewhat less poetically, the German Enlightenment philosopher Immanuel Kant, Feinstein writes that "without intuition, imagination, or esthetics, the 'scientist' is a dullard. Without rationality, discipline, or logic, the 'artist' is a dawdler" (295). Intuition here is analogous to Polanyi's concept of intuition that links data from the subsidiary with the focal pole. By itself it is insufficient as explicit knowledge, yet it is an inherent part of the process of linking tacit with explicit understanding.

What is most pertinent here, however, is the way that intuition serves for Feinstein as a cognitive element of clinical reasoning that incorporates tacit elements of clinical reasoning in a rational manner, albeit one that resists explicit formulation. Intuition, as an implicit and integral part of clinical reasoning, is associated with the way in which clinical judgment unites different elements such as deductive knowledge, information from observation, and past experience with groups of individuals, as well as statistical information. Feinstein's qualified support of intuition as an integral component of clinical judgment can be considered as the corollary of his support for the appropriate use of statistics in clinical reasoning. While intuition, as the tacit element within clinical reasoning, requires exposure to the light of explicit analysis to become rational, so too does statistics, as the explicit knowledge gained from the study of populations, require the clinical context of the individual to become real. Clinical intuition, while unreliable because of its fallibility, is nonetheless indissociable from the clinical context.

Michael Polanyi's Theory of Tacit Knowing

In the concluding section of this chapter, I wish to reflect more explicitly on Polanyi's theory of tacit knowing and its relevance for this critique of evidence-based medicine's model of clinical reasoning. According to Polanyi all human activity takes place along a continuum between its bodily and conceptual poles. The focal pole refers to the direct object of attention, whereas the subsidiary pole refers to the clues at the periphery of attention relating to the focal object we are aware of, but which are not attended to at that particular moment. Whether an object of awareness is focal or subsidiary depends on what function it fulfills. Polanyi writes that a subsidiary awareness "can have any degree of consciousness so long as it functions as a clue to the object of our focal attention" (1997, 252). Explicit knowledge is derived from the combination of focal and conceptual poles, whereas bodily and subsidiary poles combine to form tacit knowing.[34]

Tacit knowing functions at the periphery of attention and makes explicit knowledge possible. It is synonymous with practical intuition. Polanyi considers intuition to consist of an intellectual and focal awareness of an intelligible whole, which is later analyzed into its subsidiary parts. Intuition increases our epistemological horizons through its mediation between the focal and subsidiary poles. Thus, Paul Francis Wilczak notes that

> [an intuition] is attained through focal awareness. The distinction between focal and subsidiary awareness is in fact an important condition of the possibility of knowledge (*Knowing and Being*, pp. 211–24). According to Polanyi's analysis of consciousness there is a basic epistemological intention to unify the particulars of sensuous intuition into a larger pattern or focus. That focus is their interpretation, but it is not attained deductively. The focal awareness is an intuitive but intellectual integration of the particulars known at the level of subsidiary awareness. (1973, 27–28)

Since according to Polanyi our intuitive faculty works at a subsidiary level, both the clues and the principles which it integrates to become focal knowledge are not fully identifiable.

Intuition is notable because it provides the link between subsidiary and focal awareness, by bringing knowledge from the subsidiary realm into the focal, conceptual realm. It is important to emphasize that these two subsidiary and focal poles are not fixed, but are interrelated. What is subsidiary knowledge at one level may become focal at another, emphasizing processes of understanding rate and preventing any fixed hierarchy of knowledge. In *Personal Knowledge*, Polanyi provides an account of a medical student learning to read an X-ray, in order to demonstrate how tacit knowing occurs practically in the medical context:

> At first the student is completely puzzled. For he can see in the X-ray picture of a chest only the shadows of the heart and the ribs, with a few spidery blotches between them. . . . Then as he goes on listening for a few weeks, looking carefully at ever new pictures of different cases, a tentative understanding will dawn on him. And eventually, if he perseveres intelligently, a rich panorama of significant details will be revealed to him: of physiological variations and pathological changes, of scars, of chronic infections and signs of acute disease. He has entered a new world. He still sees only a fraction of what the experts can see, but the pictures are definitely making sense now and so do most of the comments made on them. He is about to grasp what he is being taught; it has clicked. (1974, 101)

Polanyi's theory of tacit reasoning is not limited to this single instance of learning to read an X-ray, but may serve as a model for clinical reasoning more generally. Tacit knowing occurs when a physician who is explicitly listening to a patient's story is simultaneously aware, but in a qualitatively different way, of the patient's tone of voice, facial expression, and choice of words,[35] or what Eric Cassell refers to as the paralanguage of the doctor-patient encounter.[36] Polanyi's theory of tacit reasoning appears to be in complete accord with Feinstein's theory of clinical reasoning.

Statistical knowledge may also be understood according to Polanyi's theory of tacit knowing. Firstly, Polanyi's theory of tacit knowing is inherently probabilistic, because scientific induction is based on clues that are not fully specifiable, on processes that are not fully definable, and on a notion of manifestations of reality that are inexhaustible.[37] Thus, Polanyi claims in his introduction to *Personal Knowledge* that "we shall find Personal Knowledge manifested in the appreciation of probability and of order in the exact sciences, and see it at work even more extensively in the way the descriptive sciences rely on skills and connoisseurship" (1974, 17). Individual intuitions are necessarily probabilistic. Additionally, the crystallization of statistical principles and data function like any other kind of scientific process through the mediation of subsidiary and focal poles of awareness. Statistical tests and data exist as explicit knowledge, yet the manner in which these tests and data are derived rely on a base of subsidiary awareness. An analogous approach to statistics has been developed in the field of connected mathematics, which argues that a statistical concept only becomes meaningful through its connections, and that this form of "connected knowing" is personal, intimate, and contextualized.[38] There is, therefore, a necessary tension arising from the realm of probability between the fact that events can be both predictable and unconstrained. While distributions are built up from individual instances, the emergence of distributions is hidden in most approaches to statistical education; this severs the connection between the micro- and macro-levels of the particular statistical phenomenon.[39] What this approach makes clear is that the achievement of a statistical insight does not preclude the use of tacit knowing in its further applications. This position, however, goes against the dominant trend in cognitive psychology that sees everyday human intuitions as poor statisticians through the application of statistical techniques.[40] It also goes against the epistemological basis of evidence-based medicine, which fails to make the link between micro- and macro-levels of emergent statistical phenomena.

Conclusion

In the light of this analysis it appears that while it is important to combine statistical epidemiology with tacit knowledge for an adequate theory of clinical reasoning, evidence-based medicine has not been able to achieve this synthesis because its epistemological foundations are constructed on the elimination of clinical intuition. Instead, this synthesis of clinical and statistical experience is present in the precursor discipline of clinical epidemiology, especially as championed by Alvan Feinstein. Feinstein's understanding of clinical judgment is synonymous with his advocating of clinical epidemiology and his critique of evidence-based medicine. His theory of clinical reasoning may be compatible with Polanyi's theory of tacit knowing. By combining precise quantitative analyses of clinical data, Feinstein managed to provide a coherent theory of clinical reasoning that did not unduly privilege either of the poles of focal or subsidiary knowledge. As Feinstein understood, mathematical statistics had a necessary place in the epistemology of clinical reasoning, provided that it derived its material for analysis from the clinical milieu. While the randomized controlled trial does elucidate causal relations and eliminate clinical biases, the manner of its application to individuals is not free from bias, but rather as clinical intuition is affected by subsidiary, and therefore unspecifiable processes. The emphasis on randomized control trials is an attempt to elicit clinical information under experimental conditions; yet its usage leads to errors because of the assumption that individual events are unchanging so that they may be correctly approximated with the epidemiological law under investigation. It is in dealing with the contingency inherent in the clinical encounter that clinical skill as a form of tacit knowledge becomes crucial, and is not adequately accounted for by proponents of evidence-based medicine. By giving a qualified place for clinical intuition, Feinstein managed to maintain the tension between clinical and statistical intuition without establishing an irresolvable dichotomy between them. This is not the case with the evidence-based medicine movement that sacrificed the epistemological nuance associated with tacit knowing in its successful attempt to become more than just a scientific medical epistemology, but a social movement.

Contingency and Correlation: The Significance of Modeling Clinical Reasoning on Statistics

Some people hate the very name of statistics, but I find them full of beauty and interest. Whenever they are not brutalized, but delicately handled by the higher methods, and are warily interpreted, their power of dealing with complicated phenomena is extraordinary. They are the only tools by which an opening can be cut through the formidable thicket of difficulties that bars the path of those who pursue the Science of man.

FRANCIS GALTON, *Natural Inheritance*

In a serious, though somewhat amusing article, David Sackett, the outspoken leader of the evidence-based medicine movement, describes a study in which he used an "evidence cart" to assist with clinical reasoning on ward rounds.[1] The tools and devices on the trolley included amongst other things a notebook computer, compact discs with Medline and other information resources, a physical-examination textbook, and compilations of the best evidence or CATs (clinically appraised topics). Starting off with the presupposition that evidence-based medicine requires the integration of patients' values and clinical expertise with the best available external evidence, the study was intended to assess the efficacy of such an evidence cart in clinical practice. Even though Sackett found the evidence cart too unwieldy to drag around on each ward round, he did conclude that the evidence made available within seconds during ward rounds did in fact alter the clinical appraisal of at least one team member about 48 percent of the time. However, the effect of evidence-based medicine on patient outcomes was not determined. Moreover, despite claiming that patients' values need to be integrated into clinical practice, this article does not indicate how the evidence cart could be used in day-to-day medicine. One unmentioned consequence of using the evidence cart was to take the attention away from the patient as the center of clinical focus. The attention to best external evidence meant eliding evidence specific to a particular patient. Sackett's evidence cart exemplifies the problem of applying statistical information about populations to the individual.

What is the philosophical significance of modeling clinical reasoning on statistics? A similar problem arises in the clinical situation to that described by John Venn in his frequency theory of probability arising from the perceived dichotomy between the individual variable and the statistical average. In his

attempt to resolve the problem of individual variability in calculating probabilities, Venn claimed that the "fundamental conception" is that of a series
which "combines individual irregularity with aggregate regularity" (1866, 4).
According to Venn, probability statements should only be interpreted as predictions of long-run frequencies rather than quantifying uncertainty about
individual cases. Because of their inherent uncertainty, clinical intuitions
pertaining to individuals are also characterized by individual variability. The
tension between statistical and clinical intuitive reasoning reformulates the
problem of relating the variability of individual behavior with the numerical
order obtaining at the level of population studies. Clinical medicine, which
is concerned with the treatment of individuals, and statistical epidemiology,
which interprets information arising from populations, appear to represent polar positions in the dichotomy of individual variability and statistical
order.

The relation between intuition and statistics can be described in terms
of a probabilistic Aristotelian model privileging clinical intuitive knowledge
of the individual versus a positivistic model claiming to attain absolute certainty from statistical data derived at the population level.[2] Yet, the startling
phenomenon to the uninitiated of statistical order arising from the apparent
chaos of individual variability indicates that there is a mysterious relation between the individual and the statistical norm—in the medical context as well
for the calculus of other probabilities. The attempt to model clinical reasoning on statistics derives its impetus from this relation. Instead of assuming
that the tension between individual variability and statistical averages pre-
cludes a relation between reasoning at the level of the individual and of the
population, the tension between these two levels of inference should be considered a live tension. This allows the possibility for bridging the dichotomy
between intuitive and statistical inference.

For reasons that will become clear, this analysis focuses on the concept of
correlation in medicine, a concept already alluded to in the context of statistics. In general, the term "correlation" refers to the process of making inferences from the comparison between two sets of data. Webster's Dictionary
defines "correlation" as a word derived from the Medieval Latin correlatio,
and referring to the relation existing between phenomena or things. This dictionary definition has become inseparable from the statistical coefficient of
correlation, referring to the measurement of the strength of association between independent variables discovered by Francis Galton and developed by
Karl Pearson. As described in the previous chapter which analyzed evidence-
based medicine, the efficacy of intuitive versus statistical inferences has been
measured according to their predictive success in correlating clinical data. In

consequence, the relation between clinical intuition versus statistics can be rephrased in terms of the concept of correlation.

I begin this study by comparing Alvan Feinstein's understanding of correlation with the statistical concept of correlation discovered by Francis Galton. Galton's achievement is contextualized by reviewing earlier attempts to incorporate statistics into medicine, and into clinical reasoning in particular. Three main historical figures, Pierre Louis, Xavier Bichat, and Claude Bernard, represent different positions on a spectrum of possibility concerning the incorporation of statistics into clinical reasoning. It is by examining their epistemologies of clinical reasoning that, I argue, the significance of the contemporary attempt to model clinical reasoning on statistics may be assessed.

Correlation

In *Clinical Judgment* Alvan Feinstein (1967) uses the term "clinical correlation" in arguing that the development of modern medical taxonomy has served to inhibit a truly scientific method of clinical reasoning derived from bedside observations of patients by the "human apparatus" of the physician. Instead, Feinstein claims that clinical data and judgment are based on the static diagnostic classification of disease derived from morbid anatomy initiated during the eighteenth century. Feinstein's critique of modern medicine crystallizes specifically around the concept of correlation, and he singles out two types of correlation: Thomas Sydenham's concept of temporal correlation, and the clinico-pathological correlate of the physicians Giovanni Battista Morgagni (1682–1771) and Xavier Bichat (1771–1802).[3] Sydenham (1624–1689) was known as the "English Hippocrates" because he shunned theoretical speculation and emphasized clinical observation, whereas Morgagni and Bichat initiated the anatomo-pathological correlate that related clinical observations with autopsy findings, still the basis of contemporary medical epistemology.

These two types of medical correlation may be associated with the beginning of the critical element in modern medicine in the seventeenth and eighteenth centuries, described by the medical historian Lester King as a new use of evidence and manner of reasoning.[4] According to King, the "medical enlightenment" between 1650 and 1695 heralded a "new critical acumen, a new regard for empiricism, a new approach to evidence and new concepts of validity" (1970, 11).[5] Under the influence of the withering critique of ancient philosophy by Francis Bacon,[6] the relation among fact, inference, and authority changed, as medicine incorporated notions of inductive science into its method. In particular, the relation between fact and inference shifted in the use of medical analogy, the form of inferential reasoning most germane to medical judgment in the eighteenth century.

King defines analogy as the process that occurs when two or more entities are brought into relation on the basis of certain observed similarities.[7] He differentiates among three types of analogies, or what he calls declarative, illustrative, and inductive analogies. Declarative analogy draws a comparison between entities but does not draw any conclusions from the comparison. Illustrative analogy draws a comparison between an object that is familiar, and one that is not but still does not draw any conclusions. Finally inductive analogy is the type of analogy that is most significant for medical judgment and is most similar to the modern use of correlation:

> The third category, that I call inductive, is by its very nature inferential. It attends to two or more events or objects or concepts; compares them; isolates and identifies certain similarities which we can observe and call "facts"; and then implies certain other similarities that we cannot directly observe but which we can infer. We might say that certain similarities perceived by the corporeal eye lead us to infer other similarities equally clear to the eye of reason. In the 18th century it was an article of faith that inference achieved by sound reasoning held all the force of facts. (1976, 178)

Sydenham's temporal correlate and the anatomo-pathological correlate of Morgagni and Bichat provided a sharpening of the inductive analogy in medicine. At the same time, however, Feinstein argues that the anatomo-pathological correlate is responsible for clinical medicine's current epistemological impasse. He claims that the emphasis on microscopic pathology at the expense of the temporal structures of diagnosis and therapy accounts for the failure of clinical reasoning to become a truly clinical science. He does not attribute the origin of this failure directly to Bichat and Morgagni, however, but rather to late nineteenth-century German pathologists, such as Wunderlich, who opposed what they considered the concept of specific entities in disease, and who posited that "pathologic physiology" should be the true foundation of medical science. In particular, Feinstein faults Rudolph Virchow, the founder of microscopic pathology, for having a "preoccupation with causes of 'disease,' a frequent lack of concern with therapy, and an absence of intensive clinical correlations" (1967, 119). Additionally, while Feinstein admits that many of the existing defective clinico-pathologic correlations occur in the natural history of disease because of the failure by clinicians and pathologists to appreciate epidemiology, most of the problems arise from a diagnostic concern that often omits the "temporal restrictions" of prognosis and therapy (114).

Feinstein argues that the problem of clinical reasoning's avoidance of the clinical context is rooted in an epistemological structure that privileges static structures such as pathology over the fluid temporal clinical context. Feinstein claims that the problem with applying statistics to medicine is not an epistemological problem inherent to statistics, but the issue is rather its application at the expense of the clinical context. Therefore, the problem of the anatomo-pathological correlate and the use of statistics as the model for clinical reasoning are related in that they both fail to incorporate temporal correlations into the structure of clinical reasoning.

This argument provides a key insight for my reevaluation of the attempt to model clinical reasoning on statistics, yet it requires further elucidation. Feinstein's argument touches on complicated philosophical questions that he does not address. For example, while clinical correlation is associated with the inductive analogy, statistical correlation in its incorporation by evidence-based medicine and decision analysis is associated with the contestation of clinical induction. Additionally, Feinstein's critique of the anatomo-pathological correlate renders problematic the epistemological and ontological foundations upon which much of modern medical epistemology is grounded. In having the discipline of pathology as the cornerstone of clinical reasoning, does medical epistemology not privilege death, rather than living clinical processes? In order to answer these philosophical questions, it is necessary to reevaluate the statistical concept of correlation developed by Francis Galton in relation to the development of modern statistical epidemiology.

Galton's Discovery of Correlation

Galton's concept of correlation encapsulated the novel understanding that statistics could be used to measure the strength of association between two independent variables. By the late 1880s Galton's work on heredity and statistics led him to formulate the concept of regression. In today's statistical language, "regression towards the mean" refers to the fact that the average measurement of a particular variable if represented by a graph will have a tendency to refer to the mean rather than to the extremities. This insight is the basis for the insight underlying the discovery of correlation, that is, that if two regression lines had the same slopes, the common slope could be used to determine the strength of the relationship between the variables in question.[8]

As Stigler has emphasized, Galton's discovery of correlation was key to the successful transmission of statistics to medicine and the social sciences. The discovery of regression, Stigler writes, "was a new way of thinking about multivariate data, a new set of concepts that by sheer force of intellect created

for biology and the social sciences a surrogate for the *missing universal law*"
(1986, 7–8; italics mine). The result of Galton's work was to provide the basis
for the crystallization of statistics into a real discipline by later statisticians,
such as Ysidro Edgeworth, Karl Pearson, and George Udny Yule. By developing statistical techniques based on regression and correlation, they provided the means to study and not simply measure variation, thereby allowing
for the successful transmission of statistics to medicine and the social sciences.[9] The development of evidence-based medicine is unthinkable without
this discovery.

While the extension of statistics to the human sciences is today often
taken for granted, it was a radical conceptual breakthrough that took a few
centuries to develop. Thus, between 1700 and 1900 theories of probability
were transmitted from astronomy and geodesy, to psychology, to biology,
and eventually to the social sciences.[10] The successful application of statistics
to the social sciences was not simply the development of new techniques,
but a new understanding that the statistical theories of probability or chance
could be applied equally to human, animate as well as inanimate data.[11]

It is not clear what prevented statisticians from making the breakthrough
to the social sciences earlier. Both the will and the means were present. Attempts to apply theories of probability to social data, such as legal testimony
can be traced as far back as 1699.[12] By 1776 numerous applications of probability to mortality tables and the computation of annuities existed. By 1830
statistical theory was sophisticated enough to measure social data. As Stigler
writes:

> Statistical methods, including the method of least squares and its probability-
> based expressions of uncertainty, were already in prominent use in astronomy
> and geodesy by the death of Laplace in 1827. Much of the material presented in
> modern courses on statistical methods for social sciences is superficially simi-
> lar to texts available by 1830s, and yet the adoption of these methods for the
> different purposes of the social scientists was so glacially slow that it amounted
> to a reinvention. The problems were conceptual, not narrowly mathematical,
> and they appeared gradually as scientists struggled to give meaning for the
> social world to the mathematical constructs of the astronauts, coping with
> difficulties that are inherent when interesting data observed in far-from con-
> trolled situations. (1999, 3)

It took, however, the two relative novices in statistics, Adolphe Quetelet and
Francis Galton, to overcome this chasm between statistics and the social sciences. Quetelet was instrumental in transforming statistics from a theory of
the measurement of the observation of errors to a theory of variation be-

tween individuals in biology and society. Galton, building upon the work of Quetelet, stumbled upon the statistical laws of regression and correlation in his application of statistical methods to anthropometric data relating to heredity.

While one cannot say for certain why Galton and Quetelet as amateur statisticians provided the missing link between statistics and the biological and social sciences, it is certain, however, that the medical content in their work was vital to their respective accomplishments. Physiognomy was central to both Quetelet and Galton's research in statistics. Galton's discovery of the statistical laws of regression and correlation was motivated by his obsession with understanding the laws of heredity. His early work in heredity from the 1860s progressively shifted toward statistics and anthropometry, culminating in the discovery of correlation in the fall of 1888. Thus, Cowan claims:

> That Galton was driven to proceed down this tortuous path from the rudimentary statistical techniques that he used in *Hereditary Genius* in 1869 to the more creative techniques that he discussed in *Natural Inheritance* twenty years later is a tribute to his commitment to the eugenic ideal and his compulsion to mathematize everything he studied. (Cowan 1977, 185)

The relation between Galton's discovery of correlation and medicine is not simply one-sided, but there is a mutual influence between the statistical law of correlation and medicine. Thus, medicine, or biology to be more specific, in the form of eugenic concerns was not only important in the discovery of correlation, but the discovery of correlation was important for the epistemology of medicine. Following on from the discovery of correlation, the period of statistics between 1890 and 1930 was characterized by the development of statistical techniques familiar to contemporary social scientists and medical epidemiologists. However, particularly with regard to the randomized controlled trial, one important consequence of the application of statistics to clinical reasoning has been the devaluation of clinical experience.

Contingency and Correlation

While the statistical law of correlation has been used to undermine the temporal correlate within clinical reasoning, Galton's discovery does in fact contain a temporal structure that can be mined in order to demonstrate the epistemological connection between statistical and intuitive reasoning.

The association between statistics and temporal uncertainty or chance is made apparent in a text of Karl Pearson, Galton's friend and biographer and an important statistician in his own right. Pearson brought these two terms together in his chapter entitled "Contingency and Correlation: The Insufficiency of Causation," included in the 3rd edition published in 1911 of his *The Grammar of Science.* Here Pearson advocated contingency tables based on Galton's law of correlation as a replacement for the inductivist theory of causation.[13] In other words, Pearson argued that there was no need for an independent concept of causal relation beyond the statistical concept of correlation. Contingency for Pearson referred to the strength of association or degree of dependency between variables measured through correlation. Summarizing this, he wrote that

> no phenomena are causal; all phenomena are contingent, and the problem
> before us is to measure the degree of this contingency, which we have seen
> lies between the zero of independence and the unity of causation. (Pearson
> 1911, 174)

Pearson's desire to remove causality from scientific explanation was motivated by his statistical conception of the cosmos as variable, unpredictable, and indeterminist. His use of contingency accords with its common dictionary definition as the unpredictability of future chance events. That which is contingent is unpredictable in the sense that it is dependent on something else. Yet, there is a paradox inherent in this usage of contingency, similar to that encapsulated by Ian Hacking in his term the "taming of chance," which refers to the paradox that the greater the indeterminism resolved by modern statistics, the greater its control. Similarly, the recognition of a contingent universe as probabilistic is a necessary step in predicting future probabilistic events. The use of correlation by Pearson was not only intended to replace the inductive model of causation with a probabilistic one, but also to provide the means to decrease or even eliminate contingency from social data by a method of numerization, allowing for the measurement of the strength of association between any two objects.

Pearson's conjunction of the concepts of correlation and contingency brings to the surface the subterranean connection between the desire to eliminate contingency through statistics and that to resolve the philosophical question of scientific inductivism. His example also demonstrates how the statistical concepts of correlation and contingency have become intertwined in their popular usage. Correlation today is inseparable from statistical correlation, as well as from its connotation of temporal uncertainty or contingency.

There is a common desire to eliminate contingency in the scientific concept of statistical correlation and uncertainty in the clinical situation that motivates proponents of evidence-based medicine to debunk clinical intuition. In contrast, the acceptance of the necessity of chance among experienced physicians explains the persistent clinical resistance to evidence-based medicine. Both these approaches to probability are present in the attempt to model clinical reasoning on statistics. Thus, Sackett[14] advocated a "hypothetico-deductivist" model compatible with probabilistic reasoning as a replacement for the error-prone inductive reasoning of clinicians. By contrast, Feinstein has advocated a structure of clinical reasoning intended to account for contingency and which includes temporality in its epistemological apparatus.

Despite the use that correlation has had in undermining the intuitive dimension of clinical reasoning, the fact that the discovery of correlation grew out of a medical concern, albeit Galton's morally controversial one (i.e., Galton's obsession with eugenics), suggests that the relation between intuitive and statistical reasoning is not an absolute dichotomy but a living tension. This claim may be analyzed further through a philosophical analysis of the historical application of statistics to clinical reasoning.

Statistical Epidemiology

While Galton's law of correlation provided the necessary breakthrough for the successful application of statistics to the medical sciences, it was by no means the first attempt to apply statistics to medicine. Attempts both to apply and to resist the application of probabilistic methods to medicine occurred almost as soon as they were invented.[15] A cursory review of the most noteworthy examples in the history of medical statistics demonstrates the complicated dynamic between statistical and clinical reasoning. Medicine at once offers a tempting terrain upon which to apply statistics to society—it presents the possibility of empirical verification as well as the promise of social amelioration—and yet, because clinical medicine treats individuals, the epistemology of clinical reasoning resists any straightforward application of statistical data derived at the population level. The main problem in applying statistics to the social sciences rests on the complicated relation between individual human events and the statistical law of large numbers.

BERNOULLI AND LAPLACE

In the eighteenth century two important statisticians, Daniel Bernoulli (1700–1782) and Pierre S. Laplace (1749–1827), both sought ways of applying statistical methods to the fields of medicine and public health. In 1760 Bernoulli, a physician and member of a family famous for its mathematicians, presented a memoir entitled "An Attempt at a New Analysis of the Mortality

Caused by Smallpox and the Advantages of Inoculation to Prevent It" to the Royal Academy of Sciences in Paris.[16] In his memoir, Bernoulli attempted to demonstrate the advantages of smallpox inoculation through calculations based on a priori assumptions about the prevalence and fatality of this contagious disease.

Laplace, the most important statistician in the classical period of statistics, argued in his *Essai philosophique sur les probabilities* for the broad application of the new calculus of probabilities:[17]

> Strictly speaking it may even be said that nearly all our knowledge is problematical; and in the small number of things which we are able to know with certainty, even in the mathematical sciences themselves, the principal means for ascertaining truth—induction and analogy—are based on probabilities; so that the entire system of human knowledge is connected with the theory set forth in this essay. ([1814] 1951, 2)[18]

Laplace considered medicine as a particularly fertile terrain for theories of probability, claiming that the best method of treatment "will manifest itself more and more in the measure that the number [of observations] is increased" (105–6). He approved of Bernoulli's research on smallpox, which justified the use of inoculation on the basis of statistical calculation.

Bernoulli and Laplace's endeavors to apply probabilistic reasoning to medicine are important for the history of statistical epidemiology, and their concerns have a surprising currency today. Of greater clinical relevance, however, is the application of statistics to clinical reasoning by nineteenth-century physicians, notably Philippe Pinel (1745–1826) and Pierre Louis (1787–1872). Between 1809 and 1820, Pinel attempted to apply Laplace's calculus of probabilities in a study of mental-hospital populations.[19] It was Louis, however, who pioneered the numerical method as an important component of clinical reasoning. The two most important opponents of the statistical method in medicine include Xavier Bichat and Claude Bernard (1813–1878). The positions of these three latter individuals, Louis, Bichat, and Bernard, pioneers in the birth of modern medicine, represent positions on the spectrum of opinion regarding statistics and therefore deserve to be examined further.[20]

PIERRE LOUIS

Pierre Louis is remembered for having been an early ardent proponent of statistical medicine as a key element of his *médicine d'observation*.[21] Around

1830 Louis presented a controversial statistical analysis of bloodletting to treat pneumonia, from which he concluded that early bloodletting appears to reduce the duration of disease in patients with pneumonitis, but also may increase the short-term mortality.[22] As a pioneer in the use of statistics in medicine and in his regard for the clinical context, Pierre Louis was an exemplary representative of the statistical conception of health and disease. While for Louis, variability pertaining to individual patients needs to be assessed in terms of statistical data at the population level, the task for the medical empiricist was to observe clinical phenomena at the bedside. As J. Rosser Matthews notes in this regard, "science" only emerged "when these observations were numerically collected and represented in tabular form" (1995, 74). For Louis, mathematics provided a powerful method to combine with empirical observation of individuals rather than as a replacement for clinical experience.

Louis's understanding of the relevance of the clinical context meant a subtle application of statistics to clinical reasoning.[23] In the 1836 preface to the English translation of Louis's *Researches on the Effects of Bloodletting in Some Inflammatory Diseases*, J. Jackson conveniently summarized Louis's method:

> First, we must be careful as to our diagnosis; and second, we must be accurate as to the period of disease; third *we must be minute in noting the particulars*, in which amendment is produced; and fourth, we must be precise in stating the extent and the manner, in which the remedy is employed. (Louis 1836, "Preface," vii; italics mine)

It is evident that Louis conceived a productive tension between the particular nosological data arising in the individual context and statistical data derived at the population level. Anne Fagot-Largeault has stated this well in her study of the causality of death:

> Thus, the causal explanation of Louis oscillates between two poles: on one side, the reconstruction, as detailed as possible, of the "process," or the history, of phenomena; on the other, the comparative evaluation of frequencies. The two are related, because the identification in the individual history of significant events for the explanation of death is done through the occurrences taken into consideration in the type-history by the comparison of cases, and the statistical generalization necessitates the identification of significant events in individual cases. (Fagot-Largeault 1989, 5.4.4; translation mine)

While this tension between clinical variability and statistical frequencies was celebrated by Pierre Louis, it was resisted by Bichat and Bernard.

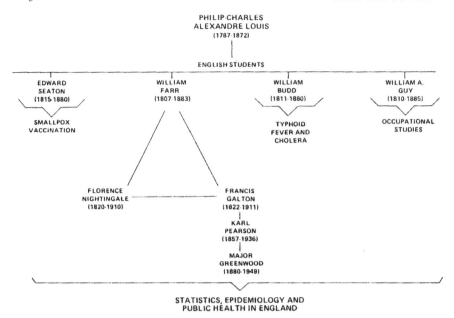

PHILIP-CHARLES
ALEXANDRE LOUIS
(1787-1872)

ENGLISH STUDENTS

| EDWARD SEATON (1815-1880) | WILLIAM FARR (1807-1883) | WILLIAM BUDD (1811-1880) | WILLIAM A. GUY (1810-1885) |

SMALLPOX VACCINATION

TYPHOID FEVER AND CHOLERA

OCCUPATIONAL STUDIES

FLORENCE NIGHTINGALE (1820-1910) ———— FRANCIS GALTON (1822-1911)

KARL PEARSON (1857-1936)

MAJOR GREENWOOD (1880-1949)

STATISTICS, EPIDEMIOLOGY AND
PUBLIC HEALTH IN ENGLAND

FIGURE 20. The influence of Pierre Louis on the development of statistics and epidemiology through some of his students in England. From Lilienfeld (1980, 33). Reproduced by kind permission of Johns Hopkins University Press.

XAVIER BICHAT

Xavier Bichat resisted the application of statistics to medicine in the name of biological variability. Bichat has already been mentioned for his initiation of the anatomo-clinical method. His contribution is most often described in terms of the development of tissular pathology. Bichat was the first to consider the anatomical body according to tissue planes and no longer in terms of spatial distributions. His understanding that particular lesions related to particular tissues resulted in the consequent development of anatomical pathology.[24] In his *Recherches physiologiques sur la vie et la mort* (1800) Bichat put forward two other novel conceptions of biological life for which he is also remembered. Firstly, he defined life as the "totality of those functions that resist death" (1809, vol. 1, art. 1). Secondly, Bichat divided living function into "organic life" centered on the self (e.g., respiration and digestion) and "animal life," where the living organism exists in relation with its external milieu (e.g., sensation and locomotion).[25] Bichat summarized these two conceptions by stating that "the measure of life then, in general, is the difference which exists between the effort of external powers and of internal resistance" (ibid.).

Bichat's opposition to statistics was derived from the theory of organic life associated with his anatomo-pathological research. He believed, like the later founder of positivism, Auguste Comte (1798–1857), that knowledge of primary causes eludes human understanding. In retracing the causes of individual deaths through cadaveric dissection, Bichat was not interested in primary causes, but rather in the impact of external agents in disease processes. He stated, therefore, that we should "observe the phenomena, and analyze the connexions which unite one to the other, without endeavouring to trace them to their first causes" (vol. 1, art. 6).[26] Additionally, Bichat opposed the use of mathematical knowledge to study the human organism on the basis that organic life is not subject to the constancy of physical laws. He wrote that vital functions "defy every calculation, for it would be necessary to have as many different rules as there are different cases" (Bichat 1801, liii; quoted in Hacking 1990, 14). In summary, for Bichat statistics provided a false knowledge of causation of individual function, which is intrinsically variable in nature.

CLAUDE BERNARD

Claude Bernard, the nineteenth-century father of modern physiology, also vehemently opposed the use of statistics in clinical medicine.[27] As an experimental physiologist Bernard's subject matter was vital phenomena, which, Bernard maintained, could only be studied through direct observation and not through the averaging of variety provided by the law of large numbers.[28] "It is easier to count the case for and against than to do a sound experiment," he wrote (Bernard 1947, 74; translation mine); and, "the numerical method, statistics, only leads to conjectures, of probabilities, and does not say anything, does not learn anything about individuals" (1947, 71). Thus, Bernard, satirized the physiologist who attempted to discern the "average European urine" through a collection taken from a railroad station urinal. For Bernard, the statistical method did not render explicit what was too small to observe with the naked eye, but rather caused the "true relations of phenomena" to "disappear in the average" (1927, 135).

Bernard opposed statistical medicine as a strict medical determinist opposed to probabilistic knowledge in medicine, and not from a sense of the inapplicability of mathematics to medicine. As a determinist Bernard believed that "there are no events without causes, and that under the same conditions, the same causes always lead to the same effects" (Fagot-Largeault 1989, 5.3.1). He argued that "the admission of a fact without cause, that is to say indeterminable in the conditions of existence, was neither more nor less than the negation of science" (1865, 1:2; translation mine). Additionally, for Bernard, the scientific method of experimental medicine provided "not only the laws of classification or the species of disease," but also the "mechanistic laws of their evolution with the knowledge of their etiological and curative determinism" (1947, 7; translation mine).

In emphasizing the experimental method as the key to determining specific mechanisms of causation, Bernard was close to the etiological theory of disease developed between 1830 and 1860, which posited that specific diseases require causes that are universal (where in any given disease, the same cause is common in every instance) and necessary (where a disease does not occur in the absence of its cause).[29] The etiological standpoint, requiring necessary and sufficient causation, is best represented by the postulates published in 1884 by the bacteriologist Robert Koch. Koch's postulates have three steps that must be fulfilled in order to prove necessary and sufficient causation. Firstly, the parasite must be present in every case of the disease under appropriate circumstances. Secondly, it should occur in no other diseases as a fortuitous and nonpathogenic parasite. Finally, the parasite must be isolated from the body in pure culture, be repeatedly passed, and induce the disease anew.[30] In the same vein, Bernard argued that physiological medicine is based on necessary and sufficient causation. He argued for the stability of the cause-effect relation in clinical medicine, despite the regular observation by physicians that similar external agents have very diverse effects on individuals.

The true reason for particular reactions are due to what Bernard called from 1851 the "internal milieu."[31] This concept refers to the intermediary between organs and the external milieu and determines the expression of particular diseases. "The medicine of antiquity," Bernard wrote, "was founded on the external milieu; experimental medicine is founded on the internal milieu" (1865, chap. 10). For Bernard, the method of experimental physiology operated at the level of the internal milieu. The importance of this concept was to provide the conceptual structure to support Bernard's belief in scientific determinism and the possibility of individual variation. This is because, as Philippe Huneman has noted, Bernard's concept of the internal milieu is constituted and manifests according to the same physico-chemical laws of all brute bodies, but its intervention produces the appearance that the organism does not obey these laws.[32] As such, the experimental method is the corollary of the principle of determinism: "The scientific law gives the necessary reason of a phenomenon in a precise circumstance and determines what may apply to a case, to an individual given. . . . Scientific laws . . . do not entail exceptions" (Bernard 1865, chap. 6). It is not sufficient to know that in general (in the majority of cases) inoculation protects against smallpox; one must explain why (through which mechanisms) it protects and identify the specific causes (the perturbations) that fail in particular cases. This signifies that medicine may not be satisfied to be free from general laws. The complexity of biological phenomena necessitate that in order to treat a particular malady scientifically it is necessary to enter into a special "etiological determinism," so that what is healing for one patient is toxic for another in apparently similar circumstances (chap. 7; adapted from Fagot-Largeault 1989, 0.2–7; translation mine). While Bernard's experimental physiology could not have been conceived without the earlier work of Bichat, his emphasis on finding direct causation in individuals led him to oppose Bichat's conception of the irregularity of vital phenomena. Bernard, while continuing the tradition of Bichat in his internal milieu, could not reconcile the two traditions issuing from Bichat—that of experimental physiology with anatomo-clinical medicine.[33]

Causality

The three positions regarding statistics in clinical medicine, articulated by Louis, Bichat, and Bernard, represent three fundamental positions on a spectrum of possibility. Thus, Louis initiated the method of clinical reasoning based on the calculus of probabilities; Bichat argued that vital phenomena are necessarily invariable and resistant to absolute mathematical comprehension; and Bernard posited an experimental determinism, rejecting statistics and arguing that the internal milieu provides the structure to reconcile general laws with individual biological irregularity. The tension among these three models can be framed in the language of causality. Bichat represents a positivism willfully ignorant of primary causes relating to the variability of vital function. On either side of him one finds a model of clinical reasoning based on an inductive (Bernard) or probabilistic (Louis) structure of causality. According to this general framework, etiological causation may be linked with models of inductive reasoning, whereas epidemiological reasoning is assessed in terms of strength of association described by Pearson's indices of correlation.

While it is tempting to analyze the tension between statistics and clinical reasoning in terms of the relation between inductive versus probabilistic theories of causality, or a determinist versus a probabilistic conception of reality, a review of these forms of causal reasoning in medicine yields a more complicated picture. As Fagot-Largeault points out, the development of a calculus of probabilities was chronologically simultaneous with the development of the anatomo-clinical method. She notes, furthermore, that the simultaneous development of these two investigative approaches of causality is not unrelated. The anatomo-clinical method and epidemiological statistics are linked in medicine's move away from a mechanistic emphasis on refined causal distinctions to precise etiological diagnostics, in which causal distinctions are nevertheless fluid.[34]

Bichat initiated this phenomenon in medical epistemology by tracing causative factors leading to the deaths of individuals, without presuming to understand the actual direct mechanism involved. Thus, in discussing how the injection of air into veins results in death, Bichat claims that "whatever may be the mode by which it destroys life, the air is certainly mortal upon getting to the brain, and that is the essential point. The manner is unimportant to our considerations, the fact alone interests us" (1809, Art. 2, sec. 2). Bichat was interested in establishing here the point of impact of the external causal agent—in this case the air injected into the circulatory system, resulting in cerebral death.[35] Bichat thereby distinguishes the primary cause of brain death from the secondary indirect effect of the intermediary organ (the lung) resulting in death of the heart (ibid.). Bichat's attempt to establish direct and indirect causal pathways for the interruption of the functions of "animal life" (psychosensorial functions) contrasts with the interruption of "organic life," which is not directly effected by cerebral death. This distinction between organic and animal life is stated clearly toward the end of Bichat's *Physiological Researches*:

> Upon calling to mind in this place the division of the organs into two great classes, namely, into those of animal, and into those of organic life, it will be seen at once that the functions of the organs of the first class must be interrupted the very moment the brain dies. Indeed, all these functions either directly or indirectly have their seat in this organ. Those which only indirectly belong to it, are the sensations, locomotion and voice, functions which are executed by other organs, it is true, but which, having their centre in the cephalic mass, cannot continue to act after the latter has ceased. On the other hand, whatever, in animal life, depends immediately upon the brain, as imagination, memory judgment, etc. can evidently never be exercised but when this organ is in activity. The great difficulty therefore rests upon the functions of organic life. (Art. 12)

In section 2 of Article 12, Bichat summarizes this essential duality within life-processes, stating that "since organic life does not immediately cease by the cessation of cerebral action, there must therefore be some intermediate agents which by their death produce this cessation."

Because of the impossibility of establishing primary causation regarding organic life, it was no problematic, but rather necessary, for Bichat's neovitalistic theory and those medical epistemological theories consequent to it to incorporate a multifactorial explanation of causality. This tendency to combine etiological and probabilistic explanations of causation of death continues up to the present. Fagot-Largeault's (1989) important study of causal reasoning related to death demonstrates convincingly that physicians from the nineteenth century to the present combined inductive and probabilistic reasoning without any real sense of logical contradiction. The twentieth century was no better than the nineteenth, she concludes, in requiring a strict diagnostic etiology of death, formulating it in a causal vocabulary that was "eclectic, lax, and sometimes with audacious intrepidity [5.2.0]. . . . In practice, physicians admitted without much difficulty that the same cause may lead to different effects and that one effect may result from different causes" (5.3.2; translation mine).

This laxness in diagnostic etiology applies not only to death certification but also to theories of disease. As they have evolved away from the bacterial model, clinical models have incorporated both etiological and probabilistic forms of reasoning. As Alfred S. Evans has emphasized, despite Koch's criteria becoming the touchstone for disease causation, their nonfulfillment was not intended by Koch to exclude the possibility of a causal relationship.[36] Moreover, other types of disease processes, such as viruses, immunology, cancer, and chronic disease, have required shifts away from rigid etiological principles of causation.

The viral example demonstrates this quite clearly. The presence of many viruses, even in healthy people, made problematic the requirement for the presence of an infective agent as the sole basis for etiology. It became evident with time that the viral agent alone was a necessary but not sufficient factor required to cause most diseases. Faced with this dilution of direct causation, Robert Huebner introduced epidemiologic principles by longitudinal and cross-sectional studies as an element of proof in causation.[37] Thus, causality in viral illnesses came to be assessed both through etiological criteria of direct causation as well as probabilistic criteria of strength of association. Karl Pearson's strength of association or correlation, derived from Francis Galton, is the first and probably most important of the criteria for epidemiological causality, which was notably presented in a celebrated paper by Bradford Hill in 1965.[38]

One cannot disassociate pathological and epidemiological models of causation from models of clinical reasoning concerning individuals. Rather than being mutually exclusive, etiological and probabilistic theories of causality were able to combine with each other, even though logically contradictory, because of the particularity of clinical medicine as practical knowledge of the individual. Thus, Canguilhem in a discussion about epistemology of medicine claims that "calculated uncertainty, it turned out, is not incompatible with etiological hypotheses and rational diagnosis based on data gathered with the aid of suitable instruments" (2000, 154). As he makes clear, it is the structure of individuality, the perennial concern of medical practice that requires its own scientific methodology:

> Why should it [medicine] feel the need for a consecration of its status within the scientific community? Might it be that medicine has preserved from its origins a sense of the uniqueness of its purpose, so that it is a matter of some interest to determine whether that sense is a tenuous survival or an essential vocation? To put it in somewhat different terms, are what used to be acts of diagnosis, decision and treatment about to become ancillary to some computerized medical program? If medicine cannot shirk the duty to assist individual human beings whose lives are in danger, even if that means violating the requirements of the rational, critical pursuit of knowledge, can it claim to be called a science? (154–55)[39]

Michel Foucault, following on from Canguilhem, states that Bichat and his successors were liberated from the causal problematic, that is, the limitation of etiological reasoning.[40] Foucault's comment about Bichat is part of his more general analysis of the influence of modern pathology on clinical medicine. For Foucault, the importance of Bichat's anatomo-pathological correlate was to situate the disciplinary construction of individuality in the concrete material of human bodies. Referring to Bichat's causal inquiries into the processes of death, Foucault writes:

> This structure, in which space, language, and death are articulated—what is known, in fact, as the anatomo-clinical method—constitutes the historical condition of a medicine that is given and accepted as positive. . . . It is when death became the concrete a priori of medical experience that death could detach itself from counter-nature and become embodied in the living bodies of individuals. (1973, 196)

These comments suggest that Bichat's incorporation of death into his analysis of the living organism both gave rise to a science of the individual and liberated it from the determinism of natural processes.[41]

This analysis explains why both Bernard and Bichat opposed statistics on the basis of biological variability. Both Bichat's concept of organic life and Bernard's concept of the internal milieu p 'sent living structures that resist the traditional scientific paradigms upon w ich mathematical statistics is founded. Feinst in, too, alludes to this comple ity of the organic realm in

his claim that the clinical context presents an exponentially complicated terrain resistant to the ready incorporation of statistics. According to Feinstein
the problem with contemporary medical epistemology arises from the fact
that the pathological correlate developed by Rudolph Virchow replaced the
temporal correlate of the clinic with the pathological correlate. Thus, clinical
reasoning came to be modeled on processes of death, rather than on life. For
Feinstein, the unthinking use of statistics in clinical reasoning is associated
with this epistemological failure resulting from the pathological correlate,
whereas clinical intuition, because of its connection with the individuality of
both clinician and patient, forms part of the epistemological solution provided by the temporal correlate.

Statistics and the Individual

What then does happen to the individual when the statistical method is applied to clinical reasoning? While Bradford Hill avoided philosophical speculation in his article about causality in epidemiology, one finds an initial attempt to address the question of the individual in statistics by Mervyn Susser
in his analysis of the foundations of causal reasoning in epidemiology. Susser
writes:

> The level of organization of populations and societies introduces a set of vari-
> ables over and above those germane to individuals. . . . The spectrum to be
> comprehended starts with the antecedent factors that cause disease, moves to
> the precursors that may enable us to predict and prevent disease, and passes
> through the full span of clinical manifestations, course, and eventual out-
> come. (1973, 7)

Susser readily acknowledges the difference between the individual and the
group in epidemiological reasoning about causation. Epidemiological variables associated with disease causation occur at a level different from the
individual. This is most evident from the ecological fallacy, the error that
results from confusing inferences at the individual and group level:

> The fallacy is to infer that a *correlation* [italics mine] between variables de-
> rived from the attributes of ecological units, that is data grouped in social or
> other aggregates, will also hold between variables derived from the attributes
> of individual units, such as persons. An association at one level may disappear
> at another, or it may even be reversed. . . . The statistical source of the dispari-
> ties is not the same in all instances, for the shift from one level to another may
> conceal linking variables of different types. (60)

The ecological fallacy consists of both the aggregative and atomistic fallacy. The former associates attributes of groups with individuals, whereas the latter makes inferences about ecological relationships from observations of individuals (59).[42] This association of statistics with the abstraction of the individual to the average, central to epidemiological reasoning, forms the basis of the difficulty in applying statistics to clinical reasoning.

How does this abstraction of the individual in statistics occur? While statistical reasoning is valuable in evaluating disease causation that cannot be determined at the individual level—for example, the correlation of smoking with lung cancer—this causation is not simply "over and above those germane to individuals," but occurs via these individuals. In other words, the statistical individual is an average of individuals who become subsumed by the group. Mary Poovey has argued, in consequence, that "the application of mathematical probability to human behavior requires a conceptual move from the empirically observable individual to an abstracted concept like Quetelet's average man or William Farr's 'human aggregate'" (1994, 414).[43] According to Poovey this type of abstraction of human nature by statistical thinking contains a double paradox, in that statistics deduces general laws through a "frightful empiricism." In the process, the individual human being "who gathers statistical data, forms the basis of statistical representation, and presumably constitutes the beneficiary of statistical knowledge, is obliterated by the numerical average or aggregate that replaces him" (ibid.).[44]

Poovey's critique of the statistical individual can be deepened at one level and challenged at another. It can be extended by incorporating the structure of nosology and challenged by examining the process through which statistics eliminates individuality. Besides the abstraction of the individual in statistics, nosology, or the classification of specific disease entities, presents an additional structure of abstraction that is unique to the epistemological structure of medical diagnostics.

The more precise use of analogy, associated with the emergence of critical medicine, allowed for the emergence of nosology as the second great seventeenth-century medical innovation. Thomas Sydenham is regarded as the founder of nosology.[45] Sydenham insisted that particular diseases were specific and not just the "confused and irregular operations of disordered and dehabilitated nature" (Faber 1923, 15). Each disease according to Sydenham has its own "natural history" that can be observed clinically in individual patients (ibid.). His categorization of disease species was akin to that "which we see exhibited by botanists in their description of plants" (ibid.). King argues that the purpose of nosology was to bring order and precision into the study of medicine and to "exhibit the deeper relationships and inner nature of diseases states' by grouping together those states that had some essential similarity" (1958, 204). Nosology, thus characterized, was an essential element in the emergence of modern medicine in the eighteenth century. It could only have occurred, however, once the usage of analogy had been pruned to concur with the data of observation.

Yet nosology, akin to statistics, eliminates the individual. This is because the emergence of a universal categorization of disease species renders the individual less important in the diagnosis and treatment of disease. This characteristic of seventeenth-century nosology in reducing the importance of the individual subjective in medicine has not disappeared but has become reinforced through the technical and scientific success of twentieth-century medicine.

Nosology is not limited to clinical medicine but is found in epidemiology, too. As with its clinical counterpart, the success of statistical epidemiology in determining disease causation is associated with the development of a statistical nosology or nosometry. This latter term was coined by William Farr (1897–1883), who realized that the ability to develop epidemiological data on particular diseases required the creation of a statistical nosology comparable to the nosology of disease in particular patients.

When individual nosology is transcribed onto a statistical nosology, the problem of abstracting the individual into a general law is encountered doubly, even exponentially. This is because the direct encounter with individual patients that restricts the abstraction that otherwise occurs through clinical reasoning is no longer present in statistical reasoning. In statistics, therefore, the individual is abstracted both through the statistical method and through statistical nosology or nosometry.

Despite this double abstraction of the individual through statistics and nosometry, it would be a mistake to conclude that the individual is completely eliminated. Rather, the individual or a number of individuals becomes hypostatized at the group or the population level. If the individual is totally eliminated, there can be no relation at all between what happens at the individual and the group level. More significantly, the hypostasis of an anthropomorphic essence through statistics establishes the relation between intuitive and statistical inferential processes. Galton's work on heredity analyzed in chapter 5 indicates how this corporeal substance became hypostatized into the abstract computations of statistical reasoning. The consequence of this claim is that there is, as with Aristotelian *phronesis*, an essentially anthropomorphic structure to statistical reasoning, particularly in its application to clinical reasoning.

Conclusion

Based on this analysis it is possible to answer the question posed at the beginning of this chapter about what the philosophical significance of modeling clinical reasoning on statistics is. The attempt to model clinical reasoning on statistics is significant in the manner in which statistical correlation transmutes an individual essence taken from the inductive analogy into a statistical association. This process allows for an apparent liberation from inductive causation as well as from the anthropomorphic substrate upon which statistical reasoning is based. My reading suggests, however, that clinical reasoning presents a more nuanced epistemological framework that allows the incorporation of both etiological and probabilistic theories of disease. Also, the relation between intuition and statistics is not one of inherent opposition, but it is a living tension brought together by their common foundation in the living tissue of the individual.

Abduction: The Intuitive Support of Clinical Induction

In this analysis of clinical reasoning I have traced the tension between the two realms of statistical mathematics and human clinical experience back to Francis Galton's important statistical discovery of correlation. Galton's law of correlation was crucial in the transmission of statistics to the social and biological sciences, culminating in the form of the randomized controlled trial. This discovery of correlation has also led to the dichotomy between intuitive and statistical reasoning, a consequence of which is to relegate intuition to a form of irrationalism. In an 1872 article entitled "Statistical Inquiries into the Efficacy of Prayer," Galton drew the association between intuition and irrationalism, arguing that prayer as an intuitive religious belief is indistinguishable from irrational categories, such as "auguries," "ecclesiastical blessings," "cursings," and "demoniacal possession," the inefficacy of which is demonstrated by statistical tests. Curiously, despite this critique of religious intuition, it is possible to detect a moment of intuitive reasoning in Galton's own scientific method, or at least an admission of a moment of intuitive clarity in his scientific reflection. In his personal memoirs Galton famously described an epiphanic moment regarding the idea of a statistical scale, falsely ascribed by Pearson to Galton's discovery of correlation:[1]

> As these lines are being written, the circumstances under which I first clearly grasped the important generalisation that the laws of Heredity were solely concerned with deviations expressed in statistical units, are vividly recalled to my memory. It was in the grounds of Naworth Castle, where an invitation had been given to ramble freely. A temporary shower drove me to seek refuge in a reddish recess in the rock by the side of the pathway. There the idea flashed across me, and I forgot everything else for a moment in my great delight. (1908, 300)

While probably not referring to the moment of Galton's discovery of correlation in the late fall of 1888, this passage is still significant for the strength of its autobiographical account of an intuitive process associated with Galton's decades-long research and reflection into the laws of heredity, from which the discovery of correlation did develop.

The contrast between Galton's critique of religious intuition as soothsaying and his own use of creative intuition in scientific reasoning nicely crystallizes the tension that animates debates about the human faculty's ability to make sense of the external world. What faculty of reason enables us to expand our knowledge to include external facts? In a word, this is the philosophical problem of induction. As described in the previous chapter, Karl Pearson believed that Galton's discovery of correlation signaled the end of inductive causation and provided the means of diminishing contingent uncertainty. The problem of induction was posed most famously and forcibly by the Scottish Enlightenment philosopher David Hume in both his *Treatise of Human Nature* (1739) and *An Enquiry into Human Understanding* (1748). In this latter work, an abridged version of the *Treatise*, Hume noted that deductive inferences do not obtain from the observed to as yet unobserved phenomena: "That there are no demonstrative arguments in this case seems evident; since it implies no contradiction that the course of nature may change" (1963, 35). The radical consequence of Hume's simple observation is that the use of inductive reasoning to predict future events based on the observation of previous events has no inferential basis. The inductive foundations of scientific reasoning are fundamentally placed in question by this observation. In his analysis in *Hume's Problem*, Colin Howson argues that the devastating nature of Hume's argument lies in his further claim that even probable inferences cannot be justified without circularity.[2] Probabilistic inferences are therefore included in Hume's circularity thesis that "all inferences from experience suppose, as their foundation, that the future will resemble the past" (Hume 1962, sec. 37; Howson 2000, 11).

The problem of induction then is the problem about the justification of induction, which in turn is a problem about the nature of human rationality. Hence, Peter Strawson justifies induction by considering it an inalienable part of human cognition.[3] Induction and intuition are analogous in that both are justified through an appeal to circularity. It is standard justificatory practice to use intuitions evidentially.[4] Similarly, Rudolf Carnap, who espouses a probabilistic view of induction, argues that it is indispensable to defend inductive reasoning through an appeal to inductive reasoning, or what he calls "inductive intuition":

But I believe all procedures of self-clarification, of making clear to ourselves what it is we have in mind, are in a way circular. We clarify *B* through *A*, and then we turn around and explain *A* with the help of *B*. I think we cannot do without it. If a person were able to distinguish valid from invalid steps in inductive reasoning, even in the simplest cases, in other words, if he were inductively blind, then it would be hopeless to try and convince him of anything in inductive logic. In order to learn inductive reasoning, we must have what I call the ability of *inductive intuition*. (1968, 265)

The intuitive support of induction was posited earlier by another Victorian gentleman, William Whewell (1794–1866), as a central component of his philosophy of the inductive sciences.[5] For Whewell inductive truth occurs via intuition when the individual scientist becomes attuned to the underling laws within the cosmos. Induction serves as the mediating link between the realms of personal experience and rational thoughts, which Whewell referred respectively to as "Sense" and "Reason" (1840, 6).[6] The intuitive support for induction is encapsulated in Whewell's notion of consilience.[7] In *The Philosophy of the Inductive Sciences* Whewell argues that "the Consilience of Inductions takes place when an Induction obtained from one class of facts, coincides with an Induction, obtained from another different class" (Whewell 1847, 469). "Consilience," then, is a term that encapsulates the notion that in order to be justified, induction requires an added intuitive assumption.[8] Intuition according to the model of consilience enables the rationality of inductive inference.

Because of its circularity, intuition, at least for its antagonists, possesses an element of irrationality. At best this is a philosophical problem of foundationalism, that is, the thesis that the justification of a proposition depends on nothing other than itself.[9] At worst this is an issue of the irrationality of human reasoning. Consider the recent adaptation of consilience by the sociobiologist E. O. Wilson. Borrowing the term from Whewell, Wilson refers to consilience as the synthetic tie between different kinds of knowledge. Consilience is the "'jumping together' of knowledge by the linking of facts and fact-based theory across disciplines to create a common groundwork of explanation" (1998, 8). For Wilson, consilience encompasses a religious sentiment in being desirous of explaining our significance in the universe. Unlike religion, however, consilience relies only on human understanding, and particularly on science, to achieve this metaphysical end. In order to attain this scientism, Wilson strips consilience of its purported irrational content. His concept of consilience, therefore, ties different sciences together, yet without the intuitive support that girds Whewell's theory of the inductive sciences. In

this regard, Wilson's conception of consilience is continuous with his reduc-
tionist thesis in his main discipline, sociobiology, where he argues that social
norms are to be completely explained by biological structures.[10]

This reductionism is further evident in the use Wilson makes of the imagery of Ariadne's thread derived from the Cretan myth of Theseus and the
Minotaur. In order to add literary weight to his argument about consilience,
Wilson refers to the mythic imagery of Ariadne's thread as the tie that binds
the sciences with the humanities. Intuition, as an element of human rationality that is not fully exposed to the light of explicit reason, is often associated
with the image of Ariadne's thread.[11] We pick up the story, as told by the
Victorian storyteller Charles Kingsley, when Theseus, armed with a sword
and a "clue of thread" provided by Ariadne, is led into the labyrinth:

> And he went down into that doleful gulf, through winding paths among the
> rocks, under caverns, and arches, and galleries, and over heaps of fallen stone.
> And he turned on the left hand, and on the right hand, and went up and
> down, till his head was dizzy; but all the while he held his clue. For when he
> went in he had fastened it to a stone, and left it to unroll out of his hand as
> he went on; and it lasted him till he met the Minotaur, in a narrow chasm be-
> tween black cliffs. And when he saw him he stopped awhile, for he had never
> seen so strange a beast. His body was a man's; but his head was the head of
> a bull, and his teeth were the teeth of a lion, and with them he tore his prey.
> And when he saw Theseus he roared, and he put his head down, and rushed
> right at him. (1902, 211)

The outcome of the story is well-known:

> Like a matador goading a bull Theseus stabbed the monster and followed him
> at full speed, holding the clue of thread in his left hand. Then on, through
> cavern after cavern, under dark ribs of sounding stone, and up rough glens
> and torrent-beds, among the sunless roots of Ida, and to the edge of the eter-
> nal snow went they, the hunter and the hunted, while the hills bellowed to the
> monster's bellow. (211–12)

Because of its subterranean associations Ariadne's thread has become symbolic of an intuitive ability, akin to a sixth sense, more commonly ascribed to
feminine cognition. The Minotaur, too, still fascinates in its allusion to the
animal underbelly of human cognition. However, Wilson's scientific allusion
to Ariadne's thread strips this literary image of much of its mythic content.[12]
Wilson explains that the labyrinth is a "fitting image of the uncharted material world in which humanity was born and which it forever struggles to understand" (1998, 73). Consilience is the "Ariadne's thread needed to traverse

it;" while the Minotaur is "our own dangerous irrationality" (ibid.). Physics stands "near the entrance of the labyrinth of empirical knowledge"; and "in the deep interior is a nebula of pathways through the social sciences, humanities, art and religion." The thread of consilience allows one to follow any pathway quickly in reverse, "back through the behavioral sciences to biology, chemistry, and finally physics" (ibid.).

Wilson's explanation provides a sanitized reading of the mythic imagery of Ariadne's thread, according to which human irrationality, represented by the Minotaur, may be swept away by the rational force of science. In his reductionism Wilson breaks the association of Ariadne's thread with intuition. His account of the myth of the Minotaur and Ariadne's thread in relation to science is as arid as his account of consilience, stripped as it is of its intuitive foundations, and instead grounded on a mixture of reductionism and syncretism. In freeing Ariadne's thread from its mythopoietic substrate, Wilson also removes precisely that which makes it valuable for the scientific imagination, that is, the intuitive foundations of inferential reasoning. In this manner Wilson perpetuates the false dichotomy between intuition and the inductive or probabilistic sciences that is also discernible in Galton's conception of statistical correlation.

What does this introductory review of the relation between intuition and induction signify for the larger analysis of clinical reasoning? I have argued throughout this book that clinical experience rooted in the face-to-face encounter presents an ethical structure that grounds medical epistemology. The relation between intuition and induction also needs to be analyzed in the light of the moral image of the individual human face. In the remainder of this chapter I shall follow this thread in analyzing the role of inductive reasoning in two influential twentieth-century philosophers of science, Hans Reichenbach and Charles Sanders Peirce. In his quest to resolve the scientific problem of induction, Reichenbach provides an illuminating frequentist theory relating statistical and inductive reasoning, but which is demonstrably flawed in its application to the clinical context. Peirce's model of abductive reasoning is particularly instructive in relating statistical facts to epistemological norms. Peirce's theory of abduction has particular relevance in explaining the underlying mechanism of clinical equipoise, a key concept in clinical research ethics. Additionally, the discussion of Peirce unites many of the aspects of clinical reasoning examined throughout this book, such as *phronesis*, physiognomy, and intuition. Hence, this discussion of Peirce provides a useful conclusion to this book-length analysis of the epistemological, ontological, and ethical dimensions of clinical reasoning.

Hans Reichenbach (1891–1953)

The logical empiricist philosopher Hans Reichenbach's position on induction in science is laid out in his 1938 book *Experience and Prediction*,[13] which deals with the problem of how we can build knowledge from what we know ("experience") to what we do not know ("prediction").[14] This project of Reichenbach's was meant to evade the Kantian a priori. He did not think that we could have absolute certainty from a priori intuitions of the type formulated by Immanuel Kant. For Kant, a priori intuitions were primarily of space and time, but also of causality, which Reichenbach contested. Like Hume, Reichenbach was skeptical of the validity of induction. He summarized Hume's problem with induction by claiming that

1 We have no logical demonstration for the validity of inductive inference.
2 There is no demonstration a posteriori for the inductive inference; any such demonstration would presuppose the very principle which it is to demonstrate. (Reichenbach, 1938a, 342)

Despite these insurmountable problems, Reichenbach was reluctant to dispense with induction, because he thought that inductive reasoning was necessary for human action. The central importance Reichenbach accorded induction in scientific reasoning is clear from the following two statements of his quoted by Popper, and published in 1930 in the Vienna Circle's journal *Erkenntnis*:

> This principle determines the truth of scientific theories. To eliminate it from science would mean nothing less than to deprive science of the power to decide the truth or falsity of its theories. Without it, clearly, science would no longer have the right to distinguish its theories from the fanciful and arbitrary creations of the poet's mind. (Popper [1939] 1959, 28–29)

And,

> the principle of induction is unreservedly accepted by the whole of science and . . . no man can seriously doubt the principle in everyday life either. (Ibid.)[15]

Reichenbach's approach to the question of induction is in line with his approach to philosophical questions more generally, which as Alberto Coffa (1991) notes was inspired by the "postulate of utilizability." This refers to Reichenbach's proposition that the most productive method in analyzing a particular concept is to give an account of what would in actual practice make this notion seem rational and justified.[16] Reichenbach argued that induction does not demonstrate direct causation, but is rather probabilistic in nature. As such, induction is a form of "probabilistic empiricism" (1938a, viii). In light of this probabilistic reconceptualization of induction, Reichenbach wrote that the Humean justification of induction should not be contested because "*we do not know whether we shall have success,*" but rather that "a justification of induction could not be given if *we knew that we should have no success*" (362). In other words, a modified form of induction based on probabilism should be retained, because we might have success in making predictions, and have had success in previous predictions.

Reichenbach called his probabilistic approach the pragmatic justification of induction. Accordingly, not only induction, but also probabilism is justified on a pragmatic basis and is an essential component of everyday reasoning. Thus, Reichenbach states that "*the meaning of probability statements is to be determined in such a way that our behavior in utilizing them for action can be justified*" (309). Similarly, in a 1931 paper entitled "The Problem of Causality in Physics,"[17] Reichenbach claimed that it is impossible to disabuse ourselves of the daily conviction that reinforces the justification of probability predictions as a fundamental fact of human cognition. Induction is justified through this concept of probabilism, because it provides the best method to limit the relative frequency in probability statements.[18]

Another ambition of Reichenbach's inductive-probabilistic model was to take account of the process of scientific discovery, including creative intuitions. A central feature of Reichenbach's conception of the process of scientific discovery is its lack of any anthropomorphism, that is, the modeling of scientific conceptions on human features. While Reichenbach admits that scientific knowledge arises through testing knowledge obtained through commonsense reasoning, the result of this testing establishes a break between common sense and scientific knowledge. For example, Reichenbach notes in his analysis of time that the importance of the physics of Galileo and Newton was to reveal that many more events could be predicted than are foreseeable to commonsense reasoning.[19] This critique of commonsense reasoning is associated with the distinction Reichenbach makes between the context of discovery and the context of justification, arguing that the analysis of science is not directed toward actual thinking processes but toward the rational reconstruction of knowledge. Reichenbach relegated scientific genius to an absolutely unknowable realm, writing that "the obscurity of the birth of great ideas will never be satisfactorily cleared up by psychological investigation" (1938a, 381). For Reichenbach the characteristic mark of an idea of genius is to be "unjustifiable a priori," but to be justified later through the success of its predictions. There is a tension between Reichenbach's acknowledgment of the existence of an a priori intuition and his reluctance to justify its role as evidentiary support for inductive-probabilistic inferences. Reichenbach's concern was to justify inductive reasoning in the face of an apparent a priori intuition. Because of the perceived difference between the context of discovery that might entail intuition and the context of justification entailing induction, Reichenbach did not think that the fact of genius presented an obstacle to his justification of induction. Moreover, Reichenbach conceived that induction itself was the essential component of scientific discovery. Referring again to the scientific genius, Reichenbach states:

> What makes the greatness of his work is that he sees the inductive relations between different elements in the system of knowledge where other people did not see them; but it is not true that he predicts phenomena which have no inductive relations at all to known facts. Scientific genius does not manifest itself in contemptuously neglecting inductive methods; on the contrary, it shows its supremacy over inferior ways of thought by better handling, by more cleverly using the methods of induction, which always will remain the genuine methods of scientific discovery. (382–83)

This statement is important for the place that induction has in associating data in the cosmos to that previously held by intuition. Reichenbach accordingly strips scientific knowledge of its anthropomorphism associated with intuition and replaces it with induction.[20] This conceptual move puts forward inductive-probabilistic inference as its own support, in the place of intuitive support for induction. However, the problems associated with Reichenbach's elimination of the intuitive support for induction becomes obvious in the clinical context.

The relation between intuition and induction in Reichenbach's inductive-probabilistic model whereby scientific inference is stripped of its possible anthropomorphic features reoccurs in Reichenbach's conception of the application of statistical probability to clinical reasoning. Reichenbach's conception of inductive probabilism espouses a frequency understanding of probability, defined as the degree of probability determined from the frequency of observations in a series of events. As Reichenbach notes, this interpretation presupposes that the individual event is not described as an individual happening, but as a member of a class: The "repetition of the event means its inclusion with a class of similar events" (1938a, 307). Medicine is exemplary for Reichenbach in providing a context where it is unnecessary to introduce a "single-case meaning" of probability statements. As an example Reichenbach refers to the physician prognosticating the mortality outcome for a certain case of tuberculosis. This instance of individual reasoning is not an isolated individual case, but is rather the "frequency of death in the class of similar cases which is meant by the degree of probability occurring in the state-ment" (308). A "class meaning" is sufficient, because "it suffices to justify the application of probability statements to actions concerned with single events" (312). While class events are significant at a population level for epidemiol-ogy, clinical reasoning relies on clinical intuition to make sense of soft data pertaining to individuals. Clinical reasoning requires the intuitive support of probabilistic induction. However, because it subsumes individual events into class events Reichenbach's frequentist inductive-probabilistic model fails to take adequate account of the individual.

The implications of Reichenbach's inductive-probabilistic model for clini-cal reasoning have been drawn in an influential paper by Kurt Lewin—widely recognized as the founder of social psychology—published in the journal of the logical empiricist movement *Erkenntnis* in 1931.[21] In this paper extending Reichenbach's insights Lewin compared Aristotelian and Galileian modes of thought in the contemporary psychology of his time, and argued that mod-ern logic accounts for individual variation better than Aristotle's philosophy of practical reasoning. This is because, as Lewin notes, Aristotelian phys-ics is replete with concepts that would today be considered valuative. Yet, like Reichenbach, Lewin opposed anthropomorphism in science, and con-sequently questioned the reliance on Aristotelian reasoning in psychology for its inexactitude. In particular Lewin argued that Aristotle's conception of lawfulness and chance in his prevents the model of Aristotelian reasoning from being able to take account of individual variation:

> For Aristotle those things are lawful, conceptually intelligible, which occur *without exception*. Also, and this he emphasizes particularly, those are lawful which occur *frequently*. Excluded from the class of the conceptually intelli-gible as mere chance are those things which occur only *once*, individual events as such. Actually since the behavior of a thing is determined by its essential nature, and this essential nature is exactly the abstractly defined class (i.e., the sum total of the common characteristics of a whole group of objects), it follows that each event, as a particular event, is chance, undetermined. For in these Aristotelian classes individual differences disappear. (1935, 5)

For Lewin, Aristotle's concept of lawfulness has a quasi-statistical char-acter. Lawfulness is equivalent to extreme regularity, as well as the highest degree of generality. As such, Lewin derides Aristotelian empiricism for excluding individual events from scientific rationality. In contrast, Lewin argues that Galileian physics "tried to characterize the individuality of the total situation concerned as concretely and accurately as possible" (30). It achieves this by focusing on the dynamics of a process, dependent not only on the inner force of an object, as characteristic of Aristotelian teleology, but primarily on the relation of forces between the object of focus and its external situation. According to this understanding there is no opposition between the general validity of a scientific law and the specifics of individual cases. Instead of determining the "abstract average of as many historically given cases as possible," scientists should first focus on "those situations in which the determinative factors of the total dynamic event are most clearly, distinctly and purely to be discerned" (31). Paradoxically, scientific laws for the new physics refer only to cases "that are never realized, or only approximately realized, in the actual course of events" (12). It is only through experimentation, that is, under artificially constructed conditions in which cases occur, that approximate the event with which the particular scientific or psychological law is concerned.

Lewin's analysis, contrasting between algorithmic knowledge and statistical probabilism in terms of Aristotelian and Galileian conceptions, highlights implicit conceptual elements of Reichenbach's inductive-probabilistic model in relation to clinical reasoning. However, there are a number of important differences between my own and Lewin's analysis of Aristotle for clinical reasoning. Firstly, Lewin errs in associating Aristotelian reasoning with statistics, rather than probabilism, since the former is a modern discipline developed for purposes of social control.[22] More importantly, while Lewin's critique of Aristotle might be insightful in terms of Aristotle's conception of scientific reasoning, or *epistemé*, it does not apply to Aristotelian practical wisdom, or *phronesis*, which is preeminently concerned with individual variation. As detailed in chapter 4, it is precisely the use of intuition, or *nous*, in Aristotle's conception of *phronesis* that makes it valuable as a model for clinical reasoning. In contrast, Reichenbach's frequentist model of probabilistic induction, upon which Lewin's critique is based, fails to take adequate account of the individual variation, and particularly in the clinical context.

C. S. Peirce (1839–1914)

The key clinical-ethical question of relating a single event concerning an individual to a statistical series of events, addressed but not resolved in Reichenbach's attempt to solve the problem of induction, finds a novel formulation in the philosophy of the American pragmatist philosopher C. S. Peirce. Peirce is celebrated as being an early proponent of a totally random or indeterministic universe. His importance for this discussion on induction and clinical reasoning derives, however, from the related model of abductive reasoning, which for Peirce provides the only form of logical and probabilistic reasoning that can make sense of our chaotic cosmos. Peirce's theory of abduction combines intuition and induction in a manner that is most promising in resolving the problem of probabilistic induction regarding individuals in the clinical context.

Abduction, which Peirce refers to at different times as hypothesis, hypothetic inference, retroduction, or presumption, is concerned with the type of reasoning that starts from hypotheses and moves toward facts.[23] In originating from a creative hypothesis, abduction provides another form of human reasoning besides the traditional inferential processes of induction and deduction. The different logical structures associated with induction, deduction, and abduction are illustrated in Peirce's well-known syllogistic schema:

> Deduction: Rule—All the beans from this bag are white.
> Case—These beans are from this bag.
> Hence, Result—These beans are white.
> Induction: Case—These beans are from this bag.
> Result—These beans are white.
> Hence, Rule—All the beans from this bag are white.
> Abduction: Rule—All the beans from this bag are white.
> Result—These beans are white.
> Hence, Case—These beans are from this bag. (1960 2.623)

Abduction starts from a particular fact, though it is motivated by the feeling that the surprising fact requires a theory to explain it. Induction, on the other hand, starts with a hypothesis, and then searches for the facts to support this theory. In abduction the consideration of the facts suggests the hypothesis. In induction the study of the hypothesis suggests the experiments which bring to light the very facts to which the hypothesis had pointed (Peirce 1960, 7.218). Deduction simply draws an internal logical conclusion from the facts at hand.

Two important points result from this theory of abduction. Firstly, abduction does not conflict with induction; rather they are parallel and complementary processes of logical reasoning. Abduction is essential because it generates imaginative hypotheses that require verification at a factual level by induction. Secondly, both induction and abduction are notable in being fundamentally probabilistic. The probabilistic nature of logical reasoning is implicitly suggested by Peirce's example of drawing beans from a bag, the favored example in the classical era of probability. Peirce explicitly connected inductive with statistical reasoning, defining induction as "an argument which assumes that the whole collection of which a number of instances have been taken at random, has all the common characters of those instances"

(2.515). Peirce understood inductive inferences as a kind of statistical argument in which inductive inferences in the long run generally afford correct conclusions from the premises (Fann 1970). Induction works "by taking the conclusion so reached as major premise of a syllogism," together with "the proposition stating that such and such objects are taken from the class in question as the minor premise." In consequence, the "other premise of the induction will follow from them deductively" (Peirce 1960, 5.274). Abduction, in its relation to induction, also possesses a probabilistic structure. Thus, abduction works by jumping to an imaginative conclusion on the basis of two conclusions derived, firstly, from the major premise about a group in question (e.g., beans from a bag) and, secondly, from the minor premise about an object from a class in question (e.g., white beans) (2.624). This imaginative conclusion needs to be verified by induction and so becomes the major premise of the inductive syllogism. The imaginative leap unique to abduction enables abduction to enlarge our knowledge of the world.[24] A valid induction about an external fact already presupposes as a hypothesis the law or general rule it is intended to infer.

An additional and generally unremarked element of abduction is the manner in which it provides an intuitive support of induction and thereby provides a means of dealing with individuality, as exemplified in clinical reasoning. Like Reichenbach, Peirce resolves the tension between inductive inferences pertaining to single events and a statistical series by claiming that a single random instance already possesses the common character of the sum of the instances, or class to which these instances belong. The genius of abduction as emphasized, however, is in detecting this common character through an imaginative leap. In this manner abduction provides intuitive support for induction. This inductive-abductive theory finds a practical exemplar in medicine. As a number of authors have commented, there is a strong link between Peirce's theory of abductive reasoning and medicine.[25] Commentators on Peirce have not to my knowledge, however, perceived Peirce's singularity in resolving the tension between the individual clinical event and the statistical series. Thus, in comparing his structure of practical reasoning with clinical reasoning, Peirce singled out medical reasoning for its complexity in combining inductive with statistical reasoning. "The medical men," Peirce writes, "deserve special mention for the reason that they have had since Galen a logical tradition of their own," and, "in their working against reasoning '*post hoc, ergo propter hoc,*'" recognize, "however dimly," the rule of induction that states that "we must first decide for what character we propose to examine the sample, and only after that decision examine the sample"; thus, "we must not take a sample of eminent men, and studying over them, find that they have certain characters and conclude that all eminent men will have those characters" (1.95–97).

These sentences bear closer analysis. At one level Peirce simply restates his general insight that induction via abduction already presupposes the law or general rule it is intended to infer, thereby relating inductive inferences to a larger class or series of events. The tension between individual events and a statistical series is removed, because an individual event already presupposes a statistical series through abductive imagination. At another level, Peirce hints at the role of character, or ethos, in abductive imagination. Clinical reasoning is exemplary for abduction because it revolves around decision making about individual persons, and not simply inorganic objects. In its concern with human characteristics, abduction is concerned with both normative and factual data.[26] Peirce's theory of abduction is novel in the way in which it ties single events to a statistical class and links statistical facts to epistemological norms. This insight, of singular importance for reconciling individual events with statistics in clinical reasoning, is most evident in relation to the concept of clinical equipoise, a key concept for the ethics of clinical research. Abduction is important for clinical equipoise, because it demonstrates the latter's inner mechanism that reconciles epistemological and moral intuitions.

Clinical Equipoise

The notion of equipoise was first developed by Charles Fried (1974), who attempted to address the question of when it is ethical to enroll a patient into a randomized controlled trial, and thereby sacrifice the physician's fiduciary duty to her patient.[27] Fried's well-known answer to the conflict between the therapeutic imperative and the epistemological imperative of randomization is to state that there is no ethical problem to randomizing patients, so long as both arms of the trial are in equipoise. The epistemic and moral aspects of equipoise are thus in alliance. Through equipoise the moral intuitions of clinical investigators are not violated, and randomized trials can continue. This notion was subsequently expanded by Benjamin Freedman in the notion of community or clinical equipoise to include the community of clinical researchers.[28] Freedman noted that Fried's notion of "theoretical equipoise" was not sufficiently robust because it would be swayed by incorporating evidence from a variety of sources, including, "data from the literature, uncontrolled experience, considerations of basic science and fundamental physiological processes, and *perhaps a 'gut feeling' or 'instinct' resulting from (or superimposed on) other considerations*" (1987, 43; italics mine). As Freedman understood, theoretical equipoise possesses a fragile epistemic threshold, becoming disturbed by even a slight accretion of evidence favoring one arm of the trial, including clinical intuitions:

> Progress in medicine relies on progressive consensus within the medical and research communities. The ethics of medical practice grants no ethical or normative meaning to a treatment preference, however powerful, that is based on a hunch or on anything less than evidence publicly presented and convincing to the clinical community. Persons are licensed as physicians after they demonstrate the acquisition of this professionally validated knowledge, not after they reveal a superior capacity for guessing. (144)

In ruling out the epistemic validity of clinical intuitions Freedman granted that clinical equipoise could still exist when a physician has a clear treatment preference, provided that there is conflict within the medical community about the preferred treatment, since, Freedman argued, "it is largely a matter of chance that the patient is being seen by a clinician with a preference for B over A, rather than by an equally competent clinician with the opposite preference" (19). Crucially, for Freedman, informed treatment preferences do not include intuitions, which do not possess normative value at the level of the Institutional Review Board where decisions are made about the inclusion criteria for particular trials. However, even though Freedman did not consider the presence of a clear treatment preference by a physician in the presence of clinical conflict sufficient basis to exclude the ethical validity of randomization, he allowed for this treatment bias to be disclosed to the patient, and considered it acceptable for a patient to decline to participate in a trial on this basis (144–45).

While it has been subject to numerous critiques, clinical equipoise remains the most important framing concept in clinical research ethics. There have been in the main two modes of attack against clinical equipoise. Firstly, it has been criticized for ignoring the clinician's therapeutic responsibility toward individual patients, epitomized by the fact that Freedman does not consider clinical intuitions or "rational hunches" as valid scientific evidence.[29] Secondly, those who wish to separate research ethics from therapy have opposed clinical equipoise for maintaining the therapeutic imperative in clinical research.[30] Far from eliminating the importance of clinical equipoise, the fact that clinical equipoise is simultaneously attacked for not being therapeutic enough and for being too therapeutic, indicates the tension within clinical equipoise in balancing between the ethics of research and therapy. In this manner clinical equipoise functions as a "decision rule" that provides moral justification to randomize subjects in trials, yet also maintains the therapeutic imperative in research.[31]

This quality of clinical equipoise can be described in terms of its mediation of divergent intuitions. Thus, in their article "Rehabilitating Equipoise," Paul Miller and Charles Weijer note that rather than referring to a precise concept Fried's and Freedman's respective notions of equipoise are intended to "elicit intuitions about inherently imprecise and multifaceted concepts" (2003, 100). For Miller and Weijer, equipoise functions in terms of mediating between divergent moral intuitions. Specifically equipoise helps to answer the question that arises out of the moral tension between the physician's commitment to individual care and broader social commitment to a program of research. However, clinical equipoise not only links different kinds of moral intuitions, but also links moral intuitions with epistemological concepts. For this reason the ethics of clinical trials, as Richard Ashcroft notes, "depends absolutely on getting the epistemology right" (1999, 315). The moral question about whether to enter a patient into a trial arises consequent to the epistemological benefit for randomization in clinical research. This benefit includes the obvious aim to eliminate researcher bias, but also relates to the moral desire to develop therapeutic interventions to eliminate the burden of disease and human suffering. The link between values and beliefs in clinical equipoise occurs through interpreting it in terms of belief rather than knowledge.

For Ashcroft and others, this insight predisposes clinical equipoise to be more compatible with subjectivist Bayesian than frequentist statistics and provides the bridge between clinical and epidemiological facts and social norms.[32] However, Freedman's notion of clinical equipoise is framed in terms of frequentist statistics. In terms of the more classical frequentist interpretation, Deborah Hellman (2002) argues that clinical equipoise pertains to the realm of beliefs and not that of decision making and action. Whereas Ashcroft concludes that clinical equipoise is incoherent because of the gap between its cognitive function and social management, Hellman criticizes it for rejecting the epistemic validity of clinical intuitions. As noted, Freedman emphasizes that the ability of clinical equipoise to extend its concerns to the community of clinical investigators is premised on discounting the clinical intuitions of individual investigators as possessing epistemic validity. The robustness of clinical equipoise, as well as its maintenance of the elastic tension between research and therapy, is achieved through this move. If intuitions do have epistemological validity with respect to clinical decision making then clinical equipoise is open to the "therapeutic critique," because clinical intuitions would comprise an important element of the fiduciary responsibility of clinicians to patients.[33] On the other hand, if clinical intuitions are not part of clinical equipoise, then therapy is arguably a separate enterprise from research, and the moral justification of clinical equipoise is undermined.

Yet, Freedman's critique of clinical intuitions is more nuanced than many of his critics allow. Freedman agreed with Alvan Feinstein's criticism of clinical investigators who excessively narrowed the conditions and hypotheses of their trial in order to ensure the validity of the trial's results.[34] The problem with this fastidious approach was that it purchased scientific manageability at the expense of being able to apply the results to the messy conditions of clinical practice. Overly fastidious trials designed to resolve some theoretical question fail to satisfy the second ethical requirement of clinical research, that is, that the results of the trial are intended to influence clinical decisions (1987, 145). For Freedman, clinical equipoise was intended to help trials to be designed "in such a way as to maximize clinical relevance and the goals of medical practice rather than methodological rigor and the goals of theoretical science" (21).[35]

Freedman's nuanced approach to clinical intuitions is evidenced from the fact that even though he does not consider the presence of a clear treatment preference by a physician in the presence of clinical conflict to exclude the ethical validity of randomization, he does allow for this treatment bias to be disclosed to the patient, and considers it acceptable for a patient to decline to participate in a trial on this basis (1987, 144–45). There is therefore a gap between the moral justification of randomization on the basis that clinical intuitions are not epistemically valid at the community level of clinicians and accepting a patient decision to abstain from enrolling in such a trial because of a clinical hunch by her practitioner toward a particular treatment. While it might seem obvious that a trial participant may withdraw from a trial for any reason whatsoever, rational or irrational, I believe that Freedman's explicit mentioning of the acceptability for a patient to withdraw from a trial on the basis of a physician hunch serves more than a rhetorical purpose. Freedman's explicit rejection of clinical intuitions was intended to demonstrate the robustness of clinical equipoise in moving beyond the fragile epistemic threshold of Freed's therapeutic equipoise. This did not necessarily obviate Freedman's sensitivity to the use of clinical intuitions in everyday clinical practice. This ambiguous space between the individual and the population level of clinical reasoning in clinical equipoise is not merely idiosyncratic, but is a clue to clinical equipoise's conceptual foundations, enabling it to effectively mediate between the binary related spheres of therapy and research, of belief and action, of epistemological and moral intuitions, and of facts and values.

Peirce's theory of abduction linking statistical facts to epistemological norms provides a theoretical framework with which to render explicit and clarify the tacit mechanisms that allow clinical equipoise to function as a decision rule, balancing the tension between therapy and research. This role of abduction is apparent from a closer examination of Deborah Hellman's previously mentioned frequentist critique of clinical equipoise.[36] Like other therapeutic critiques, Hellman takes issue with Freedman's concept of equipoise for not incorporating clinical judgment about a particular treatment for an individual that would sway the arm of one side of a clinical trial. She claims that the concept of equipoise relates to the question of belief and not to that of decision making and action. Hellman supports her critique of clinical equipoise by using the epistemology of statistical epidemiology, particularly Steven Goodman's critique of the p value fallacy. The p value was first posited by R. A. Fisher and refers to the probability of a particular event that is statistically significant and does not result from chance alone. The lower the p value, the less likely the result will be statistically significant. While controversial, statistical significance is generally associated with a p value of 0.05. Goodman claims, however, that the use of the p value in clinical trials is based on the fallacy that "an event can be viewed simultaneously both from a long-run and a short run perspective" (1999, 999). The result is that researchers commit the "p value fallacy," whereby they draw conclusions about the truth of a hypothesis from a single piece of evidence. Whereas the "short run" perspective is evidential and inductive and relates to a single experiment, the "long run" perspective is error-based and deductive, and allows the observed results to be combined with other outcomes from hypothetical repetitions of the experiment. Goodman observes that "the hypothesis test approach offered scientists a Faustian bargain—a seemingly automatic way to limit the number of mistaken conclusions in the long run, but only by abandoning the ability to measure evidence and assess truth from a single perspective" (ibid.). By combining the long- and short-run perspectives and ignoring the trade-off, the use of hypothesis tests in clinical science does more than the statisticians R. A. Fisher, Jerzy Neyman, and Egon Pearson—who devised and refined the p value—intended.

In her critique of clinical equipoise, Hellman argues that researchers make an unjustified leap from statistical data to hypotheses on the basis of the p value fallacy. Since belief as a form of knowledge is only one factor involved in a patient's decision about what to do, Hellman claims that equipoise is not capable of resolving the ethical dilemma about how to treat a patient. The move from belief to action is dependent on adding moral reasoning about action to the clinical equation. Hellman's argument claims that through the p value fallacy clinical researchers erroneously move from objective frequentist statistical data to include the kinds of subjective beliefs prevalent in nonfrequentist Bayesian statistical reasoning. Because Hellman does not support this epistemological move, she claims that clinical equipoise is established on a fallacy and delegitimizes individual clinical decisions based on experience. Rather, Hellman argues that clinical reasoning, including clinical intuition, is essential in navigating the individual circumstances leading to the correct treatment decision for a particular patient.

Hellman's critique of clinical equipoise is based on an interpretation of Goodman's p value fallacy. Her critique of clinical equipoise, therefore, falls away with the resolution by Peirce's theory of abduction of the p value fallacy. Thus, Peirce's inclusion of a third category of probabilistic reasoning demonstrates the validity of drawing a creative hypothesis based on a single piece of evidence that will then be inductively validated through a statistical series. Clinical equipoise is justified in moving from belief to action because of its basis in abduction, which links epistemological and moral concepts. Clinical intuitions arising from individual clinical interactions are then not antithetical to the larger statistical arithmetic conducted by the architects of clinical research. In linking epistemological facts and norms, abductive reasoning provides the epistemological and moral foundations of clinical equipoise at a tacit or subconceptual level, yet still requires further inductive and deductive processes of inferential reasoning in order to render this knowledge explicit and valid at an epidemiological level. While abduction is paradigmatic for clinical reasoning, its relevance for clinical research is superseded by statistical tools that demonstrate causal relations at the population level. Nonetheless, the subconceptual foundations of clinical equipoise in abduction remain. Clinical equipoise's function as a heuristic that balances the tension between therapy and research has its roots in abduction. The stated goal of clinical equipoise is to move beyond equipoise when the benefit of one arm of a research trial clearly outweighs the other. At this point the preferred therapeutic treatment is again applied to the individual by clinicians. The abductive reasoning occurring at this level becomes the terrain for the clinical observations leading to further clinical trials when an alternative treatment promising greater efficacy arises.

Conclusion

Peirce's theory of abduction provides a modern reworking of Aristotelian *phronesis*. Peirce himself claimed that abductive reasoning improves chapter 25 of Aristotle's *Prior Analytics*, a book in which significant attention is paid to the physiognomic syllogy.[37] This relation between abductive reasoning and the Aristotelian syllogism seems to suggest that there is a cosmological connection between abductive reasoning and Aristotelian *nous* of practical reasoning. Earlier I claimed that Galton's work in statistical physiognomy inverted an anthropocentric structure within Aristotelian practical reasoning, that is, that intellectual *nous* of Aristotelian *phronesis* became disembodied through a transmutation into a mathematical grid. Peirce, by contrast, develops a kind of Aristotelian intellectual *nous* in his concept of abductive reasoning, a development that succeeds in maintaining the Aristotelian respect for contingency within a probabilistic model.

This claim requires some demonstration, because Peirce, especially in his early writing, denies any place for intuitive cognition. In an article published in 1868 in the *Journal of Speculative Philosophy*, Peirce defined and rejected intuition as "a cognition not determined by a previous cognition of the same object, and therefore so determined by something out of consciousness" (5.213). As noted by K. T. Fann, Peirce's denial of intuition was a stroke against Cartesianism and British empiricism, in that both assume the dyadic (object-subject) theory of cognition and require the existence of intuition (of "innate ideas" in the former and "sense data" in the latter) as an axiom. Fann claims that the denial of intuition is associated with the denial of particular intuition of one's self and of the subjective element of cognition.[38] Thus, Peirce argues that the conception of self may be regarded as a hypothesis to explain ignorance and error, and no faculty of introspection need be postulated.[39] Yet, Peirce's theory of hypothesis or abduction can also be understood as a revision of the Aristotelian syllogism and its associated *nous*, which is not jettisoned along with intuition as Cartesian infallible certainty. Abduction requires an imaginative leap that could be considered a type of intellectual *nous*, since it is not founded on any further inferential process. It seems acceptable to consider abduction a kind of intuition, provided it is not intended to reify the subject-object relation. Thus, knowledge of the individual particular is not necessarily opposed to inductive and abductive reasoning, which Peirce regarded as species of "reduction of a manifold to unity" (5.276).

This reading of Peirce is further supported by the fact that he considered his theory of reasoning to be anthropomorphic. Against the objection that his objective idealism was too anthropomorphic, Peirce replied:

> I hear you say: "This smacks too much of anthropomorphic conception." I reply that every scientific explanation of a natural phenomenon is a hypothesis that there is something in nature to which the human reason is analogous; and that it really is so all the successes of science in its applications to human convenience are witnesses. (1.316)

Peirce's anthropomorphism can be ascribed to his belief that the human mind evolved under the same conditions as its objects of inquiry, and in consequence, the structure of human reasoning imitates its cosmic context. According to Peirce ideas may become readily apparent to the mind, because they themselves played an important part in the evolutionary unfolding of mind.[40] Abductive reasoning along with causality, force, space, and time is a preeminent example of this type of cosmic idea. Statements of this genre equating abductive reasoning as a kind of natural communication with the divine are scattered amongst Peirce's writings. For example, in one statement Peirce writes that "retroduction goes upon the hope that there is sufficient affinity between the reasoner's mind and nature to render guessing not altogether hopeless, provided each guess is checked by comparison with observation" (1.121). And elsewhere, Peirce claims:

> It is evident, that unless man had had some inward light tending to make his guesses . . . much more often true than they would be by mere chance, the human race would long ago have been extirpated for its utter incapacity in the struggle for existence. (MS 692)

Even though Peirce ascribed abductive reasoning to a kind of intuitive divination, he did not consider its results infallible. The correctness of abductive conclusions was only a surmise or a hope that needs to be further justified through the process of induction.

This reading of Peirce suggests that despite incorporating probabilistic reasoning into the structure of logical reasoning, he continued a kind of embodied intellectual reasoning that I have traced back to Aristotle and that is deeply associated with clinical reasoning. The anthropocentric structure of abductive reasoning makes it possible to find an unforced link between abduction's epistemological and normative content. Peirce's modification of the Aristotelian syllogism for an indeterminist age also confronts the question of the individual that Aristotle attempts to reconcile with universal reason. Unlike Galton, Peirce's advocacy of statistical probabilism sought to maintain an Aristotelian structure of practical reasoning that is not disconnected from the practical context. His theory, however, has a striking resonance with the argument developed earlier that the modeling of clinical reasoning on *phronesis* needs to take account of a notion of an embodied *nous* of practical reasoning. An image of what it means to be human, Peirce seems to indicate, is central for our most basic cognitive processes. Finally, Peirce's theory of abduction presents a reinterpretation of the notion of consilience remodeled for a probabilistic universe. Despite, or because of its uncertainty, the ability of the human mind to make sense and regularity from indeterminism remains a source of wonder for Peirce. Where Whewell posits intuition in the inductive sciences, Peirce speaks of the imaginative leap linking hypotheses and inferences provided by abduction. In both cases the image of the human *anthropos* is important in structuring our conceptions of science and of self. In dealing with the individual, medical science, as the discipline or art that deals most directly with the individual, remains for Peirce the most difficult of all sciences. In dealing with individual variability, we have to forego the desire for absolute certainty. Abductive reasoning recognizes this by being both fallible and indispensable at the same time. While this makes abduction appear irrational, it in fact grounds our all-too-human rationality.

Medical Ethics beyond Ontology

Intuition as it is used in clinical reasoning is a cognitive process that is at once intellectual and corporeal. While intuition is not infallible and does not necessarily participate in final conclusions, it does appear to be fundamental for human judgment. Aristotle's concept of intuition and practical reasoning has proven to be central for this understanding of clinical reasoning. Clinical reasoning combines Aristotelian *aesthesis* or sensory perception with an intuitive faculty able to extract universals from the particular. Aristotle's insight that practical reasoning requires a different form of proof from mathematical reasoning is most pertinent in relation to clinical reasoning about individuals.[1]

A central aim of this study has been to demonstrate how uncertainty is intrinsic to clinical reasoning. In order to comprehend the epistemological and moral basis of clinical reasoning, it is important to acknowledge the necessary contingency of human experience. To admit the impossibility of absolute certainty in medicine does not invalidate a conception of human rationality, or what Stephen Toulmin has expressed as "reasonableness."[2] In this vein, I do not consider this present analysis by any means conclusive, but part of an ongoing process of professional and personal self-reflection in medicine. Besides the particular analyses concerning the role of intuition in medical and moral reasoning, the different analyses of intuition in this book indicate a common thread that connects some general insights regarding human judgment in the medical context. Three general metaphysical ideas that are of central importance for a theory of clinical reasoning, but which have not been discussed directly, include temporality, following clues, and the face-to-face relation.

At certain moments of this analysis I have alluded to the presence of a neglected temporal dimension that is crucial for medical ethics reasoning. For example, I argued in chapter 2 that a theory of moral intuitionism needs to incorporate awareness of a temporal and narrative structure in end-of-life decision making. As expressed by Alvan Feinstein, in addition to the anatomo-pathological correlate, our medico-moral epistemology requires the addition of a temporal correlate.

As highlighted in the comparison between *phronesis* and clinical reasoning, clinical intuition may also be understood as a system of following clues. This image of a clue was exemplified by Peirce's theory of abduction. Abduction as a method of clues is illustrated in the following paragraph of Peirce's, which explains the difference between abductive and inductive reasoning:

> A certain anonymous writing is upon a torn piece of paper. It is suspected that the author is a certain person. His desk, to which only he has had access, is searched, and in it is found a piece of paper, the torn edge of which exactly fits, in all its irregularities, that of the paper in question. It is a fair hypothetic inference that the suspected man was actually the author. The ground of this inference evidently is that two torn pieces of paper are extremely unlikely to fit together by accident. Therefore, of a great number of inferences of this sort, but a very small proportion would be deceptive. (2.632)

In Peirce's example, the haphazard sawtooth pattern created by the rip in the paper serves as an ontological clue that can be traced by abduction to the personal authorship of a certain piece of writing. The ripped paper is metonymic for the larger cosmos, which bears the marks of human or natural activity. Abduction provides the link between an anonymous natural event, and one bearing human values. The importance of personal characteristics in abduction also suggests the importance of human values in our scientific epistemologies. Medicine is iconic as a discipline bridging the human and social sciences. The ethical concern for individuals, as argued by medical historians Georges Canguilhem and Michel Foucault, has allowed medicine to liberate itself from etiological chains of causality. This study has emphasized how clinical reasoning encompasses facts and values together in physicians' medical management of the health and well-being of individuals. Ontological and epistemological structures within clinical reasoning are often not fully explicable without the ethical dimension that is derived from the doctor-patient relationship.

Finally, the moral image of the human face is vital for structuring medical and moral reasoning. The analyses of moral intuitionism, *phronesis*, and medical statistics have all demonstrated the centrality of the individual for clinical reasoning. Each of these analyses has attempted to elicit from within the particular epistemological and ontological structures pertaining to clinical reasoning the presence of a moral dimension that resides in the human face. For example, Galton's discovery of statistical correlation was premised on his previous eugenic concern and photographic composites of human familial faces.

Phenomenology

While much of medical ethics is rooted in an analytic philosophical tradition, the three themes of temporality, clues, and the moral image of the human face are better dealt with through phenomenological, rather than analytic, philosophy. Even though my philosophical discussion has related primarily to analytic philosophy, the predominant philosophy in Anglo-American medical ethics, this reading of intuition in medical and moral reasoning has been deeply informed by phenomenology. At the conclusion of this study it is time to bring this phenomenological influence into the foreground. A complete phenomenological examination of each of these themes would require an extensive investigation. An overarching phenomenological theory is, however, not even possible, since the phenomenological movement initiated by Edmund Husserl is characterized by adherence to a series of methods rather than a set of fixed philosophical principles or categories.[3] For this reason, I shall, therefore, focus in this brief, concluding discussion on the most relevant aspects of phenomenology for clinical reasoning, that is, the relation between intuition and correlation in the phenomenological investigations of Edmund Husserl and the questioning of an ontological ethics rooted in being in the thought of Emmanuel Levinas.

EDMUND HUSSERL (1859–1938)

As mentioned in chapter one, a theory of intuition was central for Husserl's project in phenomenology. There are a number of ways in which this project intersects with the major themes analyzed in this study of clinical reasoning.

Firstly, Husserl's concept of intuition retrieved and revitalized premodern notions of formal causality and eidetic intuition of essences, as against the analytic tradition, which has a tendency to endorse modern notions of rational calculation.[4] Similarly, this analysis of practical and philosophical intuition has contested positivist approaches that only recognize as valid what can be numerically quantified.

Secondly, Husserl's phenomenological method validates prephilosophical life and thought. For Husserl, the "natural attitude," the realistic assumptions that underlie everyday life as well as the positive sciences, must be tested via the phenomenological method. In particular, Husserl proposed the phenomenological *epoché* that suspends a naïve metaphysical attitude toward the world and the phenomenological reduction that brackets off realms of consciousness, two phenomenological methods intended to thematize the correlation between the outside world and subjectivity.[5]

Husserl's critical attitude toward everyday assumptions was not meant to undermine their validity but rather to enlarge our understanding of how knowledge, including scientific knowledge, is obtained. Thus, Husserl differentiated between the "lifeworld," in which objects are characterized by their "relative, approximate, and perspectival givenness,"[6] and modern naturalistic science, which attempts to construct knowledge of the world free from first-person experience. While science attempts to overcome the naïve attitude associated with commonsense reasoning, for Husserl the world of the scientist only exists in relation to this prior naïve experience.[7] This study of clinical intuition has, similarly, privileged commonsense experience as the foundation of scientific and moral reasoning in medicine. It has contested a naïve positivist view of clinical reasoning modeled on a mechanistic model of science and a dualist concept of the human being.

Husserl's privileging of subjectivity and his validation of naïve commonsense reasoning established a positively anthropological view of human reasoning conditioned by "empirical man."[8] This philosophical anthropology is most obvious in relation to Husserl's concept of intuition as the "principle of principles" in phenomenology. Phenomenological intuition is the primary means through which objects are presented to consciousness. Thus, Levinas states in his early study of Husserlian intuition, "The phenomenological reduction is precisely the method by which we are going back to concrete man"; and, "because of it, we discover the field of pure consciousness where we can practice philosophical intuition" (1973, 146). Even though phenomenological intuition is a philosophical abstraction, it is so by bracketing off and investigation of concrete experience. Hence Husserl's clarion calls for philosophers to return "back to the things themselves!" The phenomenological method is intrinsically concerned with discovering the essence of the human through its critique of empiricism and naturalism. Phenomenology shares this epistemological concern with medicine. If phenomenology revives in a modern form Aristotelian intuitive reasoning, phenomenology of medicine revives the Hippocratic synthesis of empirical observation, clinical intuition, and holism. The shared concern by phenomenology and medicine with "empirical man" explains the importance of phenomenology for medicine, and medicine for phenomenology. While phenomenology provides the method for the critique of scientific empiricism through a philosophical anthropology, medicine, taking the human condition as its central concern, provides the natural field par excellence where this method can be tested.

Richard Zaner has already drawn out many of these implications in his phenomenological study of medicine entitled *The Context of Self: A Phenomenological Inquiry Using Medicine as a Clue.*[9] Medicine, for Zaner, provides clues for the phenomenological investigation of subjectivity:

> How does it happen, it was asked, that objects of any particular type have the sense they have been described as having? . . . By explicating the context of meanings a particular type of object has *for or through consciousness*, the critical philosopher has before him a crucial set of *"clues"* (*Leitfaden*), which "point back" (*zuwenden*) to the various typical sets or modes of consciousness having that specific type of object as their noematic correlates. *The intended object functions as a clue to the synthetic processes which intend it, and tracing out the kinds of syntheses we have mentioned* (and other besides) *is what is strictly meant by phenomenological "constitution."* (1981, 173)

Medicine as a clue is then intended as a specific "noematic correlate" of the mode of consciousness relating to the self. The shared use of correlation in medicine and phenomenology provides, perhaps, the most important association in determining the nature of clinical reasoning. While correlation generally refers to the association between two entities, such as the statistical correlation between independent variables or the anatomo-pathological correlate of Bichat, for Husserl correlation occurs fundamentally in the realm of consciousness via intentionality. Husserl describes in a major work of his, *Krisis*, how his phenomenological breakthrough was arrived at through the realization that there was a "universal *a priori* of correlation between experienced object and manners of givenness" (*Krisis*, sec. 48; quoted in Moran 2005, 18–19). In other words, everything must henceforth be understood as "an index of a subjective system of correlations" (*Krisis*, sec. 48; cited in Moran, 19). Phenomenology is nothing other than the "systematic study of the essential correlation of subjectivity with objectivity" (ibid., 7). Additionally, the phenomenological *epoché*, by bracketing off realms of consciousness, is "the way of uncovering judgments about correlation, of uncovering the reduction of all unities of sense to me myself and my sense-having and sense-bestowing subjectivity with all its capabilities" (*Hus.* 15/366; quoted in Zahavi 2003, 46).

A fundamental relation exists between phenomenological intuition and correlation. Intuition provides the means of establishing phenomenological correlations between subject and object. However, within this fundamental phenomenological structure of the noematic correlate structure one finds a contestation of ontology by ethics. Thus, another phenomenologist, Jean-Luc Marion, drawing on the work of Emmanuel Levinas, claims that between 1900 and 1901, Husserl referred to another correlate that suggests a realm beyond ontology. Marion calls this "the correlation between *appearing and that which appears as such*" (Marion 2002, 32). The significance of this correlate is that it does not conceive of that which appears as a ' "given *of* consciousness, but indeed as the givenness *to* consciousness (or even *through* consciousness) of the thing itself, given in the mode of appearing and in all of its dimensions (intuition, intention, and their variations)" (ibid.). By this means, this third concept of correlation presupposes a phenomenological relation that is no longer dependent on personal intuitions as a mastery over otherness, but rather on an openness to what is. Thus, the ethical encounter presents an ethical structure that is not contained within phenomenological intuitions.

Husserl's conception of intuition has important implications for a theory of clinical reasoning. His phenomenological concept of intuition is analogous to Aristotelian *nous* of *phronesis* in relating contingent experience to universal categories. Yet the aspect of "givenness" within Husserl's concept of correlation indicates that the question of the individual in medicine is ultimately not adequately resolved through an anthropomorphism that is primarily ontological. It is important, therefore, to ask whether there is not another way of rethinking the relation between ontology, epistemology, and ethics in clinical reasoning. An ethical critique of ontology based on the face-to-face relation appears in the writing of Emmanuel Levinas, who thereby provides a novel way to rethink the foundations of clinical reasoning.

EMMANUEL LEVINAS (1906–1995)

Emmanuel Levinas, often described as the most influential moral philosopher of the twentieth century, argued for the primacy of ethics over ontology. The three themes that have emerged in this discussion—the face-to-face relation, temporality, and the trace—are all important for Levinas's ethical theory.

The Face-to-Face Relation

In his *Cartesian Meditations* Husserl addressed the question of empathetic understanding of another person. If phenomenological intuition grasps objects through subjective intentionality, how is it possible to comprehend another person, who him- or herself possesses subjective consciousness? In his first major work, *Totality and Infinity*, Levinas addresses this question through a phenomenological description of the human face that posits an ethical responsibility to another individual. This ethical responsibility to the Other is distinguished from other philosophical categories that may be confused with this primordial face-to-face encounter, such as epistemological understanding or ontological being. The force of the face-to-face relation arises from the fact that it eludes the power of the Husserlian phenomenological reduction to render it intelligible as an object of consciousness:

> The presence of the Other, or expression, source of all signification, is not contemplated as an intelligible essence, but is heard as language, and thereby is effectuated exteriorly. Expression, or the face, overflows images, which are always immanent to my thought, as though they came from me. This overflowing, irreducible to an image of overflowing is produced commensurate with—or in the inordinateness of—Desire and goodness, as the moral dissymmetry of the I and the other. The eye can conceive it only by virtue of position which, as an above-below disposition, constitutes the elementary fact of morality. Because it is the presence of exteriority the face never becomes an image or an intuition. (1991, 297)

Levinas associates Husserl's concept of phenomenological intuition with the primacy of vision for thought. Yet the face-to-face relation is characterized not by sight, but by speech, which enacts an ethical relationship, because it maintains a structure of alterity:

> If the transcendent cuts across sensibility, if it is openness preeminently, if its vision is the vision of the very openness of being, it cuts across the vision of forms and can be stated neither in terms of contemplation nor in terms of practice. It is the face; its revelation is speech. The relation with the Other alone introduces a dimension of transcendence, and leads us to a relation totally different from experience in the sensible sense of the term, relative and egoist. (193)

As Levinas emphasizes, the Other, through the face-to-face relation, maintains a relation through the face that remains absolutely distinct and is not subsumed in a "discourse of the same" that would include professional structures of medical and moral reasoning. As developed in Levinas's last major work, *Otherwise than Being*, this is the problem, or rather impossibility, of capturing the enunciative essence of another person through formal descriptions; it is what Levinas refers to as the tension between the "saying" and the "said."[10] The relation with the Other is not a horizontal one, but one of transcendence, in which the Other's presence commands responsibility from the "height of the Good." The presence of the Other forms the basis

of the commandment "not to kill." Murder for Levinas results in total negation of another person, yet it does not succeed in subsuming or dominating
the face, but "merely" its annihilation. Murder is "senseless" and impotent,
because "the face rends the sensible" (198).

In an essay on suffering, Levinas suggests that the *techné* of medicine used
to pursue its traditional goals of healing and alleviating suffering originate
as a response to the cry of the suffering flesh.[11] This cry for help is a primordial call for interhuman solidarity and is answered by medical care. Thus,
for Levinas the exposure to being is not an ecstatic experience, but rather
the fact of suffering to which medicine necessarily responds. Medical power
and authority are, therefore, organized structures that form secondarily as a
response to the prior human suffering cry or groan. Similarly in *Totality and
Infinity* Levinas writes that

> the solitude of death does not make the Other vanish, but remains in a con-
> sciousness of hostility, and consequently still renders possible an appeal to the
> Other, to his friendship and his medication. The doctor is an a priori principle
> of human mortality. (1991, 234)

The medical injunction *primum non nocere*, or "first do no harm," is a
negative formulation of the positive principle of medical beneficence that is
derived from this structure of responsibility, arising from the vulnerability of
patients. The radical imperative to respond to human suffering with beneficence explains why beneficence, and not autonomy, is the fundamental ethical
principle inherent to medical practice. Yet, at the same time there is a danger
that medical authority once organized becomes forgetful of the ethical imperative at the heart of medical practice. This arises when medicine becomes
primarily a form of social control arranged into a network of power, for example, as analyzed in minute detail by Michel Foucault.[12] Even medical ethics
can become implicated in this program through an overarching emphasis on
ethical rules and principles or an uncritical acceptance of medical authority.

Temporality

The ethical structure within medicine is inconceivable without a sense of human finitude. A concept of time occupies a central place in Levinas's ethical
theory, where it is defined as "the very relationship of the subject with the
Other" (1987, 39). Time introduces ethical responsibility into human encounters because of its diachronicity, that is, the inability to render subjective experience of time into universal categories. Thus, in his study of the
intersubjectivity of time, *Time and the Other*, Levinas writes:

Time signifies this always of noncoincidence, but also the always of the relationship, an aspiration and an awaiting, a thread finer than an ideal line that diachrony does not cut. Diachrony preserves this thread in the paradox of a relationship that is different from all the other relationships of our logic and psychology, which, by way of an ultimate community, at the very least confer synchrony on their terms. (32)

Time itself establishes an ethical relation because the solitary instant of the existent being immured in itself becomes hypostatized into the present through the presence of the Other:

The present is the event of hypostasis. The present leaves itself—better still, it *is* the departure from self. It is a rip in the infinite beginningless and endless fabric of existing. The present rips apart and joins together again; it begins; it is beginning itself. It has a past, but in the form of remembrance. It has a history, but it is not history. (52)

In other words, one finds with Levinas's analysis of time, as with his other phenomenological analyses, a radical structure of alterity upon which the individual self is constructed. Time, like the face-to-face relation, for Levinas speaks of human experience that establishes alterity and thereby ethical responsibility beyond and prior to epistemological understanding and ontological categories. Furthermore, as Richard Cohen writes in his preface to *Time and the Other*, Levinas's description of the instant in terms of existential "conquest"—the subject's escape from anonymous existence—and existential fatigue differs from the classical account of time in terms of knowledge and causality (ibid., preface, 4–5).

In relation to Bichat, medicine pertaining to individuals is not limited by etiological determinism. This is explained at one level by the development of statistical correlation, particularly in epidemiological causation, that ruptures models of direct causation in medicine. Yet, as Canguilhem and Foucault have noted, this rupture of the chain of causality arises specifically in the clinical context.[13] Levinas's conception of temporality as irreducible alterity provides an ethical, albeit transcendental, explanation for the failure of chains of causality in the clinical encounter.

The Trace

Following clues is the third theme pertaining to clinical reasoning, or using Levinas's term, the trace. The method of following clues is classically illustrated by Peirce's method of abduction or the investigative ability of Sherlock

Holmes. Levinas, too, acknowledges this kind of epistemological method. In a paper entitled "Is Ontology Fundamental?" Levinas writes:

> The comedy begins with our simplest gestures. They all entail an inevitable awkwardness. Reaching out my hand to pull a chair toward me, I have folded the arm of my jacket, scratched the floor, and dropped my cigarette ash. In doing what I willed to do, I did a thousand and one things I hadn't willed to do. The act was not pure; I left traces. Wiping away these traces, I left others. Sherlock Holmes will apply his science to this irreducible coarseness of each of my initiatives, and thus the comedy may take a tragic turn. When the awkwardness of the act is turned against the goal pursued, we are in the midst of tragedy. Laius, in attempting to thwart the final predictions, undertakes precisely what is necessary to fulfill them. Oedipus, in succeeding, works towards his own misfortune. It is like an animal fleeing in a straight line across the snow before the sound of the hunters, thus leaving the very traces that will lead to its death. (1998, 3)

This use of following traces was described by Voltaire and expounded on by Thomas Huxley as the method of Zadig, in reference to a character from Babylonian legend. The "rigorous application of Zadig's logic to the results of accurate and long-continued observation," Huxley writes, "has founded all those sciences which have been termed historical or palaetiological, because they are retrospectively prophetic and strive towards the reconstruction in human imagination of events which have vanished and ceased to be" (1894, 9). All sciences, such as history, anatomy, archaeology, and paleoanthropology, rely on the method of following traces to conjure up past events, or to determine future ones. While Zadig's method appears magical in conjuring to presence what was previously invisible, it possesses inherent rationality, and has been regarded as the defining methodology of the late nineteenth-century human sciences.[14] Ariadne's thread has come to represent this combination of rational science with mythic substrate. Indeed the archaeologist of Ariadne, Arthur Evans, combined Zadig's method with a "passionate identification with the mythic exploits of the ancient Cretans" in a thoroughly modernist reconstruction of Bronze Age civilization (Gere 2009, 10).

For Levinas, however, the concept of the trace lies precisely in evading this ontological history. The ethical significance of the trace occurring in the face-to-face relation lies in the fact that it arises from an originary past that cannot be fully recalled to the present. Its positivity is not that of a scientific positivism, but of infinity:

> The infinite cannot be tracked down like game by a hunter. The trace left by the infinite is not the residue of a presence; its very glow is ambiguous.

Otherwise, its positivity would not preserve the infinity of the infinite any more than negativity would. (Levinas 1998, 12)

The "signifyingness" of the trace, Levinas writes in "The Trace of the Other," consists in "signifying without making appear" (1986, 356). Whereas clues are a sign of a person's worldly activity, the trace refers only to one's pure and simple passage. In this manner, the trace is disassociated from its signatory function.[15] It achieves this because the trace is primarily, if not primordially, an ethical relationship—in this case referring to the third person, or what Levinas calls "illeity." As with time and the face, the trace ruptures intuitive self-certainty through the question of the Other. Accordingly, Levinas claims that "in a trace the relationship between the signified and the signification is not a correlation, but an *unrightness* itself" (355). It is an "unrightness" because it disturbs the ipseity of self through the "*beyond* from which a face comes" (356). While an anthropological substrate is hypostatized in Galton's concept of statistical correlation and an image of the human *anthropos* is present in Peirce's probabilistic theory or hypothesis of abduction, the moral imperative behind these human images lies beyond ontology in the ethical trace associated with the temporal and corporeal presence of another sentient person. Levinas's notion of the trace also explains the possible limits of Aristotelian *phronesis*. Even though Aristotle argues that practical wisdom requires different levels of proof to suit its particular context, the philosophical temptation always exists to abstract the particular into universal philosophical categories, to remove singular terms or premises from syllogistic reasoning—an overstepping of reason in the role of intellectual *nous* in *phronesis*. Levinas's radical contribution to philosophy is to demonstrate that the ethical imperative arising from the face-to-face relation cannot be reduced to abstract philosophical concepts, even those related to *phronesis*. Before it becomes established as a philosophical medical ethics principle, beneficence is first and foremost the immediate imperative to respond to human illness and suffering.

Conclusion

Levinas's ethical analyses of time, the face, and the trace present a transcendental ethics beyond ontology that is of great importance for a theory of moral reasoning in medicine. Levinas's ethical philosophy helps explain the ethical structures that underlie the epistemological and ontological structures that exist in clinical reasoning. Levinas is also important in helping to explain the rupture in clinical reasoning's linear causality from an ethical perspective. What appears to be the result of variability within complex biological structures might also be associated with an originary ethic that grounds clinical reasoning as much as it does "first philosophy." Levinas's philosophical trajectory moves from Husserlian intentional consciousness, associated with phenomenological intuitions, to preconscious sensing or sentience. Despite its transcendentalism, Levinas's philosophy is rooted in corporeal sensibility. There is, thus, an irrevocable ambiguity within Levinas's work between the ethical imperative of responsibility arising from a transcendental height and its foundations in immanent worldliness.[16] The trace coincides with phenomenological clues as well as the passage from infinity.

A tension exists, therefore, between the infinite obligation to relieve suffering in medicine and its finite medical correlates. Similarly, there is a necessary dialectical relation, therefore, between the ethical and ontological-epistemological structures that constitute clinical reasoning. As the philosopher Adi Ophir claims in his study of the order of human evils, the transcendence within the realm of human experience extends only beyond the "is" to an "ought."[17] The gap between "is" and "ought" "appears every time someone is in distress, suffers, experiences loss, cries for help—and can be assisted without unbearably increasing the suffering and loss of others" (2005, 15):

> Concrete others are morally relevant only because, and to the extent that, they are vulnerable, prone to suffering and already suffering concrete evils. What guides moral knowledge (or practical reason, phronesis) is the interest in superfluous evils that befall particular and concrete others or to threaten them. What guides moral judgment and the intention of a moral act is the care for those others whom evil befalls. (15–16)

Intuition in its various forms—philosophical, phenomenological, practical, and clinical—provides the means of linking the phenomenal with the noumenal. As a form of direct perception it is associated with absolute certainty; as an element of practical reasoning it is inherently fallible. It links preconscious sensibility with more explicit forms of cognition. An all-too-human element of practical and moral reasoning, intuition is exemplified through clinical reasoning, concerned as it is with contingency, and responds morally to the human predicament of individuals with a human face.

Notes

Introduction

1. Franz Rosenzweig, *Understanding the Sick and the Healthy: A View of World, Man, and God* (Cambridge, MA: Harvard University Press, 1999).

2. Jan Lukasiewicz points out that this syllogism has important logical differences from the Aristotelian syllogism. Lukasiewicz claims that Aristotle does not introduce singular terms or premises, such as "Socrates is a man," into his philosophical system. *Aristotle's Syllogistic* (Oxford, Clarendon Press, 1951), 1.

3. Edward Shorter, *Bedside Manners: The Troubled History of Doctors and Patients* (New York: Simon & Schuster, 1985).

4. Hans Jonas, "Technology and Responsibility: Reflections on the New Tasks of Ethic," in *Philosophical Essays: From Ancient Creed to Technological Man* (Englewood Cliffs, NJ: Prentice-Hall, Inc., 1973), 3–20.

5. Michael Taussig, "Reification and the Consciousness of the Patient," in *The Nervous System* (London: Routledge, 1992), 83–109.

6. It is a commonly accepted truism that this unification of medicine and the humanities is the best strategy to overcome the objectification of the human being resulting from a Cartesian dualism separating body and mind/soul. The works of Eric Cassell, Edmund Pellegrino, and David Thomasma exemplify this endeavor to unite medicine and the humanities. See, for example, Eric Cassell, *The Nature of Suffering and the Goals of Medicine* (New York: Oxford University Press, 1991); Edmund Pellegrino and David Thomasma, *A Philosophical Basis of Medical Practice: Toward a Philosophy and Ethics of the Healing Professions* (New York: Oxford University Press, 1981). For an analysis of Descartes from the perspective of philosophy of medicine, see Stuart F. Spicker, ed., *The Philosophy of the Body: Rejections of Cartesian Dualism* (Chicago: Quadrangle Books, 1970).

7. Al Jonsen has traced the beginning of clinical medical ethics in the United States to discussions around the first renal transplantation in 1954, while for David Rothman it occurred slightly later with the 1975 Karen Quinlan case. See David J. Rothman, *Strangers at the Bedside* (New York: Basic Books, 1991); and Al R. Jonsen, *A Short History of Medical Ethics* (New York: Oxford University Press, 2000).

8. For a comprehensive review of the Nuremberg Code and its influence on contemporary bioethics, see George J. Annas and Michael A. Grodin, eds., *The Nazi Doctors and the Nuremberg Code* (New York: Oxford University Press, 1992).

9. Human right abuses pertaining to medical research have occurred in the United States as well. Most well-known is the infamous Tuskegee syphilis study. For an analysis of this dark period in American medicine, see Susan M. Reverby, ed., *Tuskegee's Truths: Rethinking the Tuskegee Syphilis Study* (Chapel Hill: University of North Carolina Press, 2000).

10. The practice of medicine under the Third Reich was not simply a moral aberration and poor science, but developed out of a certain medical logic. Thus, the Nazi program of killing was envisaged as a necessary means of "healing" the body politic, and as such may be considered a consequence of an Enlightenment ideal of rationality. See Gerhaard Baader, "Heilen und Vernichten: Die Mentalitat der NS-Arzte," in *Vernichten und Heilen*, ed. Angelika Ebbinghaus and Klaud Dorner (Berlin: Aufbau-Verlag, 2001), 275–95.

11. Paul Komesaroff, "Medicine and the Ethical Conditions of Modernity," in *Ethical Intersections*, ed. Jeanne Daly (Sydney, Australia: Allen & Unwin, 1996), 34–48.

12. Rothman, *Strangers at the Bedside*.

13. Ludwig Edelstein, "The Relation of Ancient Philosophy to Medicine," in *Ancient Medicine*, ed. Owsei Temkin and C. Lilian Temkin (Baltimore, MD: Johns Hopkins University Press, 1967), 349–66.

14. It is a matter of debate where contemporary technological medicine stands in relation to its traditional concern with healing. See, for example, Leon Kass, "Regarding the End of Medicine and the Pursuit of Health," *The Public Interest* 40 (1975): 11–42; Christopher Boorse, "Health as a Theoretical Concept," *Philosophy of Science* 44 (1977): 73; Lennart Nordenfelt, *On the Nature of Health: An Action-Theoretic Approach* (Dordrecht: Reidel Publishing, 1987); Fredrik Svenaeus. *The Hermeneutics of Medicine and the Phenomenology of Health: Steps Towards a Philosophy of Medical Practice* (Dordrecht: Kluwer Academic Publishers, 2000).

15. Another important aspect of medicine not directly addressed in this study concerns medicine's role in a discipline of power and the production of modern notions of subjectivity. This "genealogical" approach has been most fully developed by historian Michel Foucault. See Michel Foucault, *The Birth of the Clinic* (New York: Vintage Books, 1973). Foucault's class study of the development of modern medicine is important for my analysis of statistical reasoning in chapter six. While this study is "genealogical," investigating the effects of practice on philosophical categories of medical epistemology and ethics, it differs from Foucault in affirming the importance of a philosophical moral image for informing and structuring a medical humanism.

16. By referring to human nature I am not claiming that human nature is static. This is implicit in claiming that support for human intuitions is not necessarily to support for essentialism.

17. Lewis Wolpert, *The Unnatural Nature of Science* (London: Faber and Faber, 1992).

18. Aristotle, *Nichomachean Ethics*, 1094b.

Chapter One

1. For an analysis of the relation between medicine and philosophy and in particular the use of medical metaphors in ancient philosophy, see Werner Jaeger, "Greek Medicine as Paideia," in *Paideia: The Ideals of Greek Culture* (New York: Oxford University Press, 1944), 3: 3–45; Werner Jaeger, "Aristotle's Use of Medicine as Model of Method in His *Ethics*," *Journal of Hellenistic Studi*ς 7, (1957): 54–61; W H. S. Jones, *Philosophy and Medicine in Ancient Greece* (Baltimore, MD: Johns Hopkins University Press, 1946); I S. Hutchinson, "Doctrines of the Mean and the Debate Concerning Skills in Fourth-Century Medicine, Rhetoric and Ethics," *Apeiron* 2 (Summer 1988 17–52; Martha Nussbaum, *The Therapy of Desire: Theory and Practice in Hellenistic*

Ethics (Princeton, NJ: Princeton University Press, 1994); and Jacques Jouanna, *Hippocrates* (Baltimore, MD: Johns Hopkins University Press, 1999).

2. Jaeger, "Greek Medicine as Paideia," 5–7.

3. It is necessary to distinguish between the terms medical ethics and bioethics. While the use of these two terms is generally interchangeable, by *bioethics* I refer to questions regarding the use of biotechnologies. By *medical ethics* I refer to the discipline dealing with ethical questions in the context of day-to-day clinical practice. My concern in this book is primarily with the domain of clinical medical ethics.

4. Hanna Arendt, "Metaphor and the Ineffable: Illumination on "The Nobility of Sight," in *Organism, Medicine and Metaphysics,* ed. Stuart. F. Spicker (Dordrecht: D. Reidel Publishing Co., 1978), 303–16.

5. Victor Kal, *On Intuition and Discursive Reasoning in Aristotle* (Leiden: E. J. Brill, 1988).

6. Adapted from Mario A. Bunge, *Intuition and Science* (Englewood Cliffs: NJ, Prentice-Hall, 1962).

7. Immanuel Kant, *Critique of Pure Reason,* trans. Norman Kemp-Smith (New York: St. Martin's Press, 1965).

8. The meaning of intuition in Kant is a matter of philosophical contention, and a more detailed analysis will not be presented here. For a detailed analysis of the place of intuition in Kant, see Lorne Falkenstein, *Kant's Intuitionism: A Commentary on the Transcendental Aesthetic* (Toronto: University of Toronto Press, 1995).

9. I shall argue through this analysis that a phenomenological approach at times provides a method to describe and understand clinical experience better than analytic philosophical approaches. The importance of Husserlian phenomenology for this analysis will be discussed in greater detail in the concluding chapter.

10. For an investigation of phenomenology in relation to medicine, see Richard Zaner's classic study, *The Context of Self : A Phenomenological Inquiry Using Medicine as a Clue* (Athens: Ohio University Press, 1981).

11. Husserl's philosophical output stands between his first magnum opus, *Logical Investigations,* and his final work, *Cartesian Meditations,* as well as a large number of unpublished manuscripts. A number of introductory texts to Husserl include: Herbert Spiegelberg, *The Phenomenological Movement: A Historical Introduction,* vols. 1 and 2 (The Hague: Martinus Nijhoff, 1965); Richard Zaner, *The Way of Phenomenology: Criticism as a Philosophical Discipline* (New York: Pegasus, 1965); Emmanuel Levinas, *The Theory of Intuition in Husserl's Phenomenology* (Evanston, IL: Northwestern University Press, 1973); David Carr, *Interpreting Husserl: Critical and Comparative Studies* (Dordrecht: Martinus Nijhoff Publishers, 1987); and Dan Zahavi, *Husserl's Phenomenology* (Stanford, CA: Stanford University Press, 2003).

12. Levinas, *Theory of Intuition,* 69.

13. Ibid.

14. Ibid., 65.

15. This quote is particularly interesting, in light of Levinas's later conception of the ethical face-to face relation that is not contained by intentionality and phenomenological intuitions. This Levinasian ethical insight informs much of my own analysis of clinical reasoning, as will become apparent in the concluding chapter.

16. Section 24, of *Ideen I,* cited in Zahavi, *Husserl's Phenomenology,* 44–45.

17. *Husserliana* 19/539, 566; cited in Zahavi, *Husserl's Phenomenology,* 31–32.

18. As has been observed by others, Husserl's concept of intuition undermines the correspondence theory of truth, since it defines truth in terms of the coincidence between two

intentions, and not between two separate ontological domains. See Levinas, *Theory of Intuition,* 69; Richard Cobb-Stevens, *Husserl and Analytic Philosophy* (Dordrecht: Kluwer Academic Publishers, 1990); and Zahavi, *Husserl's Phenomenology.*

19. Feinstein's theory of clinical judgment is of central importance for the theory of clinical reasoning that I lay out in this book. Feinstein's epistemology of clinical reasoning will be examined in greater detail in chapters five, six, and seven.

20. Jerome Groopman, "Second Opinion," *New Yorker,* January 24, 2000.

21. Carl Ginzburg, "Clues: Roots of an Evidential Paradigm," in *Clues, Myths and the Historical Method* (Baltimore, MD: Johns Hopkins University Press, 1989), 96–125.

22. Henri Poincaré similarly distinguishes between two different types of mathematical intuition, an analytical sensible intuition and an inventive intuition, responding to different faculties of the soul. See *The Value of Science* (New York: Dover Publications, [1913] 1958), 25.

23. Leon R. Kass, "The Wisdom of Repugnance: Why We Should Ban the Cloning of Humans," *New Republic* 216, no. 22 (1997): 17–26.

24. James Q. Wilson, *The Moral Sense* (New York: Free Press, 1993); Jon Haidt, "The Emotional Dog and Its Rational Tail: A Social Intuitionist Approach to Moral Judgment," *Psychological Review* 108, no. 4 (2001): 814–34.

25. Tom L. Beauchamp and James F. Childress, *Principles of Biomedical Ethics* (New York: Oxford University Press, 1979).

26. Evaluating the influence of individual personalities is an important, but perhaps neglected approach to evaluate the discipline of medical ethics. Especially in its early years the discipline was shaped by the influence of strong personalities. In this regard secular medical ethics is closer to religious authority, in which charismatic leadership has an important role, than many ethicists might care to acknowledge. Incidentally, this is not the only place in which medical ethics and religion share a close resemblance. It has been noted that medical ethics provides a secular pluralistic ethics in the place of religious authority. Certainly in the United States, theologians such as Paul Ramsey and Joseph Fletcher provided key early contributions to medical ethics, though this was fairly rapidly superceded by secular approaches. Moreover, medical ethics provided a type of professional sanctuary for ethicists trained in religion, but who did not wish to be constrained by religious tenets.

27. Certainly this list is not exhaustive. Another important figure from this period, Edmund Pellegrino, will be discussed separately in chapter three as part of my analysis of clinical reasoning and *phronesis.*

28. Additional articles advocating a medical perspective include: Colleen D. Clements and Roger C. Sider, "Medical Ethics' Assault Upon Medical Values," *JAMA* 250, no. 15 (1983): 2011–15; Robert L. Holmes, "The Limited Relevance of Analytical Ethics to the Problem of Bioethics," *Journal of Medicine and Philosophy* 15 (1990): 143–59.

29. Mark Siegler, "Medical Ethics as a Medical Matter," in *The American Medical Ethics Revolution,* ed. Robert B. Baker et al., (Baltimore, MD: Johns Hopkins University Press, 1999), 171–79.

30. Albert R. Jonsen, Mark Siegler, and William J. Winslade, *Clinical Ethics: A Practical Approach to Ethical Decisions in Clinical Medicine,* Sixth Edition (New York: McGraw-Hill, 2006).

31. Leon R. Kass, "Professing Ethically: On the Place of Ethics in Defining Medicine," *JAMA* 249, n . 10 (1983): 1305–

32 "Twentieth-cen y mo al philosophers have sometimes appealed to their and our intuitions; ut one of the th s tha we ought to have learned from the history of moral philosophy is that the introductior f the word 'intuition' by a moral philosopher is always a signal that

something has gone badly wrong with an argument." Alasdair MacIntyre, *After Virtue: A Study in Moral Theory* (Notre Dame, IN: University of Notre Dame Press, 1981), 69.

33. Richard M. Hare, "Medical Ethics: Can the Moral Philosopher Help?," in *Philosophical Medical Ethics: Its Nature and Significance*, ed. Stuart F. Spicker and H. Tristram Engelhardt (Boston: D. Reidel Publishing Co., 1977), 49–62. For a similar position, see K. D. Clouser, "Bioethics," in *The Encyclopedia of Bioethics*, ed. W. Reich et al. (New York: Free Press, 1978), 114–16.

34. Baruch Brody's version of moral intuitionism is examined in greater detail in the following chapter.

35. See, for example, Stephen Toulmin, *Return to Reason* (Cambridge, MA, Harvard University Press, 2001).

36. In *Practical Reason* Pierre Bourdieu writes, that "the habitus fulfills a function which another philosophy consigns to a transcendental conscience: it is a socialized body, a structured body, a body which has incorporated the immanent structures of a world or of a particular sector of that world—a field—and which structures the perception of that world as well as action in that world." (Stanford, CA: Stanford University Press, 1998), 81.

37. That ethics is premised on the face-to-face relation between individuals was developed most strongly by the French phenomenologist Emmanuel Levinas. Levinas's ethical theory informs this study. His influence will be discussed in greater detail in the concluding chapter.

Chapter Two

1. For further elaboration of the common sense in Aristotle, see John I. Beare, *Greek Theories of Elementary Cognition from Alcmaeon to Aristotle* (Oxford: Clarendon Press, 1906); Arthur Norman Foxe, *The Common Sense from Heraclitus to Peirce: The Sources, Substances, and Possibilities of the Common Sense* (New York: Turnbridge Press, 1962); David Summers, *The Judgment of Sense* (Cambridge: Cambridge University Press, 1987).

2. See, for example, Joshua Greene, "From Neural 'Is' to Moral 'Ought': What are the Moral Implications of Neuroscientific Moral Psychology?" *Nature Reviews Neuroscience* 4 (2003): 847–50.

3. W. D. Hudson, ed., *The Is-Ought Question* (London: MacMillan, 1969).

4. MacIntyre bases his assertion on an ingenious reading of Hume's paragraph. See Alasdair C. MacIntyre, "Hume on 'Is' and 'Ought,'" in *The Is-Ought Question*, 35–50. See also Elijah Milgram, "Was Hume a Humean?," *Hume Studies* 21, no. 1 (1997): 75–93; "Hume on Practical Reasoning" (Treatise 463–69), *Iyyun: The Jerusalem Philosophical Quarterly* 46 (1997): 235–65.

5. Philippa Foot, *Virtues and Vices* (Berkeley: University of California Press), 1978.

6. The dispute as to the theoretical justification of the "is"/"ought" separation can be distinguished from its actual validity in practice. This is because even those who oppose the theoretical relation between "is" and "ought" will often concede the close relation between fact and value in day-to-day affairs. As Hilary Putnam notes, calling the gap between fact and value a dichotomy rather than a mere distinction prevents meaningful philosophical exchange. *The Collapse of the Fact/Value Dichotomy and Other Essays* (Cambridge, MA: Harvard University Press, 2002). Similarly, Hans Albert, the proponent of critical rationalism, relates "is" and "ought," while distinguishing between them, claiming that to ought to do a certain thing implies the capability of being able to do this very thing. *Kritischer Rationalismus: Vier Kapitel zur Kritik illusionaren Denkens* (Tuebingen: UTB Mohr Siebeck, 2000). Drawing on Albert, Stella Reiter-Theil has attempted to establish an empirically based method of moral reasoning in medical ethics. "Does

empirical research make bioethics more relevant? 'The embedded researcher' as a methodological approach," *Medicine, Health Care and Philosophy* 7 (2004): 17–29.

7. Robert Audi has pointed this out in writing that "many who oppose intuitionism make [such] appeals to intuitions in establishing a basis for their ethical views." *Moral Knowledge and Ethical Character* (Oxford: Oxford University Press, 1997), 33.

8. In his passage referring to the naturalistic fallacy Moore writes, "Yet a mistake of this simple kind has commonly been made about 'good.' It may be true that all things which are good are also something else, just as it is true that all things which are yellow produce a certain kind of vibration in the light. And it is a fact, that Ethics aims at discovering what are these other properties belonging to all things which are good. But far too many philosophers have thought that when they name those other properties they were actually defining good; that these properties, in fact, were simply not 'other,' but absolutely and entirely the same with goodness. This view I propose to call the 'naturalistic fallacy' and of it I shall now endeavour to dispose" (1903, 10). While Moore's naturalistic fallacy has been most influential in twentieth-century philosophy, it has been noted by A. N. Price that Moore was not in actual fact the originator of this concept, but that it can be traced to the school of eighteenth-century intuitionists. See W. D. Hudson, *Ethical Intuitionism* (London: Macmillan, 1967).

9. For a collection of philosophical papers on these subjects, see P. W. Taylor, ed., *The Moral Judgment: Readings in Contemporary Meta-Ethics* (Englewood Cliffs, NJ: Prentice-Hall, 1963).

10. The traditional distinction between consequentialists and deontologists in analytic moral philosophy is a separate issue from the distinction between naturalists and intuitionists. So Moore for example, was a consequentialist, and W. D. Ross is famous for his deontological approach to ethics; on the other hand both Moore and Ross can be considered to be intuitionists.

11. Aristotle, *Nichomachean Ethics*, 1094a.

12. W. D. Hudson, *Modern Moral Philosophy* (Garden City, NY: Anchor Books, 1970).

13. For a fuller discussion of the philosophical concept of moral supervenience, see J. Kim, "Supervenience as a Philosophical Concept," *Metaphilosophy* 21, nos. 1–2 (1990): 1–27.

14. Richard M. Hare, *The Language of Morals* (Oxford: Oxford University Press, 1952).

15. As might be expected, ethical naturalists are not hard pressed to explain the practical syllogism, since for them there is no ultimate separation between "is" and "ought." In consequence, Alasdair MacIntrye can claim there is a natural transition from "is" to "ought" in Aristotle, since 'Aristotle's examples of practical syllogism typically have a premise which includes some terms such as "suits" or "pleases."' See MacIntyre, "Hume on 'Is' and 'Ought.'"

16. In apparent agreement with Hare regarding this type of syllogism, Max Black notes that in instances of the practical syllogism where the moral premise is implicit it might appear that the facts of a case contain a moral dimension, but this type of enthymeme with an unstated premise still "smuggles" in a value dimension into a factual scenario. "The Gap between 'Is' and 'Should,'" in *Is-Ought Question*, 99–113.

17. Nicholas Rescher, "How Wide is the Gap between Facts and Values?," *Philosophy and Phenomenological Research* 50, suppl. (1990): 297–319.

18. Alan Donagan, *The Theory of Morality* (Chicago: University of Chicago Press, 1977), 17–18.

1 . Victor al, *On Intuition and Discursive Reasoning in Aristotle* (Leiden: E. J. Brill, 1988).

) For a systematic review of the history and development of moral intuitionism including the seventeenth to nineteenth centuries, see Hudson, *Ethical Intuitionism.*

l. W. D. Ross, *The Right and the Good* (Oxford: Clarendon Press, 2002).

22. John Rawls, *A Theory of Justice* (Cambridge, MA: Belknap Press, 1971), 30.

23. This collection includes Baruch Brody's early essay on moral intuitionism, republished as "Intuitions and Objective Moral Knowledge." In *Taking Issue: Pluralism and Casuistry in Bioethics* (Washington, DC: Georgetown University Press), 45–56.

24. See in particular, footnote 14, p. 15, in *Life and Death Decision Making* (New York: Oxford University Press, 1988).

25. This is exemplified by Pellegrino's claim seen earlier that the respect by physicians for patient autonomy is itself rooted in the principle of beneficence, intrinsic to the medical profession.

26. Baruch Brody, "Special Ethical Issues in the Management of PVS Patients," in *Taking Issue: Pluralism and Casuistry in Bioethics* (Washington, DC: Georgetown University Press, 2003), 173–95.

27. Baruch Brody, *Life and Death Decision Making* (New York: Oxford University Press, 1988), 87–88.

28. See, for example, Bert Broeckaert and J. M. Nunez Olarte, "Sedation in Palliative Care: Facts and Concepts," in *The Ethics of Palliative Care: European Perspectives*, ed. Henk Ten Have and Clark D. Buckingham (Philadelphia: Open University Press, 2002), 166–80.

29. Dan Sulmasy and Edmund Pellegrino, "The Rule of Double Effect: Clearing up the Double Talk," *Archives of Internal Medicine* 159 (1999): 545–50.

30. For an opinion opposing the law of double effect in medicine, see Timothy E. Quill, Rebecca Dresser, and Dan W. Brock, "The Rule of Double Effect: A Critique of Its Role in End of Life Decision-Making," *New England Journal of Medicine* 337 (1997): 1768–71. For recent discussion on this subject, see J. Boyle, "Medical Ethics and Double Effect: The Case of Terminal Sedation," *Theoretical Medicine* 25 (2004): 51–60; and Alasdair McIntyre, "The Double Life of Double Effect," *Theoretical Medicine* 25 (2004): 61–74.

31. I was present when this paper was presented at the annual meeting of the American Society for Bioethics and Humanities (ASBH) at Nashville in November 2001.

32. G. C. Sterling, *Ethical Intuitionism and Its Critics* (New York: Peter Lang, 1994).

33. This kind of phenomenological analysis of temporality in the clinical context is outlined by S. Kay Toombs, "The Temporality of Illness: Four Levels of Experience," *Theoretical Medicine* 11 (1990): 227–42.

34. H. Tristram Engelhardt, *The Foundations of Bioethics* (New York: Oxford University Press, 1996).

Chapter Three

1. Edmund Pellegrino and David C. Thomasma, *The Virtues in Medical Practice* (Oxford: Oxford University Press, 1993).

2. Aristotle, *Nich. Ethics*, 1103a6.

3. Ibid., 1094b 25ff.

4. See, for example, Hans Jonas, "The Practical Uses of Theory," in *The Phenomenon of Life: Toward a Philosophical Biology* (Evanston, IL: Northwestern University Press, [1966] 2001), 206.

5. Hans-Georg Gadamer has also developed a hermeneutic understanding of *phronesis*. *Truth and Method* (New York: Continuum, 1994), 317–29.

6. E. Gatens Robinson, "Clinical Judgement and the Rationality of the Human Sciences," *Journal of Medicine and Philosophy* 11 (1986): 167–78; I. Widdershoven-Heerding, "Medicine

as a Form of Practical Understanding," *Theoretical Medicine* 8 (1987): 179–85; E. B. Beresford, "Can Phronesis Save the Life of Medical Ethics?," *Theoretical Medicine* 17 (1996): 209–24; Kathryn Montgomery Hunter, "Don't Think Zebras": Uncertainty, Interpretation, and the Place of Paradox in Clinical Education," *Theoretical Medicine* 5 (1996): 1–17; Glen McGee, "Phronesis in Clinical Ethics," *Theoretical Medicine* 17, no. 4 (1996): 317–28; D. Davis, "*Phronesis*, Clinical Reasoning and Pellegrino's Philosophy of Medicine," *Theoretical Medicine* 18,nos. 1–2 (1997): 173–95; Kathryn Montgomery, "*Phronesis* and the Misdescription of Medicine: Against *The Medical School Commencement Speech*," in *Bioethics: Ancient Themes in Contemporary Issues*, ed. Mark G. Kuczewski and Ronald Polansky (Cambridge, MA: MIT Press, 2000), 57–66; David Thomasma, "Aristotle, *Phronesis* and Postmodern Bioethics," in *Bioethics*, 67–91; and B. Hofmann, "Medicine as Practical Wisdom (*Phronesis*)," *Poiesis Prax* 1 (2002): 135–49.

7. Stephen Toulmin, "How Medicine Saved the Life of Ethics," *Perspectives in Biology and Medicine* 25, no. 4 (1982): 736–50.

8. D. J. Allan, "The Practical Syllogism," in *Autour D'Aristote: Recueil D'Etudes De Philosophie Ancienne et Medievale offert a Mons. A. Mansion* (Louvain: Publications Universitaires De Louvain, 1955), 325–40; W. F. R. Hardie, *Aristotle's Ethical Theory* (Oxford: Clarendon Press, 1968); T. Ando, *Aristotle's Theory of Practical Cognition* (The Hague: Martinjus Nijhoff, [1958] 1971; J. M. Cooper, *Reason and Human Good in Aristotle* (Cambridge, MA: Harvard University Press, 1975); J. Leguard, "Aristotle's Practical Syllogism" (PhD diss., Department of Philosophy, University of Chicago, 1977), 129.

9. Victor Kal, *On Intuition and Discursive Reasoning in Aristotle* (Leiden: E. J. Brill, 1988).

10. Marjorie Grene, *A Portrait of Aristotle* (London: Faber and Faber Limited, 1963), 111.

11. In an earlier passage Aristotle intimated this strained analogy between *phronesis* and *nous*: "It is opposed, then, to intuitive reason; for intuitive reason is of the limiting premisses, for which no reason can be given, while practical wisdom is concerned with the ultimate particular, which is the object not of scientific knowledge but of perception—not the perception of qualities peculiar to one sense but a perception akin to that by which we perceive that the particular figure before us is a triangle; for in that direction as well as in that of the major premiss there will be a limit. But this is rather perception than practical wisdom, though it is another kind of perception than that of the qualities peculiar to each sense." Aristotle, *Nicomachean Ethics*, trans. W. D. Ross (Oxford, Clarendon Press, 1925), 1142a.

12. "If we take it that Aristotle is saying that *nous* is concerned with both extremes in both realms, practical and theoretical, then all becomes clear: we have universal speculative *nous* (the *nous 'kata tas apodēixis tōn akinetōn horon kai prō-tō-n'* of 1143b2 and 1140b31ff), particular speculative *nous* (the *nous* of particulars which is *aisth-ēsis*, of 1143b6 and 1142a29), particular practical *nous* (the *nous* which is '*en tais praktikais tou eschatou kai endechomenou*' of 143b2), and universal practical *nous* (the *nous* of the hetera protasis of 1143b11). As in speculative matters, so in practical matters, *nous* provides the starting-point and the stopping-point for reasoning. The practical reasoning which is the existence of *phronesis* begins with a conception of an end, a *hypolēpsis* about the purpose of conduct (1140b17); this right conception of an end can itself be called *phronēsis* (1140b13; 1142b34). Practical reasoning ends with a judgement about what is to be done, a self-addressed command (1143a9) or a piece of advice to another (1143a15). This too can be called *nous* (1143a27) whether or not it is backed up in a particular case by a statement of reasons (1143b14)." A. Kenny, *The Aristotelian Ethics: A Study of the Relationship between the Eudemian and Nicomachean Ethics of Aristotle* (Oxford: Clarendon Press, 1978), 171.

13. Allan argues similarly that there is an analogy "between the internal structure of the reasoning of theoretical science, which starts from self-evident principles and ends with the dem-

onstration of the properties of its subject, and that of the phronimos who starts from the highest practical principle, namely the good apprehended by him and converted . . . into an End; and who brings his reasoning down to the particular." (1955). "The Practical Syllogism," in *Autour d'Aristote: Recueil d'études de philosophie ancienne et medievale offert a A. Mansion* (1955), 329. Allan associates this analogy with two passages in Aristotle's *Ethics*, 1142a25–30 and 1143a35 ff.

14. The tension between the particular and the universal is seen clearly in the earlier paragraphs quoted regarding the *phronimos*. Whereas in the first passage Aristotle seems to say that practical reason is concerned only with universals, in the second passage he claims that practical reasoning is concerned with both particulars and universals.

15. G. Richardson Lear, *Happy Lives and the Human Good: An Essay on Aristotle's Nicomachean Ethics* (Princeton, NJ: Princeton University Press, 2004).

16. This association between *phronesis* and medicine, in fact, was already noted by the classicists Marcel Detienne and Jean-Pierre Vernant in their important study of *metis* or cunning intelligence in ancient Greece. Detienne and Vernant note the association with temporality in both ancient cunning or *metis* and *phronesis*. They point out that Aristotle wished to distinguish *phronesis* from *deinotes* or cleverness, an attribute of *metis*, since for the ancient Greeks this type of sly intelligence was associated with sly rogues. Despite this difference in social value between *phronesis* and *metis*, their temporal basis means that they both share a strong resemblance to the medical art. See *Cunning Intelligence in Greek Culture and Society* (Chicago: University of Chicago Press, 1991), 311–13.

17. See in particular Ludwig Edelstein's essay entitled "The Relation of Ancient Philosophy to Medicine," in *Ancient Medicine* (Baltimore, MD: Johns Hopkins University Press, 1967), 349–66.

18. For examinations of the Hippocratic antiphilosophical work *On Ancient Medicine*, see W. H. S. Jones, *Philosophy and Medicine in Ancient Greece* (Baltimore, MD: Johns Hopkins Press, 1946); and Jacques Jouanna, *Hippocrates*, (Baltimore, MD: Johns Hopkins University Press, 1999).

19. That Aristotle was familiar with Hippocrates is clear from the reference to Hippocrates in Aristotle's writing. Jacques Jouanna has argued that Aristotle, the son of a doctor, was obviously familiar with Hippocrates, *Hippocrates* (1999). Of course, as Owsei Temkin notes, the Hippocratic Corpus is not homogenous and was most probably not written by Hippocrates at all; *Hippocrates in a World of Pagans and Christians* (Baltimore, MD: Johns Hopkins University Press, 1991). Nonetheless, it is possible to see a shared cultural understanding amongst the Hippocratic writings that allows one to link them together.

20. The word *empeira* appears both in Plato and in the Hippocratic Corpus. Jacques Jouanna has observed: "In the *Phaedrus*, art (*technè*)—both medical and rhetorical—is opposed to empirie (*empeiria*) and to routine. By contrast, in the Hippocratic Corpus, experience (*peirè*) is the mark of the man who knows. It is synonymous with competence, and always carries a positive connotation. The point of this brief comparative sketch of Hippocratic and Platonic etymology is that it allows us to look beyond the obvious resemblances of the two accounts and actually see the emergence of a conceptual shift that was to have important implications for the theory of scientific knowledge." *Hippocrates* (1999), 257–58.

21. This point has been made by Richard Zaner. See his *Ethics and the Clinical Encounter* (Englewood Cliffs, NJ: Prentice Hall,1988), 148. Additionally, in his dissertation thesis, F. Daniel Davis argues that one can distinguish between the various schools of Hellenistic medicine according to how much emphasis they placed on the ability to learn general principles from individual cases. "Phronesis and the Physician: A Defense of the Practical Paradigm of Clinical

Rationality" (PhD diss., Department of Philosophy, Georgetown University, 1996). See Ludwig Edelstein, *Ancient Medicine* (1967) for a discussion on the three main schools of Hellenistic medicine.

22. While Edmund Pellegrino and David Thomasma have coauthored many publications together, most notably a *Philosophical Basis* and *The Virtues*, and appear to be in essential philosophical concordance with each other, there are some references to which I refer that are specific to Pellegrino. In consequence I shall refer at times both to Pellegrino and Thomasma's work, and at other times only to Pellegrino. For an overview and assessment of Pellegrino's philosophy of medicine, see *Journal of Medicine and Philosophy*, 15, no. 3, devoted to Pellegrino's work. Also see F. Daniel Davis, "*Phronesis*, Clinical Reasoning and Pellegrino's Philosophy of Medicine," *Theoretical Medicine* 18, nos. 1–2 (1997): 173–95.

23. See Edmund Pellegrino and David C. Thomasma, *The Virtues in Medical Practice* (Oxford: Oxford University Press, 1993), chap. 7.

24. Henceforth referred to as "The Anatomy."

25. "Is medicine, then, in any sense an art? Not as the term is used in the current science-art controversy. We have argued that clinical judgments must not be assigned to the realms of the intuitive and ineffable, which find their source in a presumed special intellectual light possessed by clinicians. We would prefer to reserve the word 'art' in medicine for the perfection of the things done by the physician—the craftsmanship without which the decisions taken would be improperly, unsafely, or clumsily done. The art of medicine lies in the degree of perfection each clinician exhibits in history taking, physical examination, performance of manipulative techniques such as surgery, and various diagnostic maneuevers—the work done." Edmund Pellegrino and David C. Thomasma, *A Philosophical Basis of Medical Practice* (Oxford: Oxford University Press, 1981), 147. B. Hoffmann argues that Pellegrino and Thomasma's usage of *phronesis* is more akin to a Hippocratic concept of *techné* than to Aristotelian *phronesis*. And that modeling medicine on Hippocratic *techné* would avoid many pitfalls associated with a *phronesis*-based approach. B. Hoffmann, "Medicine as Practical Wisdom (*Phronesis*)," *Poiesis and Praxis* 1, no. 2 (2002).

26. Marjorie Grene observes insightfully that Pellegrino wanted to disassociate clinical judgment from *techné*, because "many who speak of that kind of skillful performance as 'art not science' are thinking of it as 'intuitive' and so not 'rational.'" "Comments on Pellegrino's 'Anatomy of Clinical Judgment," in *Clinical Judgment: A Critical Appraisal*, ed. H. Tristram Engelhardt, Stuart F. Spicker, and Bernard Towers (Dordrecht: D. Reidel Publishing Company, 1977), 195–96.

27. A similar passage appears in Edmund Pellegrino's "The Anatomy of Clinical Judgments: Some Notes on Right Reason and Right Action," in *Clinical Judgment: A Critical Appraisal*, ed. H. T. Engelhardt et al. (Dordrecht, D. Reidel Publishing Company, 1977), 169–94.

28. "We have seen how the urge to look for clues and to make sense of them is ever alert in our eyes and ears, and in our fears and desires. The urge to understand experience, together with the language referring to experience, is clearly an extension of this primordial striving for intellectual control. The shaping of our conceptions is impelled to move from obscurity to clarity and from incoherence to comprehension, by an intellectual discomfort similar to that by which our eyes are impelled to make clear and coherent the things we see. In both cases we pick out clues which seem to suggest a context in which they make sense as its subsidiary particulars." Michael Polanyi, *Personal Knowledge: Towards a Post-Critical Philosophy* (Chicago: University of Chicago, 1974), 100–101.

29. For other explicit references to intuition in Polanyi, see Michael Polanyi, *Knowing and Being: Essays by Michael Polanyi* (Chicago: The University of Chicago Press, 1969), 143–44 and 201.

30. Castiglioni undoubtedly referred to intuition as an important element in Hippocratic empiricism. Yet, as Jacques Jouanna suggests, the distinction between rationalism and empiricism was foreign to Hippocratic epistemology; *Hippocrates* (1999). Intuition itself is arguably an element of cognitive reasoning that defies the neat divide between rationalism and empiricism.

31. See Michel Foucault, *The Birth of the Clinic* (New York: Vintage Books, 1973). This subject will be analyzed in greater detail in chapter 7.

32. For a brief survey of the wide literature on the question of brain death, see Henry K. Beecher, "Definitions of 'Life and Death' for Medical Science and Practice," *Annals of the New York Academy of Sciences* 169, no. 2 (1970): 471–74; Robert M. Veatch, "The Whole-Brain-Oriented Concept of Death. An Outmoded Philosophical Formulation," *Journal of Thanatology* 3, no. 1 (1975): 13–130; Robert M. Veatch, *Death, Dying and the Biological Revolution: Our Quest for Responsibility* (New Haven: Yale University Press, 1976); Hans Jonas (1978). "The Right to Die," *Hastings Center Report* 8, no. 4 (1978): 31–36; Dan Wikler and Michael B. Green, "Brain Death and Personal Identity," *Philosophy and Public Affairs* 9, no. 2(1980): 105–33; Richard Zaner, *Death: Beyond Whole Brain Criteria* (Dordrecht: Kluwer Academic Press, 1988); Baruch Brody and Amir Halevy, "Brain Death: Reconciling Definitions, Criteria and Tests," *Annals of Internal Medicine*, 119 (1993), 519–25; and Robert Truog, "Is It Time to Abandon Brain-Death?" *Hastings Center Report* 27, no. 1 (1997): 29–37.

33. See David M. Thomasma, *Theoretical Medicine* 5, no. 2 (1984): 181–96.

Chapter Four

1. See, for example, Martha Nussbaum, trans., *De Motu Animalium* (Princeton, NJ: Princeton University Press, 1978).

2. A very similar argument is developed in a recent study by Christopher P. Long. Thus, Long develops the idea that the *aisthesis* of *phronesis* is *nous. The Ethics of Ontology: Rethinking an Aristotelian Legacy* (Albany, New York: State University of New York Press, 2004). See also T. J. McPartland, *Lonergan and the Philosophy of Historical Existence* (Columbia: University of Missouri Press, 2001).

3. This analysis is important for my further philosophical critique of the application of statistics to clinical reasoning in the following chapters.

4. See, for example, J. Leguard, "Aristotle's Practical Syllogism" (PhD diss., Department of Philosophy, University of Chicago, 1977), 7.

5. W. F. R. Hardie, *Aristotle's Ethical Theory* (Oxford: Clarendon Press, 1968), 268.

6. Ibid., 268–69.

7. Hardie, for example, has claimed that "any report of what Aristotle has to say about practical thinking must find a place for the doctrine of the so-called 'practical syllogism'" (ibid., 228).

8. There are, of course, many different interpretations of Aristotle's practical syllogism. My reading relies mainly on Hardie's analysis of the practical syllogism. Hardie has summarized his own position as well as those of his antagonists regarding the practical syllogism as follows: "Yet commentators commonly assert or assume that Aristotle regards the practical syllogism as the proper form of all deliberation and practical reasoning. Burnet says that the analysis of the Good for Man, 'though it is deliberative and not demonstrative will proceed through middle terms

and can only be expressed adequately in the form of a series of practical syllogisms.' Joachim speaks of practical wisdom (*phronesis*) as 'an established power of reasoning or deliberating which expresses itself in syllogisms whose conclusions are . . . actions.' This makes it natural for him to say, since deliberation starts from the thought of an end, that the major premiss 'defines the nature of the end or of some constituent of the end.' Ando takes the standard of moral value' to be 'the highest major premiss' and proposes to study 'the practical syllogism as the form of deliberation.' One conclusion to which the study leads him is that 'the practical syllogism consists of the major premiss which orders one to purpose a value in general, and the minor premiss which recognizes the presence of a value in a particular case.' But in Aristotle's scheme the minor premise does not recognize a value; it merely states a fact. The practical syllogism has to be inflated in order to do the work expected by commentators, and its shape gets distorted in the process, Grant suggests as a form of the practical syllogism: such and such an end is desirable; this step will conduce to the end; taking of the step" (ibid., 249–50).

9. For J. M. Cooper the practical syllogism is only a way of expressing the content of the intuitive perceptual act, and thus does not participate in deliberation. *Reason and Human Good in Aristotle* (Cambridge, MA: Harvard University Press, 1975).

10. Hardie, additionally, takes issue with D. J. Allan's position that the practical syllogism may take either two forms, depending on whether the major premise refers to a rule or and end. Allan's position regarding the practical syllogism is summarized in the following paragraph from his essay, entitled "The Practical Syllogism": "As has been observed above, the practical syllogism may take either of two forms, according as what is expressed in the major premises is a rule or an end (see Sir Alexander Grant, *The Ethics of Aristotle*, (1874), vol. 1, 264–5). In some contexts, actions are subsumed by intuition under general rules, and performed or avoided accordingly; not, I may be added, only by the wise man, but also by the φαῦλος, and in a certain sense by the ἀχρατής. In other contexts, it is said to be a distinctive feature of practical syllogisms that they start from the announcement of an end (*Ethics* 6, 1144a31); and the same view is implied in book 8 (1151a15–19) and in *Eudemian Ethics* (1227b28–32). A particular action is then performed because it is a means, or the first link in a chain of means, leading to the end. Such a means is said to be a 'middle term' in the practical syllogism, and it seems to be termed 'false' either because the agent is mistaken is thinking that it will conduce to the end, or because it is morally unworthy, and a good end ought not to be achieved at such a price." *Autour d'Aristote*, 336.

11. Cooper's understanding of this example of the practical syllogism is in accordance with his view, as has already been seen, that the practical syllogism is not part of actual deliberation. Cooper's full interpretation of Aristotle's paragraph reads as follows: "Now this capacity, though its proper object is the different specific kinds of things, is only exercised on particular instances of these kinds. Thus in our chicken example the agent has the capacity to recognize chicken, a certain specific kind of meat, but of course when he displays this capacity it is by recognizing some particular meat specimen *as* chicken. Hence it is entirely natural for Aristotle to say [1143b2–3] that intelligent agents have intuitive, perceptual knowledge of various types of things (*nous tou eschatou*) while adding that they know the minor premisses of practical syllogisms: it is in these syllogisms that the actual recognitions in which this capacity is exercised are recorded. One knows chicken intuitively; so one knows that *this* and *this* and *this* is chicken. The mention of the minor premiss here is therefore entirely in place, and does not have to be taken as indicating that *eschaton* in this passage refers to something different from that we have found it to refer to earlier in the sixth book. As I interpret the passage, the practical syllogism is implied to lie outside the process of deliberation proper: it enters only with the exercise of the perceptual

capacity that Aristotle says agents must have with regard to the specific types of things ultimately decided on by deliberation as the appropriate means to their ends" (1975, 43–44).

12. "Yet there are various passages which by implication give us hints concerning the several different ways employed by Aristotle when a question of evaluation is unavoidable. That such passages occur bears out our fundamental contention that being and value are actually copresent in human experience. In other words, Aristotle when he expounds his philosophy of nature as a part of his full analysis of being, cannot avoid completely the question of value." W. J. Oates, *Aristotle and the Problem of Value* (Princeton, NJ: Princeton University Press, 1963), 130.

13. "Now if the mark be noble, the cleverness is laudable, but if the mark be bad, the cleverness is mere smartness; hence we call even men of practical wisdom clever or smart. Practical wisdom is not the faculty, but it does not exist without this faculty. And this eye of the soul acquires its formed state not without the aid of virtue, as has been said and is plain; for the syllogisms which deal with acts to be done are things which involve a starting-point, viz. 'since the end, i.e. what is best, is of such and such a nature, whatever it may be (let it for the sake of argument be what we please); and this is not evident except to the good man; for wickedness perverts us and causes us to be deceived about the starting-points of action. Therefore it is evident that it is impossible to be practically wise without being good." (*Nich. Ethics* 1144a, trans. Ross)

14. "Now if what is healthy or good is different for men and for fishes, but what is different; for it is to that which observes well the various matters concerning itself that one ascribes practical wisdom, and it is to this that one will entrust such matters. This is why we say that some even of the lower animals have practical wisdom, viz. those which are found to have a power of foresight with regard to their own life." (*Nich. Ethics*, 1141a25ff, trans. Ross.)

15. Aristotle, *Generation of Animals*, 753 a7–11; *Nich. Ethics*, 1141a25ff.

16. R. B. Onians, *The Origins of European Thought: About the Body, the Mind, the Soul, the World Time and Fate* (Cambridge: Cambridge University Press, 1951), 16–17.

17. Carlo Natali, *The Wisdom of Aristotle* (New York: State University of New York Press, 2001), 74–75.

Chapter Five

1. Ludmilla Jordanova, "The Art and Science of Seeing in Medicine: Physiognomy 1780–1820," in *Medicine and the Five Senses*, ed. W. F. Bynum and R. Porter (Cambridge: Cambridge University Press, 1993), 122–34.

2. J. McMaster, *Reading the Body in the Eighteenth-Century Novel* (New York: Palgrave Macmillan, 2004).

3. Jordanova, "Art and Science of Seeing."

4. Barbara Stafford, *Body Criticism: Imaging the Unseen in Enlightenment Art and Medicine* (Cambridge, MA: MIT Press, 1991), 103.

5. Jean Bottero, "Symptômes, signes, écritures: *Divination et rationalite*" (Paris: Editions du Seuil, 1974).

6. Tamsyn S. Barton locates this phrase in a number of Hippocratic references, i.e., *Epidemics* 2.6.1. Cf. 2.5.1, 2.5.16, 2.5.23, 2.6.14, 2.6.19, 6.4.19; *On Regimen* 1.36.46., 6.15. See p. 208, n45, in *Power and Knowledge: Astrology, Physiognomics, and Medicine under the Roman Empire* (Ann Arbor: University of Michigan Press, 1994).

7. The image of the snub nose, which occurred also in the example of human reasoning cited in the previous chapter from the *De Anima* associated with the practical syllogism, suggests another shared cultural reference between Aristotle and the Hippocratic Corpus. In both cases the snub

nose is metonymic. In this example in Aristotle it stands in for the whole face, whereas for the Hippocratic physiognomist, the snub nose indicates an honest character. The snub nose occurs numerously in different places in Aristotle. See, for example, bk. 6, ch. 1 of Aristotle's *Metaphysics*.

8. The most important classical text on physiognomy is entitled *Physiognomies* and for a long time was attributed to Aristotle. There is general academic consensus that this text was not in fact written by Aristotle, and is commonly referred to as "pseudo-Aristotelian." I shall not refer to this text in my discussion of physiognomy in Aristotle.

9. Tamsyn Barton (1994) has pointed out the association between rhetoric and physiognomy in the ancient world. Thus, for the rhetor, the character of the speaker, or ethos, was revealed by his body. I am reliant here on Tamsyn Barton's discussion in her book on physiognomy that elucidates the connection between physiognomy and Aristotle's enthymeme. She in turn was indebted for her insights to an unpublished paper by Michael Burnyeat.

10. See Aristotle's *Rhetoric* 2.22.1395b21–26. Cf. 1.11.1355a, 8–14. (Cited in Barton, *Power and Knowledge*, 104–5.)

11. M. Detienne and J. P. Vernant, *Cunning Intelligence in Greek Culture and Society* (Chicago: University of Chicago Press, 1978).

12. The ambivalence toward animality within human reasoning can be traced back to a dual sense of the animal-human relation. On the one hand, as mentioned, the association of humans as animals can refer to the derogatory consideration of bestiality as monstrosity. This negative sense of animality has been traced back at least to Plato. See Mary Midgley, *Beast and Man: The Roots of Human Nature* (New York: Routledge, [1979] 2002). Secondly, animality refers simply to a class of biological beings, of which the human being is particular owing to the faculty of reason and language going back to Aristotle's famous definition of the human being as "*zoon logon ekhon*," a living being capable of speech (Aristotle, *Politics*, 1253a). See also Hanna Arendt, *The Human Condition* (Chicago: University of Chicago Press, 1958). It is this latter sense of animality that is associated with the corporeal basis of human reason, and that relates animal and human rationality in both physiognomy and *phronesis*.

13. For a more complete historical description of physiognomy, see Graeme Tytler, *Physiognomy in the European Novel: Faces and Fortunes* (Princeton, NJ: Princeton University Press, 1982); Christopher Rivers, *Face Value: Physiognomical Thought and the Legible Body in Marivaux, Lavater, Balzac, Gautier, and Zola* (Madison: University of Wisconsin Press, 1994).

14. Rivers, *Face Value*, 24.

15. Ibid.

16. Besides relating humans and animals, this syllogism is important because of its syllogistic features. The relation between physiognomy and Aristotle's rhetorical syllogism has already been referred to. Rivers cites Jacques Andre in pointing out the syllogistic structure of the ethnological principle, where "if a man looks like a hog, and if hogs are known to be gluttonous and lazy, then it follows that the man is also gluttonous and lazy" (ibid., 22–23).

17. Ibid., 29.

18. Judith Wechsler has provided the following chronology of Lavater's incredibly successful publications: "His physiognomic study first appeared in Germany in 1775–78 (J. C. Lavater, *Physiognomische Fragmente zur Beförderung der Menschenkenntnis und Menschenliebe*, Leipzig and Winterthur 1775–78). It was published in France between 1781 and 1803, under the title *Essai sur la physiognomie destine a faire connaitre l'homme at a le faire aimer*, and then in a more popular and successful edition, annotated and illustrated in four volumes in 1806–9, edited by Dr Moreau de la Sarthe, under the title *L'Art de connaitre les hommes par la physionomie*, and reissued in 1820 in ten volumes. (The English edition translated by T. Holcroft, *Essay on Physi-*

ognomy, for the Promotion of Knowledge and the Love of Mankind, first appeared in London in three volumes in 1789. There were numerous other editions in all three languages, in full and abridges and it was also widely imitated and parodied. By 1810 there were fifty-five editions, and, by the 1840s, 156 publications.)" *A Human Comedy: Physiognomy and Caricature in Nineteenth Century Paris* (Chicago: University of Chicago Press, 1982), 324. For fuller studies of Lavater, see Olivier Guinaudeau, *Jean-Gaspard Lavater* (Paris: F. Alcan, 1924); Ellis Shookman, ed., *The Faces of Physiognomy: Interdisciplinary Approaches to Johann Caspar Lavater* (Rochester, NY: Camden House, 1993).

19. Lucy Hartley, *Physiognomy and the Meaning of Expression in Nineteenth-Century Culture* (Cambridge: Cambridge University Press, 2001), 32–33.

20. Hartley, *Physiognomy and the Meaning*, 11.

21. Ibid., 29.

22. The Swiss mathematician Jacques Bernoulli (1654–1705) was the first author to devote a book wholly dedicated to establishing the fundamental principles of probability. His famous *Ars Conjectandi* was published posthumously in 1713. It already suggested the idea of inverse probability, essential to modern statistics. In the section entitled "Pars Quarta," Bernoulli attempted to prove that if the number of observations is made sufficiently large, any previously determined degree of accuracy can be achieved. For more complete discussions on Bernoulli see, H. M. Walker, *Studies in the History of Statistical Method* (New York: Arno Press, [1929] 1975); Stephen M. Stigler, *The History of Statistics: The Measurement of Uncertainty before 1900* (Cambridge, MA: Belknap Press, 1986); Gerd Gigerenzer et al., *The Empire of Chance: How Probability Changes Science and Everyday Life* (Cambridge: Cambridge University Press, 1989); Anders Hald, *A History of Mathematical Statistics from 1750–1930* (New York: John Wiley & Sons, Inc., 1998).

23. Hald, *History of Mathematical Statistics*.

24. For further analyses of Quetelet, see Theodore M. Porter, *The Rise of Statistical Thinking* (Princeton, NJ: Princeton University Press, 1988); Allan Sekula, "The Body and the Archive," *October* 39 (1986), 3–64; Stigler, *History of Statistics*.

25. "Statement of the Sizes of Men in Different Countries of Scotland, Taken from the Local Militia," *Edinburgh Medical and Surgical Journal* 13 (1817): 260–64.

26. Anders Hald notes about this table that "the text of the last column should be changed to 'Proportional Number Calculated.' The numbers in columns 3 and 8 are relative frequencies summing to 1.0000." Hald, *History of Mathematical Statistics from 1750 to 1930* (New York: John Wiley & Sons, Inc., 1998), 596.

27. Frances Clegg, in a statistical primer for students, has defined the bell-shaped curve as follows: "The normal distribution is a bell-shaped curve . . . Its main feature is that the three measures of central tendency, the mean, median and mode, all lie at the same place on the curve. That is to say, they all have the same, or nearly the same value. . . . the normal distribution is always bell-shaped. As it was 'discovered' by the mathematician Gauss, it is sometimes called the Gaussian distribution." See *Simple Statistics: A Course Book for the Social Sciences* (Cambridge: Cambridge University Press, [1982] 1990).

28. Sekula, "Body and the Archive."

29. Stephen Stigler (1986) has noted that Quetelet constructed his table based on the binomial distribution itself, rather than on the approximating normal distribution.

30. Thus one sees in Quetelet the element of social control or policing that the philosopher of science Ian Hacking claims is intrinsic to Western statistics. See *The Taming of Chance* (Cambridge: Cambridge University Press, 1990).

31. These divisions follow those laid out by Ruth Cowan, "Nature and Nurture: The Interplay of Biology and Politics in the Work of Francis Galton," in *Studies in History of Biology*, ed. William Coleman and Camille Limoges (Baltimore, MD: Johns Hopkins University Press, 1977), 1:133–208.

32. Ibid., 150.

33. Karl Pearson, *The Life, Letters and Labours of Francis Galton* (Cambridge: Cambridge University Press, 1924), 2:92.

34. Unlike Darwin, as Ruth Cowan has noted, Galton was fixed in the eugenic belief in the impossibility of inheriting acquired characteristics ("Nature and Nurture").

35. Ibid., 150.

36. Galton was acquainted with Quetelet and met with him personally in 1861. See Hans-Jorg Rheinberger and Staffan Müeller-Wille, *Heredity: History and Culture of a Biological Concept* (Chicago: University of Chicago Press, 2011).

37. Francis Galton, *Memories of My Life* (London: Methuen & Co, 1908), 304.

38. J. Herschel, "Quetelet on Probabilites," *Edinburgh Review* 92 (1850): 1–57.

39. Stephen M. Stigler, *Statistics on the Table: The History of Statistical Concepts and Methods* (Cambridge, MA: Harvard University Press, 1999), 177.

40. Ruth Cowan and Stephen Stigler have both provided excellent reviews of Galton's discovery of correlation, upon which this analysis is reliant. See Ruth S. Cowan, "Francis Galton's Statistical Ideas: The Influence of Eugenics," *Isis* 63 (1972): 509–28; Stephen M. Stigler, "Francis Galton's Account of the Invention of Correlation," *Statistical Science* 4, no. 2 (1989): 73–79; Stigler, *Statistics on the Table*.

41. Stigler, *History of Statistics*.

42. Francis Galton, "Regression towards Mediocrity in Hereditary Stature," *Journal of the Anthropological Institute* 15 (1885): 246–63.

43. See Cowan, "Francis Galton's Statistical Ideas"; Ruth S. Cowan, "Nature and Nurture"; Victor L. Hilts, "Statistics and Social Science," in *Foundations of the Scientific Method*, ed. Ronald Giere and Richard Westfall (Bloomington: Indiana University Press, 1973), 206–33; Rheinberger and Müeller-Wille, *Heredity*. Cowan refers to Galton's obsession with eugenics as an *idée fixe* that provides the key to understanding his work on heredity and statistics.

44. Stigler, "Francis Galton's Account," 73–79.

45. Galton's theories of "stirp" or germ plasm are most clearly elaborated in two articles of his: "Blood Relationship," *Proceedings of the Royal Society*, no. 20 (1872): 394–402; and "A Theory of Heredity," *Contemporary Review* (1875): 80–95.

46. Anders Hald, *History of Mathematical Statistics*, 604–5.

47. Galton's composite method has been succinctly described by Alan Sekula (1986).

48. Sekula, "Body and the Archive."

49. Porter, *Rise of Statistical Thinking*, 139–40.

50. Karl Pearson, *The Life, Letters and Labours of Francis Galton* (Cambridge: Cambridge University Press, 1924), vol. 2, 286.

51. See Pearson, *Life, Letters and Labours of Francis Galton* (Cambridge: Cambridge University Press, 1923), chap. 12, "Photographic Researches and Portraiture."

52. Lucy Hartley, *Physiognomy and the Meaning of Expression in Nineteenth-Century Culture* (2001), 14.

53. Francis Galton, "Hereditary Talent and Character," *Macmillan's Magazine* 12 (1865): 318–27.

54. Pearson, *Life, Letters and Labours*, 2:211.

55. Lucy Hartley, *Physiognomy and the Meaning*, 14.

56. Ibid.

57. Susan Buck-Morss, *The Origin of Negative Dialectics* (Sussex: Harvester Press, 1977); *The Dialectics of Seeing: Walter Benjamin and the Arcades Project* (Cambridge, MA: MIT Press, 1989).

58. Buck-Morss, *Dialects of Seeing*, 67.

59. Rivers, *Face Value*, 112.

60. Ibid., 115–16.

61. This nineteenth-century concern with gait is best exemplified in the work of the criminologist Cesare Lombroso. See *Crime: Its Causes and Remedies* (Boston: Little, Brown and Company, 1911); S. J. Gould, *The Mismeasure of Man* (New York: W. W. Norton & Company, 1981).

62. Daniel J. Kevles, *In the Name of Eugenics: Genetics and the Uses of Human Heredity* (New York: Knopf, 1985).

Chapter Six

1. The use of "clinical reasoning" in this chapter is in accordance with the definition provided by Barrows and Tamblyn as the cognitive process that is necessary to valuate and manage a patient's medical problem. *Problem Based Learning: An Approach to Medical Education* (New York: Springer, 1980).

2. Theodore Porter, *Trust in Numbers: The Pursuit of Objectivity in Science and Public Life* (Princeton, NJ: Princeton University Press, 1995).

3. Ibid. The law of large numbers was defined by the French statistician S. D. Poisson in 1837: "All manner of things are subject to a universal law that we may call the *law of large numbers*. It consists of this: if we observe a very large number of events of the same nature, dependent upon the constant causes and upon causes that vary irregularly (sometimes in one way, sometimes in another, but not in a deterministic sense), we will find the ratios between the numbers of these events are approximately constant." *Recherches sur la probabilités des jugements en matière criminelle et en matière civile: Précédées des règles générales du calcul des probabilités* (Paris: Bachelier). Quoted in Stigler, *History of Statistics*, 185.

4. This term was coined by Ian Hacking in *The Taming of Chance* (Cambridge: Cambridge University Press, 1990). This term encapsulates the seeming paradox that the greater the indeterminism determined by modern statistics, the greater its control over determinism.

5. The resistance to mathematical objectivity within clinical medicine has a long history going back to at least the thirteenth century. See Richard H. Shryock, "The History of Quantification in Medical Science," in *Quantification: A History of the Meaning of Measurement in the Natural and Social Sciences*, ed. Harry Woolf (Indianapolis, IN: Bobbs-Merrill Company, Inc., 1961), 85–107. A more detailed historical review of the history of medical statistics will be provided in the following chapter.

6. Decision analysis, for its part, refers to the statistical evaluation of the process of cognition in decision making. Clinical decision analysis refers to the application of statistical methods to evaluate the cognitive processes of decision making in medicine.

7. William Meadow and Cass. R. Sunstein, "Statistics, Not Experts," *Duke Law Journal* 51, no. 2 (2001): 629–46.

8. P. Meehl, *Clinical Versus Statistical Prediction* (Minneapolis: University of Minnesota Press, 1954), 4.

9. Stephen Henry, "Recognizing Tacit Knowledge in Medical Epistemology," *Theoretical Medicine and Bioethics* 27, no. 3 (2006): 187–213.

10. Michael Polanyi refers to intuition in his major work, *Personal Knowledge*. He also explicitly addresses intuition in his essay on intuition in scientific reasoning, "Creative Imagination," in *Society, Economics & Philosophy: Selected Papers of Michael Polanyi*, ed. R. T. Allen (New Brunswick, NJ: Transaction Publishers, 1997), 249–66; and *Science, Faith and Society* (Oxford: Oxford University Press, 1946). Polanyi does not argue for the traditional philosophical conception of intuition as incorrigible certainty, but as an element of practical reasoning. While intuition covers over hidden logical associations, this does not preclude, but rather requires that we spend time trying to ascertain the tacit elements of scientific reasoning. Clinical intuition as used in here shares this meaning with Polanyi's notion of practical intuition. As such, it must be distinguished from philosophical intuition—for example, Kantian intuition—as well as the feminist literature around intuition as a kind of sixth sense. Polanyi's theory of tacit knowing will be elucidated in more detail toward the conclusion of this chapter.

11. Tim Thornton, "Tacit Knowledge as the Unifying Factor in Evidence-Based Medicine and Clinical Judgment," *Philosophy, Ethics, and Humanities in Medicine* 1, no. 2 (2006), http://www.peh-med.com/content/1/1/2.

12. In another article, David Smith also attempts to find the balance between evidence-based medicine and Polanyi's theory of tacit knowing. "Viewpoint: Envisioning the Successful Integration of EBM and Humanism in the Clinical Encounter: Fantasy or Fallacy," *Academic Medicine* 83, no. 3 (2008): 268–73. Smith criticizes those who attempt to displace evidence-based medicine by tacit knowing. Yet, as argued in this paper, the epistemological issue is not in favoring either tacit knowing or statistical epidemiology, but in mediating between the two, a process which is better accounted for through clinical epidemiology than evidence-based medicine.

13. Sackett derives the hypothetico-deductive terminology from Peter Medawar's study on *Induction and Intuition in Scientific Thought* (Philadelphia: American Philosophical Society, 1969).

14. Evidence-based medicine was first formally conceptualized at McMaster University in Canada, which continues to be a primary center of evidence-based medical practice. For a detailed study of the evidence-based medicine movement, see Jeanne Daly, *Evidence-Based Medicine and the Search for a Science of Clinical Care* (Berkeley: University of California Press, 2005).

15. S. Buetow, "Beyond Evidence-Based Medicine: Bridge-Building a Medicine of Meaning," *Journal of Evaluation in Clinical Practice* 8, no. 2 (2002): 103–8.

16. Geoffrey R. Norman "Examining the Assumptions of Evidence-Based Medicine," *Journal of Evaluation in Clinical Practice* 5, no. 2 (1999): 139–47.

17. The opposition to evidence-based medicine by the mainstream medical establishment was not universal, and explains in part the movement's success. For example, Frank Davidoff, editor of the *Annals of Internal Medicine*, threw his weight firmly behind the new statistical clinical discipline. See "Evidence-Based Medicine: Why All the Fuss?," *Annals of Internal Medicine* 122 (1995): 727.

18. For a sociological analysis of evidence-based medicine's critique of medical authority, see Tom Marshall, "Scientific Knowledge in Medicine: A New Clinical Epistemology," *Journal of Evaluation in Clinical Practice* 3 (1997): 135–38.

19. Ross Upshur has taken Polychronis to task for mistakenly confusing probabilistic reasoning with mathematical certainty. "Certainty, Probability and Abduction: Why We Should Look to C. S. Peirce Rather than Godel for a Theory of Clinical Reasoning," *Journal of Evalu-*

ation in Clinical Practice 3, no. 3 (1997): 201–6. Yet, the mistaken assumption of attempting to found a scientific medicine based on the mathematical precision provided by statistical probabilism is precisely the error that Polychronis claims is committed by proponents of evidence-based medicine.

20. For a comparison of Fisher and Bradford Hill, see the series of papers published in the *International Journal of Epidemiology* 32 (2003): 922–48.

21. A. R. Jadad, ed., *Randomised Controlled Trials: A User's Guide* (London: BMJ Books, 1998).

22. Austin Bradford Hill, "The Clinical Trial," *British Medical Bulletin* 7 (1951): 278–82; "The Clinical Trial," *New England Journal of Medicine* 247 (1952): 113–19; "Memories of the British Streptomycin Trial in Tuberculosis: The First Randomized Clinical Trial," *Controlled Clinical Trials* 11 (1990): 77–79.

23. Richard Horton, "Common Sense and Figures: The Rhetoric of Validity in Medicine," *Statistics in Medicine* 19 (2000), 3149–64.

24. While Bradford Hill did not articulate how this would work, the problem is one of combining statistical data with tacit knowing pertaining to individuals. At the very least Bradford Hill identified the problem of applying statistical data to individual contexts, even though he did not provide a detailed solution to this conundrum.

25. He is also somewhat infamously remembered for his opposition to the first statistical study authored by Richard Doll and Bradford Hill, which unequivocally associates lung cancer with smoking.

26. Fisher's concept of specifying rigorous uncertainty is comparable with the Viennese philosopher Karl Popper's famous theory of falsifiability.

27. The uncritical reliance on randomized controlled trials has come under increased scrutiny during the last few years. For another critique of evidence-based medicine's reliance on randomized controlled trials, see J. W. Sleigh, "Logical Limits of Randomized Controlled Trials," *Journal of Evaluation in Clinical Practice* 3, no. 2 (1997): 145–48; Ted Kaptchuk, "The Double-Blind, Randomized, Placebo-Controlled Trial: Gold Standard or Golden Calf?," *Journal of Clinical Epidemiology* 54 (2001): 541–49; D. G. Altman, "Statistics in Medical Journals: Some Recent Trends," *Statistics in Medicine* 19 (2000): 3281–84; and J. Grossman and F. Mackenzie, "The Randomized Controlled Trial: Gold Standard, or Merely Standard?," *Perspectives in Biology and Medicine* 48, no. 4 (2005): 516–34.

28. Davidoff, Case, and Fried, "Evidence-Based Medicine," 727.

29. G. H Guyatt et al., "Determining Optimal Therapy: Randomized Trials in Individual Patients," *New England Journal of Medicine* 314, no. 14 (1986): 889–92.

30. John R. Paul, "Clinical Epidemiology," *Journal of Clinical Investigation* 17 (1938): 539.

31. For a more complete description of the influence on and relation between Feinstein and Sackett and the discipline of clinical epidemiology, see Daly, *Evidence-Based Medicine.*

32. Other notable publications by Feinstein on the subject of clinical judgment include: "The Basic Elements of Clinical Science," *Journal of Chronic Diseases* 16 (1963): 1125–33; "Scientific Methodology in Clinical Medicine: Introduction, Principles and Concepts," *Annals of Internal Medicine* 61, no. 3 (1964), 564–79; "Clinical Epidemiology: I–III,." *Annals of Internal Medicine:* 69, nos. 4, 5, and 6 (1968): 807–20, 1037–61, 1287–311; *Clinical Biostatistics* (Saint Louis, MO: C. V. Mosby, 1977); "An Additional Basic Science for Clinical Medicine, Pts. I-III," *Annals of Internal Medicine* 99 (1983): 393–97, 544–50, 705–12; *Clinical Epidemiology: The Architecture of*

Clinical Research (Philadelphia, PA: W. B. Saunders Company, 1985); *Clinimetrics* (New Haven, CT: Yale University Press, 1987).

33. This passage is reminiscent of the language of the "gaze" rendering the truth of visible things that Michel Foucault describes in association with the birth of clinical medicine in Paris at the beginning of the nineteenth century. *The Birth of the Clinic* (New York: Vintage Books, 1973).

34. Jerry H. Gill, *Michael Polanyi's Postmodern Philosophy* (Albany: State University of New York Press, 2000), 39.

35. Stephen G. Henry, Richard M. Zaner, and Robert S. Dittus, "Moving Beyond Evidence-Based Medicine." *Academic Medicine* 82, no. 3 (2007): 292–97.

36. Eric Cassell, *Talking with Patients*, vol. 1, *The Theory of Doctor-Patient Communication* (Cambridge, MA: MIT Press, 1985).

37. Polanyi, "Creative Imagination."

38. Uri Wilensky, "What is Normal Anyway? Therapy for Epistemological Anxiety," *Educational Studies in Mathematics: Special Issue on Computational Environments in Mathematics Education* 33, no. 2 (1997): 171–202.

39. Wilensky's approach to mathematical education is to allow the learner to make connections between the microrules of probability and the resultant macrostatistical distributions as a therapy for "epistemological anxiety" in understanding statistics.

40. Daniel Kahneman and Amos Tversky, "Judgment under Uncertainty: Heuristics and Biases," *Science* 185 (1974): 124–13.

Chapter Seven

1. D. L. Sackett and S. E. Straus, "Finding and Applying Evidence during Clinical Ward Rounds: The 'Evidence Cart,'" *Journal of the American Medical Association* 280 (1998): 1336–38.

2. This has been well described in Anne Fagot-Largeault's analysis, *Les Causes de la mort histoire naturelle et facteurs de risque* (Paris: Librairie Philosophique J. Vrin, 1989). Whereas Fagot-Largeault's work focuses on statistics in relation to the causes of death, this analysis applies a similar analysis of statistics in relation to clinical reasoning.

3. See, in particular, Alvan R. Feinstein, "The Diagnostic Taxonomy of Disease: Past and Present," in *Clinical Judgment* (Baltimore, MD: Williams Wilkins, 1967), 72–88.

4. I am reliant on the work of Lester King in this analysis of analogy in clinical reasoning. As a medical historian King has written comprehensively on the shift in thinking heralded by "critical" medicine. He provides a working definition of his use of "critical" in the following paragraph: "I do not want to offer any general definition of the word 'critical,' but I use it in this sense: What did he accept as evidence? What did he accept as valid reasoning? How aware was he of his assumptions? How much scrutiny did he devote to terms and concepts that others accepted without thought or question? How much did he doubt, and what did he take to resolve his doubts? These are particular aspects of the term 'critical' in the sense that I use it." "Empiricism and Rationalism in the Works of Thomas Sydenham," *Bulletin of the History of Medicine* 44 (1970): 9.

5. The new approach to evidence is famously illustrated in Molière's satire, *Le Malade*. In this play the foolish doctor replies when asked how a certain powder causes sleep, that it has a *virtus ¿ormativa* (i.e., the power to induce sleep). The problem with the *virtus dormativa* for Molière and other moderns is that it does not take account of the modern scientific concept of cause and effect. For a discussion of the sleep-inducing properties of opium in Molière and late

seventeenth-century medical thought, see Lester S. King, *The Philosophy of Medicine: The Early Eighteenth Century* (Cambridge, MA: Harvard University Press, 1978), 187–89.

6. Central to Bacon's philosophy was a questioning of ancient authority. Bacon famously denounced the Aristotelian concern for first principles in favor of mechanisms of immediate cause and effect. For an excellent analysis of the influence of Bacon on seventeenth-century science, see Richard Foster Jones, *Ancients and Moderns: A Study of the Rise of the Scientific Movement in Seventeenth-Century England* (Berkeley: University of California Press, 1975).

7. Lester S. King, "Evidence and Its Evaluation in Eighteenth-Century Medicine," *Bulletin of the History of Medicine* 50 (1976): 174–90. The development of analogy in medicine did not originate, however, in eighteenth-century medicine. As King notes, analogy as a form of inductive reasoning was already present in Hippocratic thinking, and analogy is the basis of many sophisticated statistical tests in modern medical science (*Philosophy of Medicine*). For a fuller discussion on the relation between analogy and inference, see Mary B. *Hesse, Models and Analogies in Science* (Notre Dame, IN: University of Notre Dame Press), 72–75.

8. Stigler, "Francis Galton's Account," 73–79.

9. Porter, *Rise of Statistical Thinking*, 4.

10. The birth of modern statistics is generally traced back to a correspondence about a gambling problem between the mathematicians Pascal and Fermat in 1654. The first stage of statistics that developed around this time, the so-called classical epoch of statistics was predominantly concerned with measuring astronomical errors of observation.

11. Like most historians and philosophers of statistics, I refer in this chapter to theories of probability and statistics interchangeably. Ian Hacking mentions two elements associated with theories of probability and statistics, respectively (i.e., "physical indeterminism" and "statistical information developed for purposes of social control"). *The Taming of Chance* (Cambridge: Cambridge University Press, 1990), 5–6. For Hacking, this political association of statistics in Western polities is indissociable from the way that these polities "make up people." This relation of statistics to individuality will be important for this evaluation of the significance of applying statistics to clinical reasoning. The element of social control that Hacking emphasizes is intrinsic to the very term "statistics." Thus, the word *statistik* is attributed to the writings of Gottfried Achenwall (1719–72). For Achenwall and other eighteenth-century statisticians, statistics did not refer to enumeration so much as to verbal description of political and social facts. See Walker, *Studies in the History*, 32.

12. Walker, *Studies in the History*, 30.

13. In his *Enquiry Concerning Human Understanding* (1748), the Scottish Enlightenment philosopher David Hume (1711–76) famously questioned the validity of induction. Thus, Hume pointed out that regarding matters of fact known from observation, there is no logical reason to infer the validity of inferential causation. Thus, simply because the sun rose today does not mean that it will necessarily rise tomorrow. While it is reasonable to accept the "authority of experience" in day-to-day life, this principle does not withstand philosophical scrutiny. Similarly, in his *Treatise of Human Nature* (1739), Hume questioned the validity of the direct relation between cause and effect pertaining to data derived from sensible perception. Hume's question regarding the place of induction and causality in science has come to be known as the problem of inductivism, and will be dealt with directly in the following chapter.

14. D. L. Sackett, R. B. Haynes, G. H. Guyatt, and P. Tugwell, *Clinical Epidemiology: A Basic Science for Clinical Medicine* (Boston: Little Brown, 1991).

15. The belief that clinical reasoning pertaining to particular individuals cannot be reduced to numerical models has been traced back as far as the thirteenth century. See Richard H.

Shryock, *The Development of Modern Medicine: An Interpretation of the Social and Scientific Factors Involved* (New York: Oxford University Press, 1948).

16. For a review of Bernoulli and Laplace's medical statistics, see Walker, *Studies in the History*, 28–29; Abraham M. Lilienfeld and David Lilienfeld, "What Else Is New? An Historical Excursion," *American Journal of Epidemiology*, 105 (1977): 169–79.

17. Lorraine Daston attributes Laplace's belief in the efficacy of probability theory in all aspects of analysis to the influence of Etienne Condillac's empiricist epistemology. *Classical Probability in the Enlightenment* (Princeton, NJ: Princeton University Press, 1988). All ideas according to this theory are derived from sense experience. Subjective beliefs could in a well-disciplined mind attain mathematical and objective order. Laplace summed this perspective up in saying that probabilistic theory was "only common sense reduced to a calculus." Pierre S. Laplace, *A Philosophical Essay on Probabilities* (New York: Wiley, [1814] 1951), 196.

18. It is interesting to note here Laplace's early critique of inductive and analogical reasoning from the perspective of probabilism, since it is precisely this critique that will resurface in the contemporary debate around the application of statistics to clinical reasoning. Laplace is unusual, however, in having argued for determinism to make sense of a probabilistic universe. Patrick Suppes has observed that Laplace dispels the illusion "that because random happenings may be found everywhere, the analysis of phenomena somehow becomes too complex, too disorderly, and consequently too difficult to leave any hope for the development of systematic theory." *Probabilistic Metaphysics* (Oxford: Basil Blackwell, 1984), 27.

19. Shryock, *Development of Modern* Medicine, 101.

20. J. Rosser Matthews provides a similar comparison between Pierre Louis and Claude Bernard in his fine study, *Quantification and the Quest for Medical Certainty* (Princeton, NJ: Princeton University Press, 1995). This present analysis extends the comparison to include Xavier Bichat.

21. J. P. Vandenbroucke, "Evidence Based Medicine and '*medicine d'observation*,'" *Journal of Clinical Epidemiology* 49, no. 12 (1996): 1335–38.

22. For discussion on Pierre Louis, see also Shryock, "History of Quantification," 85–107; Porter, *Rise of Statistical Thinking*; Edmund A. Gehan and Noreen A. Lemak, *Statistics in Medical Research* (New York: Plenum Medical Book Co., 1994); Fagot-Largeault, *Causes de la mort*; and Matthews, *Quantification and the Quest*.

23. Attributing a direct historical link between Pierre Louis and the contemporary evidence-based medicine movement is epistemologically problematic because of Louis's more nuanced application of statistics to medicine—one that took full cognizance of the clinical context. Thus, while Pierre Louis argued for a new type of medical epistemology based on the tabulation of information at a population level, he took pains to differentiate himself from the statistical anthropometry of Quetelet. See Matthews, *Quantification and the Quest*, 29. Additionally, as Alfredo Morabia has recently argued, the methodological approach of evidence-based medicine in emphasizing statistical epidemiological methods over clinical observation is not in accordance with Louis's more subtle application. (Morabia developed this argument in paper at a conference on evidence-based medicine at the College de France, Paris, which I attended. "*Pierre Louis ou l'utilisation de méthodes appropriées en médecine*," Séminaire de la Chaire: Histoire et philosophie de la médecine scientifique [2004].)

24. This analysis of Bichat draws largely on Philippe Huneman's excellent study of neovitalism in Bichat. See *Bichat, la vie et la mort* (Paris: Presse Universitaires de France, 1998). Huneman has demonstrated how Bichat's science of life posited a particular form of neovitalism that did not eschew the scientific or experimental method. Rather, Bichat's anatomo-pathological

correlate was part of an attempt to develop a science of life removed from the type of science that has inorganic bodies for objects.

25. Huneman, *Bichat.*

26. For a more extensive analysis of the relation between Bichat and Comte, see Fagot-Largeault, *Causes de la mort,* sec. 5.1.

27. It is, perhaps, not unusual that Bernard as an experimental physiologist should oppose statistics out of the same concern to protect individual clinical experience as shown by clinicians. Bernard perceived his scientific method as the assessment of the physiological function in the laboratory of individual organisms. One finds a similar resistance to mathematical theorizing in Evelyn Fox Keller's description of twentieth-century experimental biologists. See *Making Sense of Life: Explaining Biological Development with Models, Metaphors, and Machines* (Cambridge, MA: Harvard University Press, 2002).

28. An excellent analysis of Bernard's attitude towards statistics is provided by Fagot-Largeault, *Causes de la mort.*

29. K. Codell Carter, *The Rise of Causal Concepts of Disease: Case Histories* (Aldershot: Ashgate, 2003).

30. Alfred S. Evans, "Causation and Disease: A Chronological Journey," *American Journal of Epidemiology* 108 (1978): 249–58.

31. Huneman, *Bichat,* 101–2.

32. Ibid.

33. Ibid., 97.

34. Fagot-Largeault, *Causes de la mort,* 5.0.

35. Ibid., 5.1.2.

36. Alfred S. Evans, "Causation and Disease: The Henle-Koch Postulate Revisited," *Yale Journal of Biology and Medicine* 49 (1976): 175–95; "Causation and Disease: A Chronological Journey" (1978).

37. R. J. Huebner, "The Virologist's Dilemma," *Annals of New York Academy of Sciences* 67 (1957): 430–45.

38. See Austin Bradford Hill, "The Environment and Disease: Association or Causation," *Proceedings of the Royal Society of Medicine* 58 (1965): 295–300. Besides strength of association, the other criteria include consistency of observations in different places and at different times; specificity (exposure leads to a particular illness); temporality (exposure must precede illness); biological gradient (the greater the exposure the greater the risk or severity of disease); plausibility; coherence; experiment; and analogy.

39. See also Georges Canguilhem, *The Normal and the Pathological* (New York: Zone Books, [1978] 1989).

40. "For Morgagni, the seat was the point of insertion in the organism of the chain of causalities; it was identified with its ultimate link. For Bichat and his successors, the notion of seat is freed from the causal problematic (and in this respect, they are the heirs of the clinicians); it is directed towards the future of the disease rather than to its past; the seat is the point from which the pathological organization radiates. Not the *final cause,* but the *original site.* It is in this sense that the fixation onto a corpse of a segment of immobile space may resolve the problems presented by the temporal developments of a disease." Michel Foucault, *The Birth of the Clinic: An Archaeology of Medical Perception* (New York: Vintage Books, 1973).

41. Rom Harré has highlighted the difference between the two opposing paradigms of scientific knowledge (i.e., the "explanatory" biological or medical paradigm that is closer to the Aristotelian epistemology, than to "descriptive" positivism). See *The Philosophies of Science*

(Oxford: Oxford University Press, 1972), chap. 6; and Fagot-Largeault, *Causes de la mort*, A0.2–2.

42. For the original article detailing the ecological fallacy, see W. S. Robinson, "Ecological Correlations and the Behavior of Individuals," *Journal of the American Statistical Association* 30 (1950): 517–36. For a more recent evaluation of Robinson see S. V. Subramanian et al., "Revisiting Robinson: The Perils of Individualistic and Ecologic Fallacy," *International Journal of Epidemiology* 38 (2009): 342–60.

43. Farr pioneered the statistical classification of disease while working in the office of the Registrar-General for England and Wales between 1838 and 1879. For an interesting article on Farr and the individual in statistics, see V. L. Hilts, "William Farr (1807–83) and the 'Human Unit,'" *Victorian Studies* 14, no. 2 (1970): 143–50.

44. This obliteration of the empirical individual in the average was a sought after effect of nineteenth-century statistics. This is exemplified in a statistical report by four mathematicians, including the important statistician Poisson, presented in Paris, on October 5, 1835, to the French Academy of Sciences: "In statistical affairs . . . the first care before all else is to lose sight of the man taken in isolation in order to consider him only as a fraction of the species. It is necessary to strip him of his individuality to arrive at the elimination of all accidental effects that individuality can introduce into the question." Cited in Hacking, *Taming of Chance*, 80n1.

45. Knud Faber, *Nosography* (New York: Paul Hoeber, 1923). Anne Fagot-Largeault summarizes the development of nosology in the eighteenth century in the following paragraph: "The attempts of systematic classification of diseases had been numerous in the second part of the eighteenth century. We cite often the work of Sauvages as the first in this domain. In reality, if *Nosologia Methodica* of Francois Bossier de Lacroix, said Sauvages (*editio ultima*, 1768), is the major work of reference; it was not the first. The small treatise of Carl von Linné entitled *Genera morborum* was published in the same year (1763). In this thesis on 'methods of classification in nosology' (Paris, 1853), E. Bouchut attempted to show the first modern classifications to Felix Pater, and even to Jean Fernal (sixteenth century), and not to ignore that we may find the origins much further, until Hippocratic medicine." *Causes de la mort*, 89. (Translation mine.)

Chapter Eight

1. Stephen M. Stigler, "Francis Galton's Account of the Invention of Correlation," *Statistical Science* 4, no. 2 (1989): 73–79.

2. Colin Howson, *Hume's Problem: Induction and the Justification of Belief* (Oxford: Oxford University Press, 2000).

3. Peter F. Strawson, *Introduction to Logical Theory* (London: Methuen & Co. Ltd., 1952).

4. George Bealer, "On the Possibility of Philosophical Knowledge," in *Metaphysics*, ed. J. E. Tomberlin, Philosophical Perspectives 10 (Cambridge: Blackwell, 1996).

5. William Whewell, *Philosophy of the Inductive Sciences* (London: J. W. Parker & Sons, 1840). Galton was undoubtedly familiar with Whewell's writing. In *Hereditary Genius* he refers to Whewell in positive terms: "His intellectual energy was prodigious, his writing unceasing, and his conversational powers extraordinary. Also, few will doubt that, although the range of his labours was exceedingly wide and scattered, Science in one form or another was his chief pursuit. His influence on the progress of Science during the early years of his life was, I believe, considerable, but it is impossible to specify the particulars of that influence, or so to justify our opinion that posterity will be likely to pay regard to it. Biographers will seek in vain for important discoveries in Science, with which Dr. Whewell's name may hereafter be identified." *He-*

reditary Genius: An Inquiry into Its Laws and Consequences (London: MacMillan & Co., [1869] 1892), 186. There has been increased interest in Whewell following the strong critique of extreme scientific positivism. The importance of Whewell's contribution to the philosophy of science has been compared with Karl Popper and Thomas Kuhn. For recent work on Whewell, see, for example, Frederik Schipper, "William Whewell's Conception of Scientific Revolutions," *Studies in History and Philosophy of Science* 19 (1988): 43–53; Menachem Fisch, *William Whewell: Philosopher of Science* (Oxford: Clarendon Press, 1991); Richard Yeo, *Defining Science: William Whewell, Natural Knowledge, and Public Debate in Early Victorian Britain* (Cambridge: Cambridge University Press, 1993).

6. Whewell proposed a progressive version of intuition that emphasized the processes of thought as opposed to the products of scientific discovery. See William Whewell, *Astronomy and General Physics Considered with Reference to Natural Theology* (London: William Pickering, 1836), 304. In his description of the process of induction, Whewell emphasized the structure of subjective reasoning. As Lucy Hartley notes, for Whewell inductive truth is intuited over a period of time through a process of prolonged and active engagement between the cognitive framework of the individual and the worldly objects of external perception. *Physiognomy and the Meaning of Expression in Nineteenth-Century Culture* (Cambridge: Cambridge University Press, 2001).

7. Whewell's assumption of a rational order in the cosmos to which the human belongs and can make sense of through induction harkens back to the scholastic conception of *synderesis* i.e., the intuitive ability to make moral decisions. Despite Galton's statistical critique of intuitive prayer, the redefinition of direct causality through statistical correlation is an analogous, albeit scientific attempt to establish a chain of inferential order. Consilience is hence a secular analogue of synderesis.

8. As Mary Hesse observes, Whewell's notion of consilience is not very precise, in that it can either refer to the inductive support of a new conception, or else to the development of inferences by means of analogies that do not involve a new basic language or confirmation system. M. Hesse, "Consilience of Inductions," in *The Problem of Inductive Logic*, ed. Imre Lakatos (Amsterdam: North-Holland Publishing Company), 254.

9. Steven D. Hales, "The Problem of Intuition," *American Philosophical Quarterly* 37, no. 2 (2000): 135–47.

10. This reductionism extends to the realm of ethics. Thus, in his classic work in sociobiology, E. O Wilson argued that "the time has come for ethics to be removed temporarily from the hands of the philosophers and biologicized." *Sociobiology: The New Synthesis* (Cambridge, MA: Harvard University Press, 1975), 562. According to this sociobiological conception, ethics is nothing more than a product of biological mechanisms and processes. Wilson would in all likelihood agree with my claim linking reductionism in sociobiology to his conception of consilience. In *Consilience* Wilson pleads guilty to the charge of "*conflation, simplism, ontological reductionism, scientism*, and other sins made official by the hissing suffix." *Consilience* (New York: Knopf, 1998), 11. For positive and negative analyses of sociobiology, see David Barash, *Sociobiology: The Whisperings Within* (London: Souvenir Press, 1980); Philip Kitcher, *Vaulting Ambition: Sociobiology and the Quest for Human Nature* (Cambridge, MA: MIT Press, 1985); and Mary Midgley, "Darwinism and Ethics," in *Medicine and Moral Reasoning*, ed. K. W. M. Fulford, et al. (Cambridge: Cambridge University Press, 1994), 6–18.

11. As Cathy Gere has ably demonstrated, Crete and Ariadne have served a pivotal, though ambiguous, role in the birth of modernism. See *Knossos & the Prophets of Modernism* (Chicago: University of Chicago Press, 2009).

12. This reductionism is not necessary in relating myths to science. As Mary Midgley has argued, myths are not necessarily opposed to science, but "in fact they are a central part of it: the part that decides its significance in our lives." This is because for Midgley, "myths are not lies. Nor are they detached stories. They are imaginative patterns, networks or powerful symbols that suggest particular ways of interpreting the world." *The Myths We Live By* (New York: Routledge, 2003), 1.

13. Hans Reichenbach, *Experience and Prediction* (Chicago: University of Chicago Press, 1938).

14. J. Alberto Coffa, *The Semantic Tradition from Kant to Carnap* (Cambridge: Cambridge University Press, 1991), 331.

15. See also Donald Gillies, *Philosophy of Science in the Twentieth Century: Four Central Themes* (Oxford: Blackwell, 1993), 10.

16. See Hans Reichenbach, *Experience and Prediction* (Chicago: University of Chicago Press, 1938), sec. 15; and "On Probability and Induction," *Philosophy of Science* 5 (1938): 21−45.

17. Reprinted in Hans Reichenbach, "The Problem of Causality in Physics," in *Selected Writings, 1909–1953*, ed. M. Reichenbach and R. S. Cohen (Dordrecht: Reidel, 1978), 1:326−42.

18. Wesley Salmon, the most articulate exponent of Reichenbach's justification of induction, summarizes this position as follows: "There is no way to prove, either a priori or a posteriori, prior to a justification of induction, that a given empirical sequence of events will have a limit for the relative frequency of a particular attribute. Nevertheless, to attempt to establish the value of a limit of this relative frequency, it is advantageous to use the rule of induction by enumeration, for if there is a limit the rule of induction by enumeration will establish its value and if there is no limit no method can establish its value. If any rule will work, induction by enumeration will work." "The Pragmatic Justification of Induction," *The Justification of Induction*, ed. R. Swinburne (Oxford: Oxford University Press, 1974), 88.

19. Hans Reichenbach, *The Direction of Time* (Berkeley: University of California Press, 1955), 10.

20. This move critiquing anthropomorphism with the scientific tool of induction can be traced back to the philosopher Francis Bacon (1561–1626). *Novum Organon*, bk. 1, ed. Fulton H. Anderson (New York: Liberal Arts Press [1620] 1960).

21. Republished in Kurt Lewin, "The Conflict between Aristotelian and Galileian Modes of Thought in Contemporary Psychology," in *A Dynamic Theory of Personality: Selected Papers by Kurt Lewin* (New York: McGraw-Hill Book Company, 1935), 1–42.

22. Ian Hacking, *The Taming of Chance* (Cambridge: Cambridge University Press, 1990).

23. K. T. Fann, *Peirce's Theory of Abduction* (The Hague: Martinus Nijhoff, 1970).

24. Hans R. Fischer, "Abductive Reasoning as a Way of Worldmaking," *Foundations of Science* 6, no. 317 (2001): 141−45.

25. See, for example, Umberto Eco and Thomas A. Sebeok, eds., *The Sign of Three: Dupin, Holmes, Peirce* (Bloomington: Indiana University Press, 1938). In that volume, see in particular the essay by Thomas A. Sebeok and Jean Umiker-Sebeok, "'You Know My Method': A Juxtaposition of Charles S. Peirce and Sherlock Holmes," 11−54; and K. Montgomery Hunter, *Doctors' Stories: The Narrative Structure of Medical Knowledge* (Princeton, NJ: Princeton University Press, 1991).

26. Abduction's relating of facts with values occurs in C. S. Peirce's conception of three cosmological levels in our indeterministic universe to which the three kinds of inferences correspond. These levels are described by Peirce as "firstness," "secondness," and "thirdness," respectively. "Firstness" is illustrated by the property of independence, of disconnectedness.

"Secondness" refers to the feature of brute reaction, of two things coming into contact with one another. The final category, "thirdness," is the category of relationship, of mediation, and of law and regularity. Abduction, involving an imaginative guess, corresponds to the level of randomness. Deduction is associated with the second level akin to a mechanical law. Finally, induction is placed at the third level of reasoning, and occurs through the synthesis of a new law from formerly disconnected facts. At the level of randomness, to which abduction is associated, both norms and facts are not yet crystallized. *Collected Papers of Charles Sanders Peirce* (Cambridge, MA: Belknap Press, 1960–66); Andrew Reynolds, *Peirce's Scientific Metaphysics: The Philosophy of Chance, Law, and Evolution* (Nashville, TN: Vanderbilt University Press, 2002). This conflation between fact and values in abduction is further evidenced by Peirce's relating of abduction to a kind of neurophysiological emotion, or sensuous element of thought. See Peirce, *Collected Papers*, 2.711.

27. Charles Fried, *Medical Experimentation: Personal Integrity and Social Policy* (Amsterdam: North Holland, 1974).

28. Benjamin Freedman, "Equipoise and the Ethics of Clinical Research," *New England Journal of Medicine* 317 (1987): 141–45.

29. Fred Gifford, "Community-Equipoise and the Ethics of Randomized Clinical Trials," *Bioethics* 9 (1995): 127–84.

30. Frank Miller and H. Howard Brody, "A Critique of Clinical Equipoise: Therapeutic Misconception in the Ethics of Clinical Trials," *Hastings Center Report* 33, no. 3 (2003): 19–28.

31. Emily L. Evans and Alex J. London, "Equipoise and the Criteria for Reasonable Action," *Journal of Law, Medicine, and Ethics* 34, no. 2 (2006): 441–50.

32. See, for example, Richard Lilford, "Ethics of Clinical Trials from a Bayesian and Decision Analytic Perspective: Whose Equipoise Is It Anyway?" *British Medical Journal*, 326 (2003): 980–81.

33. Don Marquis, "Leaving Therapy to Chance," *Hastings Center Report* 13, no. 4 (1983): 40–47.

34. Alvan R. Feinstein, "An Additional Basic Science for Clinical Medicine: II; The Limitations of Randomized Trials," *Annals of Internal Medicine* 99 (1983): 544–50.

35. Thus, in commenting on the use of ethics and statistics in clinical research, Benjamin Freedman and Stanley H. Shapiro suggest a "'bottom-up' method, that begins with the multitude of choices posed in the process of designing and running a clinical trial, remaining alert to the potential ethical implications of each such choice." "Ethics and Statistics in Clinical Research: Towards a More Comprehensive Examination," *Journal of Statistical Planning and Inference* 42 (1994): 223–40.

36. Deborah Hellman, "Evidence, Belief, and Action: The Failure of Equipoise to Resolve the Ethical Tension in the Randomized Clinical Trial," *Journal of Law, Medicine, and Ethics* 30 (2002): 375–80.

37. See Peirce, *Collected Papers*, 2.776. Tamsyn Barton suggests that Peirce might have found something closer to his ideas in Stoic nondeductive inference. *Power and Knowledge: Astrology, Physiognomics, and Medicine under the Roman Empire* (Ann Arbor: University of Michigan Press, 1994), 136.

38. Fann, *Peirce's Theory of Abduction*, 17.

39. Peirce, *Collected Papers*, 5.225ff.

40. Reynolds, *Peirce's Scientific Metaphysics*. The analysis in the following section is heavily indebted to Reynolds's insightful study.

Conclusion

1. *Nich. Ethics*, 1094b.

2. See Stephen Toulmin, *Return to Reason* (Cambridge, MA: Harvard University Press, 2001).

3. Herbert Spiegelberg, *The Phenomenological Movement: A Historical Introduction* (The Hague: Martinus Nijhoff, 1965), 5–6.

4. Richard Cobb-Stevens, *Husserl and Analytic Philosophy* (Dordrecht: Kluwer Academic Publishers, 1990), 1.

5. For a very good discussion on Husserl's concept of the natural attitude and the *epoché*, see Dan Zahavi, *Husserl's Phenomenology* (Stanford, CA: Stanford University Press, 2003), 44–46.

6. Ibid., 126.

7. See Emmanuel Levinas, *The Theory of Intuition in Husserl's Phenomenology* (Evanston, IL: Northwestern University Press, 1973), 9.

8. Ibid.

9. For an analysis of Zaner's transition from phenomenology to clinical ethics to narrative, see my essay "Between and Beyond: Medicine and Narrative in Dick Zaner's Phenomenology," in *Clinical Ethics and the Necessity of Stories: Essays in Honor of Richard M. Zaner*, ed. O. P. Wiggins and A. C. Allen (New York: Springer Press, 2010), 119–38.

10. Emmanuel Levinas, *Otherwise than Being: Or, Beyond Essence*, trans. Lingis (The Hague: Martinus Nijhoff, 1981).

11. See Emmanuel Levinas, "Useless Suffering," in *The Provocation of Levinas*, ed. R. Bernasconi and D. Wood (London: Routledge, 1988), 156–67.

12. Michel Foucault, *The Birth of the Clinic* (New York: Vintage, 1973).

13. Foucault, *Birth of the Clinic*; Georges Canguilhem, *The Normal and the Pathological*, trans. Carolyn R. Fawcett (New York: Zone Books, [1978] 1989).

14. Carl Ginzburg, "Clues: Morelli, Freud and Sherlock Holmes," in *The Sign of Three: Dupin, Holmes, Pierce*, ed. Umberto Eco and T. A. Sebeok (Bloomington: Indiana University Press, 1983).

15. See Didier Franck, "De la trace à l'énigme," in *Levinas et la Signification* (Paris: Presses Universitaires de France, 2008), 111–23.

16. Franck, *Levinas et la signification*.

17. Adi Ophir, *The Order of Evils: Toward an Ontology of Morals* (New York: Zone Books, 2005).

Bibliography

1817. "Statement of the Sizes of Men in Different Countries of Scotland, Taken from the Local Militia." *Edinburgh Medical and Surgical Journal* 13: 260–64.

Albert, H. 2000. *Kritischer Rationalismus: Vier Kapitel zur Kritik illusionaren Denkens*. Tuebingen: UTB Mohr Siebeck.

Allan, D. J. 1955. "The Practical Syllogism." *Autour d'Aristote: Recueil d'études de philosophie ancienne et medievale*, edited by A. Mansion, 325–40. Louvain: Publications Universitaires de Louvain.

Altman, D. G. 2000. "Statistics in Medical Journals: Some Recent Trends." *Stat Med* 19: 3281–84.

Andō, T. (1958) 1971. *Aristotle's Theory of Practical Cognition*. The Hague: Martinus Nijhoff.

Annas, G. J., and M. A. Grodin, eds. 1992. *The Nazi Doctors and the Nuremberg Code*. New York: Oxford University Press.

Arendt, H. 1958. *The Human Condition*. Chicago: University of Chicago Press.

———. 1978. "Metaphor and the Ineffable: Illumination on "The Nobility of Sight." In *Organism, Medicine and Metaphysics*, edited by S. F. Spicker, 303–16. Dordrecht: Reidel Publishing Co.

Aristotle. 1925. *Nicomachean Ethics*. Translated by W. D. Ross. Oxford: Clarendon Press.

———. 1928. *Metaphysica*. Edited by W. D. Ross. Oxford: Clarendon Press.

———. 1931. *De Anima*. Translated by J. A. Smith. Oxford: Clarendon Press.

———. 1949. *Aristotle's Prior and Posterior Analytics*. Edited by W. D. Ross. Oxford: Clarendon Press.

———. 1978. *De Motu Animalium*. Translated by M. Nussbaum. Princeton: Princeton University Press.

Ashcroft, R. 1999. "Equipoise, Knowledge and Ethics in Clinical Research and Practice." *Bioethics* 13, no. 3: 314–26.

Audi, R. 1997. *Moral Knowledge and Ethical Character*. Oxford: Oxford University Press.

Baader, G. 2001. "Heilen und Vernichten: Die Mentalitat der NS-Arzte." In *Vernichten und Heilen*, edited by A. Ebbinghaus and K. Dorner, 275–95. Berlin: Aufbau-Verlag.

Bacon, F. (1620) 1960. *Novum Organon*, bk. 1. Edited by F. H. Anderson. New York: Liberal Arts Press.

Barash, D. 1980. *Sociobiology: The Whisperings Within*. London: Souvenir Press.

Barrows, H. S., and R. M. Tamblyn. 1980. *Problem Based Learning: An Approach to Medical Education*. New York: Springer.

Barton, T. 1994. *Power and Knowledge: Astrology, Physiognomics, and Medicine under the Roman Empire*. Ann Arbor: University of Michigan Press.

Bealer, G. 1996. "On the Possibility of Philosophical Knowledge." In *Metaphysics*, edited by J. E. Tomberlin. Philosophical Perspectives, vol. 10. Cambridge: Blackwell.

Beare, J. I. 1906. *Greek Theories of Elementary Cognition from Alcmaeon to Aristotle*. Oxford: Clarendon Press.

Beauchamp, T. L., and J. F. Childress. 1979. *Principles of Biomedical Ethics*. New York: Oxford University Press.

Beecher, H. K. 1970. "Definitions of 'Life and Death' for Medical Science and Practice." *Annals of the New York Academy of Sciences* 169, no. 2: 471–74.

Benjamin, W. (1955) 1968. "The Work of Art in the Age of Mechanical Reproduction." In *Illuminations*, 217–52. New York: Schocken Books.

———. 1972. *Gesammelte Schriften*. Frankfurt: Suhrkamp Verlag.

———. 1979. "A Small History of Photography." In *One-Way Street and Other Writings*. London: New Left Books.

Beresford, E. B. 1996. "Can Phronesis Save the Life of Medical Ethics?" *Theoretical Medicine* 17: 209–24.

Bernard, C. 1865. *Introduction à l'étude de la médecine expérimentale*. Paris: Éditions Garnier-Flammarion.

———. (1865) 1927. *An Introduction to the Study of Experimental Medicine*. New York: Macmillan Company.

———. 1947, posth. *Principes de médecine expérimentale*. Paris: PUF.

Bichat, X. 1801. *Anatomie générale appliquée a la médecine*. Paris: Brosson.

———. 1809. *Physiological Researches upon Life and Death*. Translated by T. Watkins. Philadelphia, PA: Smith & Maxwell.

Black, M. 1969. "The Gap Between 'Is' and 'Should.'" In *The Is-Ought Question*, edited by W. D. Hudson, 99–133. New York: Macmillan.

Bland, J. M., and D. G. Altman. 1994. "Some Examples of Regression toward the Mean." *BMJ* 309: 780.

Boorse, C. 1977. "Health as a Theoretical Concept." *Philosophy of Science* 44: 573.

Bottero, J. 1974. *Symptômes, Signes, Écritures. Divination et Rationalité*. Paris: Éditions du Seuil.

Bourdieu, P. (1977) 1999. *Outline of a Theory of Practice*. Cambridge: Cambridge University Press.

———. 1998. *Practical Reason: On the Theory of Action*. Stanford, CA: Stanford University Press.

Boyle, J. 2004. "Medical Ethics and Double Effect: The Case of Terminal Sedation." *Theoretical Medicine* 25: 51–60.

Braude, H. D. 2010. "Between and Beyond: Medicine and Narrative in Dick Zaner's Phenomenology." In *Clinical Ethics and the Necessity of Stories: Essays in Honor of Richard M. Zaner*, edited by O. P. Wiggins and A. C. Allen. New York: Springer Press.

Brody, B. 1979. "Intuitions and Objective Moral Truth." *The Monist* 62: 446–56.

———. 1988. *Life and Death Decision Making*. New York: Oxford University Press.

———. 2003. *Taking Issue: Pluralism and Casuistry in Bioethics*. Washington, DC: Georgetown University Press.

Brody, B., and A. Halevy. 1993. "Brain Death: Reconciling Definitions, Criteria and Tests." *Annals of Internal Medicine* 119: 519–25.

Broeckaert, B., and J. M. N. Olarte. 2002. "Sedation in Palliative Care: Facts and Concepts." In *The Ethics of Palliative Care: European Perspectives,* edited by H. Ten Have, and D. Clark, 166–80. Philadelphia, PA: Open University Press.

Buck-Morss, S. 1977. *The Origin of Negative Dialectics.* Sussex: Harvester Press.

———. 1989. *The Dialectics of Seeing: Walter Benjamin and the Arcades Project.* Cambridge, MA: MIT Press.

Buetow, S. 2002. "Beyond Evidence-Based Medicine: Bridge-Building a Medicine of Meaning." *Journal of Evaluation in Clinical Practice* 8, no. 2: 103–8.

Bunge, M. A. 1962. *Intuition and Science.* Englewood Cliffs, NJ: Prentice-Hall.

Bynum, W. F., and R. Porter, eds. 1993. *Medicine and the Five Senses.* New York: Cambridge University Press.

Canguilhem, G. (1978) 1989. *The Normal and the Pathological.* Translated by C. R. Fawcett. New York: Zone Books.

———. 2000. *A Vital Rationalist: Selected Writings from Georges Canguilhem.* Translated by A. Goldhammer. New York: Zone Books.

Carnap, R. 1968. "Inductive Logic and Intuition." In *The Problem of Inductive Logic,* edited by I. Lakatos, 258–67. Amsterdam: North-Holland Publishing Company.

Carr, D. 1987. *Interpreting Husserl: Critical and Comparative Studies.* Dordrecht: Martinus Nijhoff Publishers.

Carter, K. C. 2003. *The Rise of Causal Concepts of Disease: Case Histories.* Aldershot: Ashgate.

Cassell, E. J. 1985. *Talking with Patients.* Volume 1, *The Theory of Doctor-Patient Communication.* Cambridge, MA: MIT Press.

———. 1991. *The Nature of Suffering and the Goals of Medicine.* New York: Oxford University Press.

Castiglioni, A. 1934. "Neo-Hippocratic Tendency of Contemporary Medical Thought." *Medical Life* 61, no. 3: 115–46.

Chalmers, I. 2003. "Fisher and Bradford Hill: Theory and Pragmatism?" *International Journal of Epidemiology* 32: 922–24.

Clegg, F. (1982) 1990. *Simple Statistics: A Course Book for the Social Sciences.* Cambridge: Cambridge University Press.

Clouser, K. D. 1978. "Bioethics." *The Encyclopedia of Bioethics,* edited by W. Reich et al., 114–16. New York: Free Press.

Cobb-Stevens, R. 1990. *Husserl and Analytic Philosophy.* Dordrecht: Kluwer Academic Publishers.

Coffa, J. A. 1991. *The Semantic Tradition from Kant to Carnap.* New York: Cambridge University Press.

Cooper, J. M. 1975. *Reason and Human Good in Aristotle.* Cambridge, MA: Harvard University Press.

Cowan, R. S. 1972. "Francis Galton's Statistical Ideas: The Influence of Eugenics." *Isis* 63: 509–28.

———. 1977. "Nature and Nurture: The Interplay of Biology and Politics in the Work of Francis Galton." In *Studies in History of Biology,* edited by W. Coleman and C. Limoges, 1:133–208. Baltimore, MD: Johns Hopkins University Press.

Crombie, A. C. 1952. *Augustine to Galileo: The History of Science, A.D. 400–1650.* London: Falcon Press.

Daly, J. 2005. *Evidence-Based Medicine and the Search for a Science of Clinical Care.* Berkeley: University of California Press.

d'Amador, R. 1836. "Memoire sur le calcul des probabilités appliqué a la médecine." *Bulletin de l'Académie Royale de Médecine* 1: 622–80.

Damasio, A. R. 1999. *The Feeling of What Happens: Body and Emotion in the Making of Consciousness.* New York: Harcourt Brace & Co.

Daston, L. 1988. *Classical Probability in the Enlightenment.* Princeton, NJ: Princeton University Press.

Davidoff, E. 1999. "In the Teeth of the Evidence: The Curious Use of Evidence-Based Medicine." *Mount Sinai Journal of Medicine* 66, no. 2: 75–83.

Davidoff, F., K. Case, and P. W. Fried. 1995. "Evidence-Based Medicine: Why All the Fuss?" *Annals of Internal Medicine* 122: 727.

Davis, F. D. 1996. "Phronesis and the Physician: A Defense of the Practical Paradigm of Clinical Rationality." PhD diss., Department of Philosophy, Georgetown University.

———. 1997. "*Phronesis*, Clinical Reasoning and Pellegrino's Philosophy of Medicine." *Theoretical Medicine* 18, nos. 1–2: 173–95.

Descartes. 1968. "Rules for the Direction of Mind." In *The Philosophical Works of Descartes*, 1:1–77. Cambridge: Cambridge University Press.

Detienne, M., and J.-P. Vernant. 1991. *Cunning Intelligence in Greek Culture and Society.* Chicago: University of Chicago Press.

Donagan, A. 1977. *The Theory of Morality.* Chicago: University of Chicago Press.

Eco, U., and T. A. Sebeok, eds. 1983. *The Sign of Three: Dupin, Holmes, Peirce.* Bloomington: Indiana University Press.

Edelstein, L. 1967. *Ancient Medicine.* Baltimore, MD: Johns Hopkins University Press.

Editorial. 1995. "Evidence-Based Medicine, In Its Place." *Lancet* 346, no. 8978: 785.

Elstein, A. S. 2000. "Clinical Problem Solving and Decision Psychology." *Academic Medicine* 75, suppl. 10: S134–36.

Engelhardt, H. T. 1996. *The Foundations of Bioethics.* New York: Oxford University Press.

Engelhardt, H. T., Jr. et al. 1973. "The Philosophy of Medicine: A New Endeavor." *Texas Reports on Biology and Medicine* 3: 443–52.

Evans, A. S. 1976. "Causation and Disease: The Henle-Koch Postulate Revisited." *Yale J Biol Med* 49: 175–95.

———. 1978. "Causation and Disease: A Chronological Journey." *American Journal of Epidemiology* 108: 249–58.

Evans, E. L., and A. J. London. 2006. "Equipoise and the Criteria for Reasonable Action." *Journal of Law, Medicine, and Ethics* 34, no. 2: 441–50.

Evidence Based Medicine Working Group. 1992. "Evidence Based Medicine: A New Approach to the Teaching of Medicine." *JAMA* 268: 2420–25.

Faber, K. 1923. *Nosography.* New York: Paul Hoeber.

Fagot-Largeault, A. 1989. *Les Causes de la mort histoire naturelle et facteurs de risque.* Paris: Librairie Philosophique J. Vrin.

Falkenstein, L. 1995. *Kant's Intuitionism: A Commentary on the Transcendental Aesthetic.* Toronto: University of Toronto Press.

Fann, K. T. 1970. *Peirce's Theory of Abduction.* The Hague: Martinus Nijhoff.

Feinstein, A. R. 1963. "The Basic Elements of Clinical Science." *Journal of Chronic Diseases* 16: 1125–33.

———. 1964. "Scientific Methodology in Clinical Medicine." Pt. 1, "Introduction, Principles and Concepts." *Annals of Internal Medicine* 61, no. 3: 564–79.

———. 1967. *Clinical Judgment*. Baltimore, MD: Williams Wilkins.

———. 1968. "Clinical Epidemiology." Pts. 1–3. *Annals of Internal* Medicine: 69, nos. 4–6: 807–20, 1037–61, 1287–311.

———. 1973. "An Analysis of Diagnostic Reasoning." Pt. 2, "The Strategy of Intermediate Decisions." *Yale Journal of Biology and Medicine* 46: 264–83.

———. 1977a. *Clinical Biostatistics*. Saint Louis: C.V. Mosby.

———. 1977b. "Clinical Biostatistics." Pt. 39, "The Haze of Bayes, the Aerial Palaces of Decision Analysis, and the Computerized Ouija Board." *Clinical Pharmacology Therapeutics* 21: 482–96.

———. 1983. "An Additional Basic Science for Clinical Medicine." Pts. 1–3. *Annals of Internal Medicine* 99: 393–97, 544–50, 705–12.

———. 1985. *Clinical Epidemiology: The Architecture of Clinical Research*. Philadelphia, PA: W. B. Saunders Company.

———. 1987. *Clinimetrics*. New Haven, CT: Yale University Press.

———. 1994. "Clinical Judgment Revisited: The Distraction of Quantitative Models." *Annals of Internal Medicine* 1994, no. 120: 799–805.

Feinstein, A. R., and R. I. Horwitz. 1997. "Problems in the 'Evidence' of 'Evidence-Based Medicine.' " *American Journal of Medicine* 103, no. 6: 529–35.

Fisch, M. 1991. *William Whewell: Philosopher of Science*. Oxford: Clarendon Press.

Fischer, H. R. 2001. "Abductive Reasoning as a Way of Worldmaking." *Foundations of Science* 6, no. 317: 141–45.

Fisher, R. A. 1925. *Statistical Methods for Research Workers*. Edinburgh: Oliver and Boyd.

———. 1926. "The Arrangement of Field Experiments." *Journal of Ministry of Agriculture of Great Britain* 33: 503–13.

———. (1935) 1951. *The Design of Experiments*. Edinburgh: Oliver and Boyd.

Foot, P. 1978. *Virtues and Vices*. Berkeley: University of California Press.

Foucault, M. 1973. *The Birth of the Clinic*. New York: Vintage Books.

Foxe, A. N. 1962. *The Common Sense from Heraclitus to Peirce: The Sources, Substances, and Possibilities of the Common Sense*. New York: Turnbridge Press.

Franck, D. 2008. *Levinas et la signification*. Paris: Presses Universitaires de France.

Frankena, W. K. 1973. *Ethics*. New York: Prentice Hall.

Freedman, B. 1987. "Equipoise and the Ethics of Clinical Research." *New England Journal of Medicine* 317: 141–45.

Freedman, B., and S. H. Shapiro. 1994. "Ethics and Statistics in Clinical Research: Towards a More Comprehensive Examination." *Journal of Statistical Planning and Inference*, no. 42: 223–40.

Fried, C. 1974. *Medical Experimentation: Personal Integrity and Social Policy*. Amsterdam: North Holland.

Gadamer, H.-G. 1994. *Truth and Method*. New York: Continuum.

Galton, F. 1865. "Hereditary Talent and Character." *Macmillan's Magazine* 12: 318–27.

———. (1869) 1892. *Hereditary Genius: An Inquiry into its Laws and Consequences*. London: Macmillan.

———. 1872a. "Blood Relationship." *Proceedings of the Royal Society* 20: 394–402.

———. 1872b. "Statistical Inquiries into the Efficacy of Prayer." *Fortnightly* 12, n.s.: 125–35.

———. 1875. "A Theory of Heredity." *Contemporary Review* 27: 80–95.

———. 1877. "Typical Laws of Heredity," *Proceedings of the Royal Institution*, Feb. 9.

———. 1878. "Composite Portraits." *Journal of the Anthropological Institute* 8: 132–42.

———. 1879. "Generic Images." *Nineteenth Century* 6, no. 29: 157–69.

———. 1881. "Letter." *Nature* 18: 383.

———. (1883) 1951. *Inquiries into Human Faculty and Its Development.* London: Eugenics Society.

———. 1885. "Regression towards Mediocrity in Hereditary Stature." *Journal of the Anthropological Institute* 15: 246–63.

———. 1888. "Co-relations and the Measurement, Chiefly from Anthropometric Data." *Proceedings of the Royal Society* 45: 135–45.

———. 1889. *Natural Inheritance.* London: Macmillan.

———. 1908. *Memories of My Life.* London: Methuen & Co.

Gatens Robinson, E. 1986. "Clinical Judgment and the Rationality of the Human Sciences." *Journal of Medicine and Philosophy* 11: 167–78.

Gehan, E. A., and N. A. Lemak. 1994. *Statistics in Medical Research.* New York: Plenum Medical Book Co.

Gere, C. 2009. *Knossos & the Prophets of Modernism.* Chicago: University of Chicago Press.

Giampalmo, A., and A. C. Quaglia. 1990. "A Propaedeutic Concept: The Pathologic Physiognomy of Organs." *Pathologica* 82, no. 1082: 583–92.

Gifford, F. 1995. "Community-Equipoise and the Ethics of Randomized Clinical Trials." *Bioethics* 9: 127–84.

Gill, J. H. 2000. *Michael Polanyi's Postmodern Philosophy.* Albany: State University of New York Press.

Gillies, D. 1993. *Philosophy of Science in the Twentieth Century: Four Central Themes.* Oxford: Blackwell.

———. 2000. *Philosophical Theories of Probability.* New York: Routledge.

Ginzburg, C. 1983. "Clues: Morelli, Freud and Sherlock Holmes." In *The Sign of Three: Dupin, Holmes, Pierce,* edited by U. Eco and T. A. Sebeok. Bloomington: Indiana University Press.

———. 1989. "Clues: Roots of an Evidential Paradigm." In *Clues, Myths and the Historical Method,* 96–125. Baltimore, MD: Johns Hopkins University Press.

———. 2004. "Family Resemblances and Family Trees: Two Cognitive Metaphors." *Critical Inquiry* 30: 537–56.

Gould, S. J. 1981. *The Mismeasure of Man.* New York: W.W. Norton & Company.

Green, M. B., and D. Wikler. 1980. "Brain Death and Personal Identity." *Philosophy and Public Affairs* 9, no. 2: 105–33.

Greene, J. 2003. "From Neural "Is" to Moral "Ought": What are the Moral Implications of Neuroscientific Moral Psychology?" *Nature Reviews Neuroscience* 4: 847–50.

Grene, M. 1963. *A Portrait of Aristotle.* London: Faber and Faber Limited.

———. 1977. "Comments on Pellegrino's Anatomy of Clinical Judgment." In *Clinical Judgment: A Critical Appraisal,* edited by H. T. Engelhardt, S. F. Spicker, and B. Towers. Dordrecht: D. Reidel Publishing Company.

Groopman, J. 2000. "Second Opinion." *New Yorker,* January 24.

Grossman, J., and F. J. Mackenzie. 2005. "The Randomized Controlled Trial: Gold Standard, or Merely Standard?" *Perspectives in Biology and Medicine* 48, no. 4: 516–34.

Guiffrey, F., and P. Marcel. 1912–1913. *Inventaire général des dessins du Musée du Louvre et du Musée de Versailles, école française,* vols. 7–8. Paris: Musée du Louvre.

Guinaudeau, O. 1924. *Jean-Gaspard Lavater.* Paris: F. Alcan.

Guyatt, G. H., and D. Rennie, eds. 2002. *Users' Guides to the Medical Literature: A Manual for Evidence-Based Clinical Practice.* Chicago, IL: AMA Press.

Guyatt, G. H. et al. 1986. "Determining Optimal Therapy: Randomized Trials in Individual Patients." *New England Journal of Medicine* 314, no. 14: 889–92.

Habermas, J. 2003. *The Future of Human Nature.* Cambridge: Polity.

Hacking, I. 1980. "The Theory of Probable Inference: Neyman, Peirce and Braithwaite." In *Science, Belief, and Behavior*, edited by D. H. Mellor. Cambridge: Cambridge University Press.

———. 1990. *The Taming of Chance.* Cambridge: Cambridge University Press.

Haidt, J. 2001. "The Emotional Dog and its Rational Tail: A Social Intuitionist Approach to Moral Judgment." *Psychological Review* 108, no. 4: 814–34.

Hald, A. 1998. *A History of Mathematical Statistics from 1750 to 1930.* New York: John Wiley & Sons, Inc.

Hales, S. D. 2000. "The Problem of Intuition." *American Philosophical Quarterly* 37, no. 2: 135–47.

Hampshire, S. 1978. "Public and Private Morality." In *Public and Private Morality*, edited by S. Hampshire. Cambridge: Cambridge University Press.

Hardie, W. F. R. 1968. *Aristotle's Ethical Theory.* Oxford: Clarendon Press.

Hare, R. M. 1952. *The Language of Morals.* New York: Oxford University Press.

———. 1977. "Medical Ethics: Can the Moral Philosopher Help?" *Philosophical Medical Ethics: Its Nature and Significance*, edited by J. S. F. Spicker and H. T. Engelhardt. Boston: D. Reidel Publishing Co.: 49–62.

Harré, R. 1972. *The Philosophies of Science.* Oxford: Oxford University Press.

Hartley, L. 2001. *Physiognomy and the Meaning of Expression in Nineteenth-Century Culture.* Cambridge: Cambridge University Press.

Hellman, D. 2002. "Evidence, Belief, and Action: The Failure of Equipoise to Resolve the Ethical Tension in the Randomized Clinical Trial." *Journal of Law, Medicine, and Ethics* 30: 375–80.

Henry, S. 2006. "Recognizing Tacit Knowledge in Medical Epistemology." *Theoretical Medicine and Bioethics* 27, no. 3: 187–213.

Henry, S. G., R. M. Zaner, and R. S. Dittus. 2007. "Moving Beyond Evidence-Based Medicine." *Academic Medicine* 82, no. 3: 292–97.

Herschel, J. 1850. "Quetelet on Probabilites." *Edinburgh Review* 92: 1–57.

Hesse, M. B. 1966. *Models and Analogies in Science.* Notre Dame, IN: University of Notre Dame Press.

Hill, A. B. 1951. "The Clinical Trial." *British Medical Bulletin* 7: 278–82.

———. 1952. "The Clinical Trial." *New England Journal of Medicine* 247: 113–19.

———. 1965. "The Environment and Disease: Association or Causation." *Proceedings of the Royal Society of Medicine* 58: 295–300.

———. 1990. "Memories of the British Streptomycin Trial in Tuberculosis: The First Randomized Clinical Trial." *Controlled Clinical Trials* 11: 77–79.

Hilts, V. L. 1970. "William Farr (1807–1883) and the 'Human Unit.'" *Victorian Studies* 14, no. 2: 143–50.

———. 1973. "Statistics and Social Science." In *Foundations of the Scientific Method*, edited by R. Giere and R. Westfall, 206–33. Bloomington: Indiana University Press.

Hofmann, B. 2002. "Medicine as Practical Wisdom (*Phronesis*)." *Poiesis Prax* 1: 135–49.

Horton, R. 2000. "Common Sense and Figures: The Rhetoric of Validity in Medicine." *Statistics in Medicine* 19: 3149–64.

Howson, C. 2000. *Hume's Problem: Induction and the Justification of Belief.* Oxford: Oxford University Press.

Hudson, W. D. 1967. *Ethical Intuitionism.* Toronto: Macmillan.

———. 1969. *The Is-Ought Question.* London: MacMillan.

———. 1970. *Modern Moral Philosophy.* Garden City, NY: Anchor Books.

Huebner, R. J. 1957. "The Virologist's Dilemma." *Annals of New York Academy of Sciences* 67: 430–45.

Hume, D. (1739) 1962. *A Treatise of Human Nature,* edited by D. G. C. Macnabb. London: Collins.

———. (1748) 1963. "An Enquiry Concerning Human Understanding." In *Hume's Enquiries,* edited by L. A. Selby-Bigge. Oxford: Clarendon Press.

———. (1777) 1960. *An Enquiry Concerning the Principles of Morals.* La Salle, IL: Open Court.

Huneman, P. 1998. *Bichat, la vie et la mort.* Paris: Presse Universitaires de France.

Husserl, E. 1962. *Die Krisis der europaischen Wissenschaften und die Transezendentale Phanemonologie: Eine Einleitung in die phanomenologische Philosophie.* The Hague: Martinus Nijhoff.

———. 1973. *Zur Phanemonologie der Intersubjecktivitat: Texte aus dem Nachlass; Dritter Teil: 1929–1935.* The Hague: Martinus Nijhoff.

Hutchinson, D. S. 1988. "Doctrines of the Mean and the Debate Concerning Skills in Fourth-Century Medicine, Rhetoric and Ethics." *Apeiron* 2 (Summer): 17–52.

Huxley, T. H. 1894. "On the Method of Zadig." In *Science and Hebrew Tradition.* New York: D. Appleton and Company.

Jadad, A. R., ed. 1998. *Randomized Controlled Trials: A User's Guide.* London: BMJ Books.

Jaeger, W. 1944. "Greek Medicine as Paideia." In *Paideia: The Ideals of Greek Culture,* 3:3–45. New York: Oxford University Press.

———. 1957. "Aristotle's Use of Medicine as Model of Method in his Ethics." *Journal of Hellenistic Studies* 77: 54–61.

Jansen, L. A. 2000. "The Virtues in Their Place: Virtue Ethics in Medicine." *Theoretical Medicine* 21: 261–76.

———. 2003. "The Moral Irrelevance of Proximity to Death." *Journal of Clinical Ethics*: 49–58.

Jonas, H. 1966a. *The Phenomenon of Life: Toward a Philosophical Biology.* Evanston, IL: Northwestern University Press.

———. (1966b) 2001. "The Practical Uses of Theory." In *The Phenomenon of Life: Toward a Philosophical Biology,* 188–210. Evanston, IL: Northwestern University Press.

———. 1973. "Technology and Responsibility: Reflections on the New Tasks of Ethics." *Philosophical Essays: From Ancient Creed to Technological Man,* 3–20. Englewood Cliffs, NJ: Prentice-Hall, Inc.

———. 1974. "Against the Stream: Comments on the Definition and Redefinition of Death." In *Philosophical Essays: From Ancient Creed to Technological Man,* 132–40. Englewood Cliffs, NJ: Prentice Hall.

———. 1978. "The Right to Die." *Hastings Center Report* 8, no. 4: 31–36.

Jones, R. F. 1975. *Ancients and Moderns: A Study of the Rise of the Scientific Movement in Seventeenth-Century England.* Berkeley: University of California Press.

Jones, W. H. S. 1946. *Philosophy and Medicine in Ancient Greece.* Baltimore, MD: Johns Hopkins Press.

Jonsen, A. R. 2000. *A Short History of Medical Ethics.* New York: Oxford University Press.

Jordanova, L. 1993. "The Art and Science of Seeing in Medicine: Physiognomy 1780–1820." In *Medicine and the Five Senses,* edited by W. F. Bynum and R. Porter. Cambridge: Cambridge University Press: 122–34.

Jouanna, J. 1999. *Hippocrates.* Baltimore, MD: Johns Hopkins University Press.

Kahneman, D., and A. Tversky. 1974. "Judgment under Uncertainty: Heuristics and Biases." *Science* 185: 1124–31.

Kal, V. 1988. *On Intuition and Discursive Reasoning in Aristotle.* Leiden: E. J. Brill.

Kant, I. (1929) 1965. *Critique of Pure Reason.* Reprint, New York: St. Martin's Press.

Kaptchuk, T. 2001. "The Double-Blind, Randomized, Placebo-Controlled Trial: Gold Standard or Golden Calf?" *Journal of Clinical Epidemiology* 54: 541–49.

Kass, L. R. 1975. "Regarding the End of Medicine and the Pursuit of Health." *Public Interest* 40: 11–42.

———. 1983. "Professing Ethically: On the Place of Ethics in Defining Medicine." *JAMA* 249, no. 10: 1305–10.

———. 1990. "Practicing Ethics: Where's the Action?" *Hastings Center Report* 20, no. 1: 5–12.

———. 1997. "The Wisdom of Repugnance: Why We should Ban the Cloning of Humans." *New Republic* 216, no. 22:17–26.

Kay Toombs, S. 1990. "The Temporality of Illness: Four Levels of Experience." *Theoretical Medicine* 11: 227–42.

Keller, E. F. 2002. *Making Sense of Life: Explaining Biological Development with Models, Metaphors, and Machines.* Cambridge, MA: Harvard University Press.

Kenny, A. 1978. *The Aristotelian Ethics: A Study of the Relationship between the Eudemian and Nicomachean Ethics of Aristotle.* Oxford: Clarendon Press.

Ketner, K. L., ed. 1992. *Reasoning and the Logic of Things.* Cambridge, MA: Harvard University Press.

Kevles, D. J. 1985. *In the Name of Eugenics: Genetics and the Uses of Human Heredity.* New York: Knopf.

Kim, J. 1990. "Supervenience as a Philosophical Concept." *Metaphilosophy* 21, no. 102: 1–27.

King, L. S. 1970a. "Empiricism and Rationalism in the Works of Thomas Sydenham." *Bulletin of the History of Medicine* 44: 1–11.

———. 1970b. *The Road to Medical Enlightenment: 1650–1695.* London: Macdonald.

———. 1976. "Evidence and Its Evaluation in Eighteenth-Century Medicine." *Bulletin of the History of Medicine* 50: 174–90.

———. 1978. *The Philosophy of Medicine: The Early Eighteenth Century.* Cambridge, MA: Harvard University Press.

Kingsley, C. 1902. *The Heroes, or Greek Fairy Tales for my Children.* New York: Macmillan Company.

Kitcher, P. 1985. *Vaulting Ambition: Sociobiology and the Quest for Human Nature.* Cambridge, MA: MIT Press.

Komesaroff, P. 1996. "Medicine and the Ethical Conditions of Modernity." In *Ethical Intersections,* edited by J. Daly, 34–48. Sydney: Allen & Unwin.

Jonsen, A. R., M. Siegler, and W. J. Winslade. 2006. *Clinical Ethics: A Practical Approach to Ethical Decisions in Clinical Medicine.* 6th ed. New York: McGraw-Hill.

Laplace, P. S. (1814) 1951. *A Philosophical Essay on Probabilities.* New York: Wiley.

Lavater, J. C. 1804. *Essays on Physiognomy.* London: Ward, Lock, & Bowden Limited.

Leguard, J. 1977. "Aristotle's Practical Syllogism." PhD diss., Department of Philosophy, University of Chicago.

Levinas, E. 1973. *The Theory of Intuition in Husserl's Phenomenology*. Evanston, IL: Northwestern University Press.

———. 1981. *Otherwise than Being: Or, Beyond Essence*. Translated by A. Lingis. Hague: Martinus Nijhoff.

———. 1986. "The Trace of the Other." In *Deconstruction in Context: Literature and Philosophy*, edited by M. C. Taylor. Chicago: University of Chicago Press: 345–59.

———. 1987. *Time and the Other*. Pitttsburgh, PA: Duquesne University Press.

———. 1988. "Useless Suffering." In *The Provocation of Levinas*. Edited by R. Bernasconi and D. Wood, 156–67. London: Routledge.

———. 1991. *Totality and Infinity*. Dordrecht: Kluwer Academic Publishers.

———. 1998a. "Is Ontology Fundamental?" In *Entre Nous: Thinking-of-the-Other*, 1–11. New York: Columbia University Press.

———. 1998b. *Otherwise than Being*. Pittsburgh, PA: Duquesne University Press.

Lewin, K. 1935. "The Conflict Between Aristotelian and Galileian Modes of Thought in Contemporary Psychology." In *A Dynamic Theory of Personality: Selected Papers by Kurt Lewin*, 1–42. New York: McGraw-Hill Book Company.

Lilford, R. 2003. "Ethics of Clinical Trials from a Bayesian and Decision Analytic Perspective: Whose Equipoise Is It Anyway?" *British Medical Journal* 326: 980–81.

Lilienfeld, A. M., ed. 1980. *Times, Places, and Persons: Aspects of the History of Epidemiology*. Baltimore, MD: Johns Hopkins University Press.

Lilienfeld, A. M., and D. Lilienfeld. 1977. "What Else Is New? An Historical Excursion." *American Journal of Epidemiology* 105: 169–79.

Lombroso, C. 1911. *Crime: Its Causes and Remedies*. Boston: Little, Brown, and Company.

Long, C. 2002. "The Ontological Re-Appropriation of Phronesis." *Continental Philosophy Review* 35, no. 1: 35–60.

———. *The Ethics of Ontology: Rethinking an Aristotelian Legacy*. Albany: State University of New York Press.

Louis, P. C. A. 1836. *Researches on the Effects of Bloodletting in Some Inflammatory Diseases*. Translated by C. G. Putnam, with a preface by J. Jackson. Boston: Hilliard, Gray and Company.

Lukasiewicz, J. 1951. *Aristotle's Syllogistic*. Oxford: Clarendon Press.

MacIntyre, A. C. 1969. "Hume on 'Is' and 'Ought.'" In *The Is-Ought Question*, edited by W. D. Hudson, 35–50. London: Macmillan.

———. 1981. *After Virtue: A Study in Moral Theory*. Notre Dame, IN: University of Notre Dame Press.

Malterud, K. 2002. "Reflexivity and Metapositions: Strategies for Appraisal of Clinical Evidence." *Journal of Evaluation in Clinical Practice* 8, no. 2: 121–26.

Marks, H. M. 2003. "Rigorous Uncertainty: Why RA Fisher Is Important." *International Journal of Epidemiology* 32: 932–37.

Marion, J.-L. 2002. *Being Given: Toward A Phenomenology of Givenness*. Translated by J. L. Kosky. Stanford, CA: Stanford University Press.

Marshall, T. 1997. "Scientific Knowledge in Medicine: A New Clinical Epistemology." *Journal of Evaluation in Clinical Practice* 3: 135–38.

Matthews, J. 1995. *Quantification and the Quest for Medical Certainty*. Princeton, NJ: Princeton University Press.

McGee, G. 1996. "Phronesis in Clinical Ethics." *Theoretical Medicine* 17, no. 4: 317–28.

McIntyre, A. 2004. "The Double Life of Double Effect." *Theoretical Medicine* 25: 61–74.

McPartland, T. J. 2001. *Lonergan and the Philosophy of Historical Existence.* Columbia: University of Missouri Press.

Meadow, W., and C. R. Sunstein. 2001. "Statistics, not Experts." *Duke Law Journal* 51, no. 2: 629–46.

Medawar, P. B. 1969. *Induction and Intuition in Scientific Thought.* Philadelphia, PA: American Philosophical Society.

Meehl, P. 1954. *Clinical Versus Statistical Prediction.* Minneapolis: University of Minnesota Press.

Midgley, M. (1979) 2002. *Beast and Man: The Roots of Human Nature.* New York: Routledge.

———. 1989. *Wisdom, Information and Wonder.* London: Routledge.

———. 1994. "Darwinism and Ethics." *Medicine and Moral Reasoning,* edited by K. W. M. Fulford, G. Gillett, and J. M. Sosckice, 6–18. Cambridge: Cambridge University Press.

———. 2003. *The Myths We Live By.* New York: Routledge.

Milgram, E. 1995. "Was Hume a Humean?" *Hume Studies* 21, no. 1: 75–93.

———. 1997. "Hume on Practical Reasoning." Treatise 463–69, *Iyyun: The Jerusalem Philosophical Quarterly* 46: 235–65.

Miller, P. B., and C. Weijer. 2003. "Rehabilitating Equipoise." *Kennedy Institute of Ethics Journal* 13, no. 2: 93–118.

Montgomery Hunter, K. 1991. *Doctors' Stories: The Narrative Structure of Medical Knowledge.* Princeton, NJ: Princeton University Press.

———. 1996. "'Don't Think Zebras': Uncertainty, Interpretation, and the Place of Paradox in Clinical Education." *Theoretical Medicine* 17: 1–17.

———. 2000. "*Phronesis* and the Misdescription of Medicine: Against the Medical School Commencement Speech." In *Bioethics: Ancient Themes in Contemporary Issues,* edited by M. G. Kuczewski and R. Polansky, 57–66. Cambridge, MA: MIT Press.

Moore, G. E. 1903. *Principia Ethica.* Cambridge: Cambridge University Press.

Morabia, A. 1996. "P.C.A. Louis and the Birth of Clinical Epidemiology." *Journal of Clinical Epidemiology* 49, no. 12: 1327–33.

———. 2004. "Pierre Louis ou l'utilisation de méthodes appropriées en médecine." *Séminaire de la Chaire: Histoire et philosophie de la médecine scientifique.* Paris: Collège de France.

Moran, D. 2005. *Edmund Husserl: Founder of Phenomenology.* Cambridge: Polity.

Natali, C. 2001. *The Wisdom of Aristotle.* New York: State University of New York Press.

Nordenfelt, L. 1987. *On the Nature of Health: An Action-Theoretic Approach.* Dordrecht: Reidel Publishing.

Norman, G. R. 1999. "Examining the Assumptions of Evidence-Based Medicine." *Journal of Evaluation in Clinical Practice* 5, no. 2: 139–47.

Nussbaum, M. 1978. *Aristotle's De Motu Animalium.* Princeton, NJ: Princeton University Press.

———. 1994. *The Therapy of Desire: Theory and Practice in Hellenistic Ethics.* Princeton, NJ: Princeton University Press.

Oates, W. J. 1963. *Aristotle and the Problem of Value.* Princeton, NJ: Princeton University Press.

Onians, R. B. 1951. *The Origins of European Thought: About the Body, the Mind, the Soul, the World Time, and Fate.* Cambridge: Cambridge University Press.

Ophir, A. 2005. *The Order of Evils: Toward an Ontology of Morals.* New York: Zone Books.

Osler, W. 1921. *The Evolution of Modern Medicine.* New Haven, CT: Yale University Press.

Paul, J. 1938. "Clinical Epidemiology." *J Clin Invest* 17: 539.

Pearson, K. 1911. *The Grammar of Science*. London: Adam and Charles Black.

———. 1914–1930. *The Life, Letters and Labours of Francis Galton*. 3 of 4 vols. Cambridge: Cambridge University Press.

Peirce, C. S. 1960–1966. *Collected Papers of Charles Sanders Peirce*. Cambridge, MA: Belknap Press.

———. 1963–1979. *Charles S. Peirce Papers*. Cambridge, MA: Harvard University Library, Microreproduction Service with the cooperation of the Houghton Library.

———. 1976. *The New Elements of Mathematics*, edited by C. Eisele. The Hague: Mouton.

Pellegrino, E. D. 1974. "Medicine and Philosophy: Some Notes on the Flirtations of Minerva and Aesculapius." Presidential address at the Society for Health and Human Values.

———. 1977. "The Anatomy of Clinical Judgments: Some Notes on Right Reason and Right Action." In *Clinical Judgment: A Critical Appraisal*, edited by H. T. Engelhardt et al., 169–94. Dordrecht: D. Reidel Publishing Company.

———. 1979. "Medicine, Science, Art: An Old Controversy Revisited." *Man and Medicine* 4, no. 1: 43–52.

Pellegrino, E. D., and D. C. Thomasma. 1981. *A Philosophical Basis of Medical Practice*. Oxford: Oxford University Press.

———. 1993. *The Virtues in Medical Practice*. Oxford: Oxford University Press.

Poisson, S. D. 1837. *Recherches sur la probabilités des jugements en matière criminelle et en matière civil, précédés des règles générales du calcul des probabilités*. Paris: Bachelier.

Polanyi, M. 1946. *Science, Faith and Society*. Oxford: Oxford University Press.

———. 1969. *Knowing and Being: Essays by Michael Polanyi*. Chicago: University of Chicago Press.

———. 1974. *Personal Knowledge: Towards a Post-Critical Philosophy*. Chicago: University of Chicago Press.

———. 1997. "Creative Imagination." In *Society, Economics & Philosophy: Selected Papers of Michael Polanyi*, edited by R. T. Allen, 249–66. New Brunswick, NJ: Transaction Publishers.

Polychronis, A. et al. 1996. "Evidence-Based Medicine: Reference? Dogma? Neologism? New Orthodoxy?" *Journal of Evaluation in Clinical Practice* 2, no. 1: 1–3.

Poovey, M. 1994. "Figures of Arithmetic, Figures of Speech: The Discourse of Statistics." In *Questions of Evidence: Proof, Practice, and Persuasion across the Disciplines*, edited by J. Chandler, A. I. Davidson, H. D. Harootunian, 401–21. Chicago: University of Chicago Press.

Popper, K. 1959. *The Logic of Scientific Discovery*. London: Hutchinson.

Porter, T. M. 1986. *The Rise of Statistical Thinking*. Princeton, NJ: Princeton University Press.

———. 1995. *Trust in Numbers: The Pursuit of Objectivity in Science and Public Life*. Princeton, NJ: Princeton University Press.

Potter, V. R. 1971. *Bioethics: Bridge to the Future*. Englewood Cliffs, NJ: Prentice Hall, Inc.

Prichard, H. A. (1912) 1949. "Does Moral Philosophy Rest on a Mistake?" In *Moral Obligation*, edited by H. A. Prichard, 1–17. Oxford: Oxford University Press.

Putnam, H. 1987. *The Many Faces of Realism: The Paul Carus Lectures*. LaSalle, IL: Open Court.

———. 2002. *The Collapse of the Fact/Value Dichotomy and Other Essays*. Cambridge, MA: Harvard University Press.

Quetelet, L. A. J. 1835. *Sur l'homme et le développement de ses facultés, ou essai de physique sociale*. Paris: Bachelier.

———. (1842) 1969. *A Treatise on Man and the Development of His Faculties: A Facsimile Reproduction of the English Translation of 1842*. Gainesville, FL: Scholars Facsimiles & Reprints.

———. (1846) 1849. *Lettres à S.A.R. le duc regnant de Saxe-Cobourg et Gotha, sur la théorie des probabilités, appliquée aux sciences morales et politiques.* Brussels: Hayez.

Quill, T. E., R. Dresser, and D. W. Brock. 1997. "The Rule of Double Effect: A Critique of Its Role in End of Life Decision-Making." *New England Journal of Medicine* 337: 1768–71.

Rawls, J. 1971. *A Theory of Justice.* Cambridge, MA: Belknap Press.

Reichenbach, H. 1938a. *Experience and Prediction.* Chicago: University of Chicago Press.

———. 1938b. "On Probability and Induction." *Philosophy of Science* 5: 21–45.

———. 1956. *The Direction of Time.* Berkeley: University of California Press.

———. 1978a. "Induction and Probability." *Selected Writings, 1909–1953*, edited by M. Reichenbach and R. S. Cohen, 2: 372–87. Dordrecht: Reidel.

———. 1978b. "The Problem of Causality in Physics." *Selected Writings, 1909–1953*, edited by M. Reichenbach and R. S. Cohen, 1:326–42. Dordrecht: Reidel.

Reiter-Theil, S. 2004. "Does Empirical Research Make Bioethics More Relevant? 'The Embedded Researcher' as a Methodological Approach." *Medicine, Health Care and Philosophy* 7: 17–29.

Rescher, N. 1990. "How Wide is the Gap between Facts and Values?" *Philosophy and Phenomenological Research* 50, suppl.: 297–319.

Reverby, S. M., ed. 2000. *Tuskegee's Truths: Rethinking the Tuskegee Syphilis Study.* Chapel Hill: University of North Carolina Press.

Reynolds, A. 2002. *Peirce's Scientific Metaphysics: The Philosophy of Chance, Law, and Evolution.* Nashville, TN: Vanderbilt University Press.

Rheinberger, H.-J., and S. Müeller-Wille. 2011. *Heredity: History and Culture of a Biological Concept.* Chicago: University of Chicago Press.

Richardson Lear, G. 2004. *Happy Lives and the Human Good: An Essay on Aristotle's Nicomachean Ethics.* Princeton, NJ: Princeton University Press.

Ricoeur, P. 1983. *Temps et Recit.* Paris: Éditions du Seuil.

Rivers, C. 1994. *Face Value: Physiognomical Thought and the Legible Body in Marivaux, Lavater, Balzac, Gautier, and Zola.* Madison: University of Wisconsin Press.

Robinson, W. S. 1950. "Ecological Correlations and the Behavior of Individuals." *Journal of the American Statistical Association* 30: 517–36.

Rosenzweig, F. 1999. *Understanding the Sick and the Healthy: A View of World, Man, and God.* Cambridge, MA: Harvard University Press.

Ross, W. D. 2002. *The Right and the Good.* Oxford: Clarendon Press.

Rothman, D. J. 1991. *Strangers at the Bedside.* New York: Basic Books.

Rowe, C. 1971. *The Eudemian and Nicomachean Ethics: A Study in the Development of Aristotle's Thoughts.* Cambridge: Cambridge Philological Society.

Sackett, D. L. et al. 1991. *Clinical Epidemiology: A Basic Science for Clinical Medicine.* Boston: Little Brown.

———. 1997. *Evidence-Based Medicine: How to Practice & Teach EBM.* New York: Churchill Livingstone.

Sackett D. L., and S. E. Straus. 1998. "Finding and Applying Evidence During Clinical Ward Rounds: the 'Evidence Cart.'" *Journal of the American Medical Association* 280: 1336–38.

Salmon, W. C. 1974. "The Pragmatic Justification of Induction." In *The Justification of Induction*, edited by R. Swinburne, 85–97. Oxford: Oxford University Press.

Schipper, F. 1988. "William Whewell's Conception of Scientific Revolutions." *Studies in History and Philosophy of Science* 19: 43–53.

Sebeok, T., and J. U. Sebeok. 1983. "'You Know My Method': A Juxtaposition of Charles S. Peirce and Sherlock Holmes." In *The Sign of Three: Dupin, Holmes, Peirce*, 11–54. Bloomington: Indiana University Press.

Sekula, A. 1986. "The Body and the Archive." *October* 39: 3–64.

Shahar, E. 1997. "A Popperian Perspective of the Term 'Evidence-Based Medicine.'" *Journal of Evaluation in Clinical Practice* 3: 109–16.

Sheets-Johnstone, M. 1999. *The Primacy of Movement*. Philadelphia, PA: John Benjamins Publishing Company.

Shookman, E., ed. 1993. *The Faces of Physiognomy: Interdisciplinary Approaches to Johann Caspar Lavater*. Rochester, NY: Camden House.

Shorter, E. 1985. *Bedside Manners: The Troubled History of Doctors and Patients*. New York: Simon and Schuster.

Shryock, R. H. 1948. *The Development of Modern Medicine: An Interpretation of the Social and Scientific Factors Involved*. New York: Oxford University Press.

———. 1961. "The History of Quantification in Medical Science." In *Quantification: A History of the Meaning of Measurement in the Natural and Social Sciences*, edited by H. Woolf, 85–107. Indianapolis, IN: Bobbs-Merrill Company, Inc.

Sidgwick, H. 1907. *Methods of Ethics*. London: Macmillan.

Siegler, M. 1999. "Medical Ethics as a Medical Matter." In *The American Medical Ethics Revolution*, edited by R. B. Baker et al., 171–79. Baltimore, MD: Johns Hopkins University Press.

Siegler, M., and A. Dudley Goldblatt. 1978. "Clinical Intuition: A Procedure for Balancing the Rights of Patients and the Responsibilities of Physicians." In *The Law-Medicine Relation: A Philosophical Exploration*, edited by S. Spicker et al., 5–31. Dordrecht: D. Reidel Publishing Company.

Sleigh, J. W. 1997. "Logical Limits of Randomized Controlled Trials." *Journal of Evaluation in Clinical Practice* 3, no. 2: 145–48.

Smith, D. G. 2008. "Viewpoint: Envisioning the Successful Integration of EBM and Humanism in the Clinical Encounter: Fantasy or Fallacy." *Academic Medicine* 83, no. 3: 268–73.

Smolensky, P. 1998. "On the Proper Treatment of Connectionism." *Behavioral and Brain Sciences* 11, no. 1: 1–74.

Spicker, S. F., ed. 1970. *The Philosophy of the Body; Rejections of Cartesian Dualism*. Chicago: Quadrangle Books.

———. 1993. "Intuition and the Process of Medical Diagnosis: The Quest for Explicit Knowledge in the Technological Era." In *Science, Technology, and the Art of Medicine*, edited by C. Delkeskamp-Hayes and M. A. Gardell Cutter, 199–210. Dordrecht: Kluwer Academic Publishers.

Spiegelberg, H. 1965. *The Phenomenological Movement: A Historical Introduction*. The Hague: Martinus Nijhoff.

Stafford, B. M. 1991. *Body Criticism: Imaging the Unseen in Enlightenment Art and Medicine*. Cambridge, MA: MIT Press.

Stempsey, W. 1999. *Disease and Diagnosis: Value Dependant Realism*. Dordrecht: Kluwer Academic Publishers.

Sterling, G. C. 1994. *Ethical Intuitionism and Its Critics*. New York: Peter Lang.

Stigler, S. M. 1986. *The History of Statistics: The Measurement of Uncertainty before 1900*. Cambridge, MA: Belknap Press.

———. 1989. "Francis Galton's Account of the Invention of Correlation." *Statistical Science* 4, no. 2: 73–79.

———. 1999. *Statistics on the Table: The History of Statistical Concepts and Methods.* Cambridge, MA: Harvard University Press.

Straus, E. 1982. *Man, Time, and World.* Pittsburgh, PA: Duquesne University Press.

Strawson, P. F. 1952. *Introduction to Logical Theory.* London: Methuen & Co. Ltd.

Sulmasy, D., and E. Pellegrino. 1999. "The Rule of Double Effect: Clearing up the Double Talk." *Archives of Internal Medicine* 159: 545–50.

Summers, D. 1987. *The Judgment of Sense.* Cambridge: Cambridge University Press.

Suppes, P. 1984. *Probabilistic Metaphysics.* Oxford: Basil Blackwell.

Susser, M. 1973. *Causal Thinking in the Health Sciences: Concepts and Strategies of Epidemiology.* New York: Oxford University Press.

Svenaeus, F. 2000. *The Hermeneutics of Medicine and the Phenomenology of Health: Steps towards a Philosophy of Medical Practice.* Dordrecht: Kluwer Academic Publishers.

Taussig, M. 1992. "Reification and the Consciousness of the Patient." In *The Nervous System*, 83–109. London: Routledge.

———. 1993. *Mimesis and Alterity: A Particular History of the Senses.* New York: Routledge.

Taylor, P. W., ed. 1963. *The Moral Judgment: Readings in Contemporary Meta-Ethics.* Englewood Cliffs, NJ: Prentice Hall.

Temkin, O. 1991. *Hippocrates in a World of Pagans and Christians.* Baltimore, MD: Johns Hopkins University Press.

Thomasma, D. C. 1984. "The Comatose Patient, the Ontology of Death, and the Decision to Stop Treatment." *Theoretical Medicine* 5, no. 2: 181–96.

———. 2000. "Aristotle, Phronesis and Postmodern Bioethics." In *Bioethics: Ancient Themes in Contemporary Issues*, edited by M. G. Kuczewski and R. Polansky. Cambridge, MA: MIT Press.

Thornton, T. 2006. "Tacit Knowledge as the Unifying factor in Evidence-Based Medicine and Clinical Judgment." *Philosophy, Ethics, and Humanities in Medicine* 1, http://www.peh-med.com/content/1/1/2.

Toulmin, S. 1982. "How Medicine Saved the Life of Ethics." *Perspectives in Biology and Medicine* 25, no. 4: 736–50.

———. 2001. *Return to Reason.* Cambridge, MA: Harvard University Press.

Toulmin, S., and A. R. Jonsen. 1988. *The Abuse of Casuistry: A History of Moral Reasoning.* Berkeley: University of California Press.

Truog, R. 1997. "Is it Time to Abandon Brain-Death?" *Hastings Center Report* 27, no. 1: 29–37.

Tytler, G. 1982. *Physiognomy in the European Novel: Faces and Fortunes.* Princeton, NJ: Princeton University Press.

Upshur, R. 1997. "Certainty, Probability and Abduction: Why We Should Look to C. S. Peirce Rather than Godel for a Theory of Clinical Reasoning." *Journal of Evaluation in Clinical Practice* 3, no. 3: 201–6.

Vandenbroucke, J. P. 1996. "Evidence Based Medicine and '*Medicine d'Observation.*'" *J Clin Epidemiol* 49, no. 12: 1335–38.

Veatch, R. M. 1973. "The Medical Model: Its Nature and Problems." *Hastings Center Studies* 1, no. 3: 59–76.

———. 1975. "The Whole-Brain-Oriented Concept of Death: An Outmoded Philosophical Formulation." *Journal of Thanatology* 3, no. 1: 13–130.

————. 1976. *Death, Dying and the Biological Revolution: Our Quest for Responsibility.* New Haven, CT: Yale University Press.

————, ed. 1997. *Medical Ethics.* New York: Bartlett and Jones.

————. 1999. "Who Should Control the Scope and Nature of Medical Ethics?" In *The American Medical Ethics Revolution,* edited by R. B. Baker et al., 158–70. Baltimore, MD: Johns Hopkins University Press.

————. 2002. "The Birth of Bioethics: Autobiographical Reflections of a Patient Person." *Cambridge Quarterly of Healthcare Ethics* 11: 344–52.

Venn, J. 1866. *The Logic of Chance. An Essay on the Foundations and Province of the Theory of Probability, with Especial Reference to Its Application to Moral and Social Science.* London: Macmillan.

Von Neumann, J. M., and O. Morgenstern. 1947. *Theory of Games and Economic Theory.* New York: Wiley.

Walker, H. M. (1929) 1975. *Studies in the History of Statistical Method.* New York: Arno Press.

Warner, J. H. 1986. *The Therapeutic Perspective: Medical Practice, Knowledge, and Identity in America, 1820–1885.* Cambridge, MA: Harvard University Press.

Wechsler, J. 1982. *A Human Comedy: Physiognomy and Caricature in Nineteenth Century Paris.* Chicago: University of Chicago Press.

Whewell, W. (1833) 1836. *Astronomy and General Physics Considered with Reference to Natural Theology.* London: William Pickering.

————. 1847. *Philosophy of the Inductive Sciences.* 2nd ed. 2 vols. London: J.W. Parker & Sons.

Widdershoven-Heerding, I. 1987. "Medicine as a Form of Practical Understanding." *Theoretical Medicine* 8: 179–85.

Wilczak, P. F. 1973. "Faith, Motive, and Community: An Interpretation of the Philosophy of Michael Polanyi." PhD diss., University of Chicago Divinity School.

Wilensky, U. 1997. "What Is Normal Anyway? Therapy for Epistemological Anxiety." *Educational Studies in Mathematics: Special Issue on Computational Environments in Mathematics Education* 33, no. 2: 171–202.

Wilson, E. O. 1975. *Sociobiology: The New Synthesis.* Cambridge, MA: Harvard University Press.

————. 1998. *Consilience.* New York: Knopf.

Wilson, J. Q. 1993. *The Moral Sense.* New York: Free Press.

Wolpert, L. 1992. *The Unnatural Nature of Science.* London: Faber and Faber.

Yeo, R. 1993. *Defining Science: William Whewell, Natural Knowledge, and Public Debate in Early Victorian Britain.* Cambridge: Cambridge University Press.

Zahavi, D. 2003. *Husserl's Phenomenology.* Stanford, CA: Stanford University Press.

Zaner, R. 1964. *The Problem of Embodiment: Some Contributions to a Phenomenology of the Body.* The Hague: Martinus Nijhoff.

————. 1970. *The Way of Phenomenology: Criticism as a Philosophical Discipline.* New York: Pegasus.

————. 1981. *The Context of Self: A Phenomenological Inquiry Using Medicine as a Clue.* Athens: Ohio University Press.

————. 1988a. *Death: Beyond Whole Brain Criteria.* Dordrecht: Kluwer Academic Press.

————. 1988b. *Ethics and the Clinical Encounter.* Englewood Cliffs, NJ: Prentice Hall.

Index

Italic page numbers indicate an illustration.

Foot, Philippa, 19
Foucault, Michel, 144, 171, 177–78, 184n15, 202n33
Frankena, William, 20
Freedman, Benjamin, 161–65
frequentist statistics, 163, 165. *See also* Reichenbach, Hans
Fried, Charles, 161, 163

Gadamer, Hans-Georg, 189n5
Galton, Francis, xxi–xxii, 71, 77–78, 80, 84, 103, 127; composite photography, 90–98, 104, compared with Benjamin's theory of montage, 98–99, 102; conception of the stirp, 88–89; discovery of regression and correlation, 72–73, 86–91, 98, 104, 113, 128–35, 143, 149–50, 153, 172, 180; illustrations, *87–89, 91–96*; quincunx, 90; shift from physical to psychical anthropometry, 97–98; statistical physiognomy, 96–98, 166, 168; study of heredity, 85–86, 104, 131, 133, 147, 150; the transformer, 91–96; on William Whewell, 206n5
Gaussian distribution. *See* bell-shaped curve
genetics, xv–xvi
Gere, Cathy, 207n11
Ginzburg, Carlo, 72, 98
Goodman, Steven, 165–66
goodness, 19–22, 24–25, 28, 176
Greek culture, 66
Grene, Marjorie, 23, 45, 55–56, 58, 69, 192n26
Groopman, Jerome, 5
Guyatt, Gordon, 116

Habermas, Jürgen, xvi
Hacking, Ian, 134, 197n30, 199n4, 203n11
Hald, Anders, 197n26
Hampshire, Stuart, 40
Hardie, W. F. R., 62–64, 193n7
Hare, R. M., 10, 19, 24–26, 32
Harré, Rom, 205n41
Hartley, Lucy, 78, 97–98, 207n6
Haynes, Brian, 116
healing, as a goal of medicine, xiii, xvi, 1, 9, 51, 141, 177
health: as a Hippocratic goal of medicine, 12; as a metaphor, 47–48
Hellman, Deborah, 163, 165–66
Henry, Stephen, 117
heredity: laws of, 84–85, 89–90, 102; mental, 97
Herschel, John, 85
Hesse, Mary, 207n8
Hippocrates, 191n19
Hippocratic author, 1, 16, 47–48
Hippocratic Corpus, 47, 73, 191n19, 191n20
Hippocratic ethic, 11, 22
Hippocratic medicine, 48, 56, 107, 206n45
Hippocratic Oath, 8
Hoffman, B., 192n25

Homer, 66
Horton, Richard, 114
Howson, Colin, 150
Hudson, W. D., 25
Huebner, Robert, 143
human nature, xvii
Hume, David: moral theory, 18–19; problem of induction, xxii, 150, 154, 203n13 (*see also* induction); separation of "is" and "ought," 18–20, 22, 181
Huneman, Philippe, 140, 204n24
Husserl, Edmund, xxiii–xxiv, 4, 172–76
Huxley, Thomas, 179

idealism, xix, 14
induction: based on probabilism, 155–56; and intuition, 153, 159; philosophical problem of, 150–51, 153, 158–60, 168, 209n26
inductive-probabilistic model, 156–58
intentionality, 4
intuition, xvi–xx, 16, 45–46, 52–57, 107–8, 122–24, 170, 181; as the art of medicine, xxiv, 5; clinical, xxii–xxiii, 109–10, 171; as common sense, 5; in the contemporary sense, 6; and correlation, 172, 174–75; as a form of irrationalism, 6, 10, 122, 149, 151; Hippocratic, 5; inductive, 150 (*see also* induction: and intuition); mathematical, 186n22; as a moral epistemology, 29; in philosophy, 2–5; practical, 5, 18, 43, 108, 124, 200n10; in scientific reasoning, 57; and statistics, 128
intuitions: clinical, 122, 128, 162, 164, 166; moral, xvii, xx, 6–12, 15, 17, 20, 26–39, 51, 161–64; philosophical versus clinical, 7–8

Jackson, J., 137
Jaeger, Werner, 1, 47
Jansen, Lynn, 36–38
Jonas, Hans, 57–60, 65; philosophy of the organism, 58–59
Jonsen, Al, 9, 13, 183n7
Jouanna, Jacques, 191n19, 191n20, 193n30
justice, 28–29, 50

Kal, Victor, 45
Kant, Immanuel, 3, 8, 123, 154, 185n8
Kass, Leon, 6, 8–10
Keller, Evelyn Fox, 205n27
Kenny, Anthony, 46
King, Lester, 129–30, 146, 202n4
Kingsley, Charles, 152
knot of being, 58–59, 65
Koch, Robert, 140, 143
Kuhn, Thomas, 207n5

Lancet, The, 111
language: clinical, 120–22; moral, 24–26